Effect of Phenolic Compounds on Human Health

Effect of Phenolic Compounds on Human Health

Editors

Elena González-Burgos
M. Pilar Gómez-Serranillos Cuadrado

MDPI • Basel • Beijing • Wuhan • Barcelona • Belgrade • Manchester • Tokyo • Cluj • Tianjin

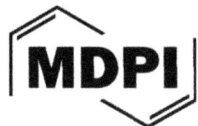

Editors
Elena González-Burgos
Universidad Complutense de Madrid
Spain

M. Pilar Gómez-Serranillos Cuadrado
Universidad Complutense de Madrid
Spain

Editorial Office
MDPI
St. Alban-Anlage 66
4052 Basel, Switzerland

This is a reprint of articles from the Special Issue published online in the open access journal *Nutrients* (ISSN 2072-6643) (available at: https://www.mdpi.com/journal/nutrients/special_issues/Phenolic_Health).

For citation purposes, cite each article independently as indicated on the article page online and as indicated below:

LastName, A.A.; LastName, B.B.; LastName, C.C. Article Title. *Journal Name* **Year**, *Volume Number*, Page Range.

ISBN 978-3-0365-2898-4 (Hbk)
ISBN 978-3-0365-2899-1 (PDF)

© 2022 by the authors. Articles in this book are Open Access and distributed under the Creative Commons Attribution (CC BY) license, which allows users to download, copy and build upon published articles, as long as the author and publisher are properly credited, which ensures maximum dissemination and a wider impact of our publications.

The book as a whole is distributed by MDPI under the terms and conditions of the Creative Commons license CC BY-NC-ND.

Contents

About the Editors . . . . **vii**

Elena González-Burgos and M. Pilar Gómez-Serranillos
Effect of Phenolic Compounds on Human Health
Reprinted from: *Nutrients* 2021, *13*, 3922, doi:10.3390/nu13113922 . . . . **1**

Aslı Devrim-Lanpir, Pelin Bilgic, Tuğba Kocahan, Gökhan Deliceoğlu, Thomas Rosemann and Beat Knechtle
Total Dietary Antioxidant Intake Including Polyphenol Content: Is It Capable to Fight against Increased Oxidants within the Body of Ultra-Endurance Athletes?
Reprinted from: *Nutrients* 2020, *12*, 1877, doi:10.3390/nu12061877 . . . . **3**

Gopalsamy Rajiv Gandhi, Alan Bruno Silva Vasconcelos, Ding-Tao Wu, Hua-Bin Li, Poovathumkal James Antony, Hang Li, Fang Geng, Ricardo Queiroz Gurgel, Narendra Narain and Ren-You Gan
Citrus Flavonoids as Promising Phytochemicals Targeting Diabetes and Related Complications: A Systematic Review of In Vitro and In Vivo Studies
Reprinted from: *Nutrients* 2020, *12*, 2907, doi:10.3390/nu12102907 . . . . **19**

Hyung-Seok Yu, Won-Ju Kim, Won-Young Bae, Na-Kyoung Lee and Hyun-Dong Paik
Inula britannica Inhibits Adipogenesis of 3T3-L1 Preadipocytes via Modulation of Mitotic Clonal Expansion Involving ERK 1/2 and Akt Signaling Pathways
Reprinted from: *Nutrients* 2020, *12*, 3037, doi:10.3390/nu12103037 . . . . **51**

Jorge Simón, María Casado-Andrés, Naroa Goikoetxea-Usandizaga, Marina Serrano-Maciá and María Luz Martínez-Chantar
Nutraceutical Properties of Polyphenols against Liver Diseases
Reprinted from: *Nutrients* 2020, *12*, 3517, doi:10.3390/nu12113517 . . . . **73**

Carme Grau-Bové, Marta Sierra-Cruz, Alba Miguéns-Gómez, Esther Rodríguez-Gallego, Raúl Beltrán-Debón, Mayte Blay, Ximena Terra, Montserrat Pinent and Anna Ardévol
A Ten-Day Grape Seed Procyanidin Treatment Prevents Certain Ageing Processes in Female Rats over the Long Term
Reprinted from: *Nutrients* 2020, *12*, 3647, doi:10.3390/nu12123647 . . . . **93**

Cindy Romain, Linda H. Chung, Elena Marín-Cascales, Jacobo A. Rubio-Arias, Sylvie Gaillet, Caroline Laurent, Juana María Morillas-Ruiz, Alejandro Martínez-Rodriguez, Pedro Emilio Alcaraz and Julien Cases
Sixteen Weeks of Supplementation with a Nutritional Quantity of a Diversity of Polyphenols from Foodstuff Extracts Improves the Health-Related Quality of Life of Overweight and Obese Volunteers: A Randomized, Double-Blind, Parallel Clinical Trial
Reprinted from: *Nutrients* 2021, *13*, 492, doi:10.3390/nu13020492 . . . . **105**

Alexandria Turner, Martin Veysey, Simon Keely, Christopher J. Scarlett, Mark Lucock and Emma L. Beckett
Genetic Variation in the Bitter Receptors Responsible for Epicatechin Detection Are Associated with BMI in an Elderly Cohort
Reprinted from: *Nutrients* 2021, *13*, 571, doi:10.3390/nu13020571 . . . . **121**

Hira Shakoor, Jack Feehan, Vasso Apostolopoulos, Carine Platat, Ayesha Salem Al Dhaheri, Habiba I. Ali, Leila Cheikh Ismail, Marijan Bosevski and Lily Stojanovska
Immunomodulatory Effects of Dietary Polyphenols
Reprinted from: *Nutrients* **2021**, *13*, 728, doi:10.3390/nu13030728 . . . . **135**

Katarzyna Kowalska, Radosław Dembczyński, Agata Gołąbek, Mariola Olkowicz and Anna Olejnik
ROS Modulating Effects of Lingonberry (*Vaccinium vitis-idaea* L.) Polyphenols on Obese Adipocyte Hypertrophy and Vascular Endothelial Dysfunction
Reprinted from: *Nutrients* **2021**, *13*, 885, doi:10.3390/nu13030885 . . . . **153**

Gustavo Ignacio Vazquez-Cervantes, Daniela Ramírez Ortega, Tonali Blanco Ayala, Verónica Pérez de la Cruz, Dinora Fabiola González Esquivel, Aleli Salazar and Benjamín Pineda
Redox and Anti-Inflammatory Properties from Hop Components in Beer-Related to Neuroprotection
Reprinted from: *Nutrients* **2021**, *13*, 2000, doi:10.3390/nu13062000 . . . . **171**

Elena González-Burgos, Isabel Ureña-Vacas, Marta Sánchez and M. Pilar Gómez-Serranillos
Nutritional Value of *Moringa oleifera* Lam. Leaf Powder Extracts and Their Neuroprotective Effects via Antioxidative and Mitochondrial Regulation
Reprinted from: *Nutrients* **2021**, *13*, 2203, doi:10.3390/nu13072203 . . . . **193**

Naila Rabbani, Mingzhan Xue, Martin O. Weickert and Paul J. Thornalley
Reversal of Insulin Resistance in Overweight and Obese Subjects by *trans*-Resveratrol and Hesperetin Combination—Link to Dysglycemia, Blood Pressure, Dyslipidemia, and Low-Grade Inflammation
Reprinted from: *Nutrients* **2021**, *13*, 2374, doi:10.3390/nu13072374 . . . . **209**

About the Editors

Elena González-Burgos is an Associate Professor in Pharmacology, Pharmacognosy and Botanical in the Faculty of Pharmacy at UCM (Spain). She received a Ph.D. in Pharmacy from UCM (2012) and graduated "Cum laude". She is a member of the research group UCM "Pharmacology of natural products" and her expertise are in the study of phytochemistry and pharmacology of natural products from medicinal plants and lichens. Her research formation has been completed in prestigious international centers (King's College, London, UK and Center for Neurosciences and Cell Biology, Coimbra, Portugal). She is the author of 46 JCR scientific publications, 15 book chapters and many communications in congress.

M. Pilar Gómez-Serranillos Cuadrado is a Professor in Pharmacology, Pharmacognosy and Botanical in the Faculty of Pharmacy at UCM (Spain). She is Director of the research group "Pharmacology of natural products". Her main research work focuses on the study of the neuroprotective activity and cytotoxic activity of natural products in cell-based models. Moreover, her research focuses on phytochemical studies (the identification, isolation, and characterization of the active principles responsible for pharmacological activities). She is the author of 122 JCR publications and 32 book chapters.

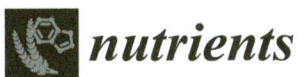

Editorial

Effect of Phenolic Compounds on Human Health

Elena González-Burgos * and M. Pilar Gómez-Serranillos

Department of Pharmacology, Pharmacognosy and Botany, Faculty of Pharmacy, Universidad Complutense de Madrid, 28040 Madrid, Spain; pserra@ucm.es
* Correspondence: elenagon@ucm.es

Citation: González-Burgos, E.; Gómez-Serranillos, M.P. Effect of Phenolic Compounds on Human Health. *Nutrients* **2021**, *13*, 3922. https://doi.org/10.3390/nu13113922

Received: 13 October 2021
Accepted: 18 October 2021
Published: 1 November 2021

Publisher's Note: MDPI stays neutral with regard to jurisdictional claims in published maps and institutional affiliations.

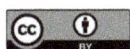

Copyright: © 2021 by the authors. Licensee MDPI, Basel, Switzerland. This article is an open access article distributed under the terms and conditions of the Creative Commons Attribution (CC BY) license (https://creativecommons.org/licenses/by/4.0/).

This book, based on a Special Issue of *Nutrients*, contains a total of 12 papers (8 original research and 4 reviews) on the effect of phenolic compounds on human health. The consumption of exogenous medicinal plants and food rich in phenolic compounds represents a promising therapeutically to prevent many chronic diseases, including diabetes, cardiovascular diseases, cancer, and neurodegenerative diseases, among others.

The original articles include three in vitro studies, one in vivo work, and four clinical trials. Regarding in vitro studies, two of them study the effect of polyphenols on obesity. Hence, *Inula Britannica* flower aqueous extract, which is rich in phenolic compounds, has shown to inhibit adipogenesis through modulation of mitotic clonal expansion and the extracellular signal-regulated kinase 1/2 and Akt signaling pathways in 3T3-L1 adipocytes [1]. Likewise, in another in vitro study, it has been shown that anthocyanin and non-anthocyanin polyphenol fractions from lingonberry fruit could help prevent and treat obesity and endothelial dysfunction by reducing oxidative stress and inflammation through enhancing antioxidant enzyme expression and inhibiting ROS production and pro-inflammatory genes expression and adhesion molecules [2]. In addition to these anti-obesity effects of polyphenols, their neuroprotective role has been demonstrated in other work. Particularly, methanol extracts of *Moringa oleifera* leaf powder, rich in polyphenols with potent antioxidant properties, protected human neuroblastoma cells from H_2O_2-induced oxidative stress. Pretreatments with concentration of 25 µg/mL of moringa extracts reduced reactive oxygen production and lipid peroxidation, as well as increasing the reduced glutathione content and antioxidant enzymatic activity. Moreover, this study revealed that moringa can act at the mitochondrial level by regulating calcium levels and increasing mitochondrial membrane potential [3].

The only in vivo study included in this book covers the preventive role of grape seed-derived procyanidins (GSPE) (500 mg/kg) in age-related processes in female rats, such as pancreas dysfunction and tumor development [4].

Finally, four clinical trials are compiled. Two of them have shown the benefits of polyphenols in overweight and obese people. Hence, supplementation with a polyphenol-rich ingredient (900 mg/day for 16-week) improved the physical and mental health of overweight and obese volunteers [5]. Moreover, a combination of trans-resveratrol and hesperetin (tRES-HESP, 90–120 mg) reduced dysglycemia, blood pressure, vascular inflammation, and dyslipidemia in healthy, overweight, and obese subjects. These beneficial effects are related to its ability to counteract methylglyoxal accumulation and protein glycation and to decrease TXNIP and TNFα expression. The study also demonstrated that these compounds exert their effects synergistically [6]. In other work, it has been seen that a diet rich in polyphenols in ultra-endurance athletes enhance both exercise performance and post-exercise recovery for balancing redox balance [7]. Furthermore, this book also included a cross-sectional study to investigate the multidirectional interactions between TAS2R genotype [TAS2R4 gene (rs2233998 and rs2234001); TAS2R5 gene (rs2227264)], epicatechin intake, and body mass index (BMI), together in an elderly cohort. This study demonstrated that there is not an association between epicatechin intake and BMI and TAS2R genotype [8].

Regarding the reviews, two general papers on the effect of dietary polyphenols as immunomodulatory and liver protector agents have been included [9,10], and two more specific papers focused on the benefits of hop components in beer, rich in flavonoids, as neuroprotective agents, based on its antioxidant and anti-inflammatory activities, and the benefits of citrus flavonoids in diabetes [11,12].

We believe that this collection includes a summary of current studies on the benefits of polyphenols and of great value for future research in this area.

Conflicts of Interest: The authors declare no conflict of interest.

References

1. Yu, H.S.; Kim, W.J.; Bae, W.Y.; Lee, N.K.; Paik, H.D. Inula britannica Inhibits Adipogenesis of 3T3-L1 Preadipocytes via Modulation of Mitotic Clonal Expansion Involving ERK 1/2 and Akt Signaling Pathways. *Nutrients* **2020**, *12*, 3037. [CrossRef] [PubMed]
2. Kowalska, K.; Dembczyński, R.; Gołąbek, A.; Olkowicz, M.; Olejnik, A. ROS Modulating Effects of Lingonberry (*Vaccinium vitis-idaea* L.) Polyphenols on Obese Adipocyte Hypertrophy and Vascular Endothelial Dysfunction. *Nutrients* **2021**, *13*, 885. [CrossRef] [PubMed]
3. González-Burgos, E.; Ureña-Vacas, I.; Sánchez, M.; Gómez-Serranillos, M.P. Nutritional Value of Moringa oleifera Lam. Leaf Powder Extracts and Their Neuroprotective Effects via Antioxidative and Mitochondrial Regulation. *Nutrients* **2021**, *13*, 2203. [CrossRef] [PubMed]
4. Grau-Bové, C.; Sierra-Cruz, M.; Miguéns-Gómez, A.; Rodríguez-Gallego, E.; Beltrán-Debón, R.; Blay, M.; Terra, X.; Pinent, M.; Ardévol, A. A Ten-Day Grape Seed Procyanidin Treatment Prevents Certain Ageing Processes in Female Rats over the Long Term. *Nutrients* **2020**, *12*, 3647. [CrossRef] [PubMed]
5. Romain, C.; Chung, L.H.; Marín-Cascales, E.; Rubio-Arias, J.A.; Gaillet, S.; Laurent, C.; Morillas-Ruiz, J.M.; Martínez-Rodriguez, A.; Alcaraz, P.E.; Cases, J. Sixteen Weeks of Supplementation with a Nutritional Quantity of a Diversity of Polyphenols from Foodstuff Extracts Improves the Health-Related Quality of Life of Overweight and Obese Volunteers: A Randomized, Double-Blind, Parallel Clinical Trial. *Nutrients* **2021**, *13*, 492. [CrossRef] [PubMed]
6. Rabbani, N.; Xue, M.; Weickert, M.O.; Thornalley, P.J. Reversal of Insulin Resistance in Overweight and Obese Subjects by trans-Resveratrol and Hesperetin Combination-Link to Dysglycemia, Blood Pressure, Dyslipidemia, and Low-Grade Inflammation. *Nutrients* **2021**, *13*, 2374. [CrossRef] [PubMed]
7. Devrim-Lanpir, A.; Bilgic, P.; Kocahan, T.; Deliceoğlu, G.; Rosemann, T.; Knechtle, B. Total Dietary Antioxidant Intake Including Polyphenol Content: Is it Capable to Fight against Increased Oxidants within the Body of Ultra-Endurance Athletes? *Nutrients* **2020**, *12*, 1877. [CrossRef] [PubMed]
8. Turner, A.; Veysey, M.; Keely, S.; Scarlett, C.J.; Lucock, M.; Beckett, E.L. Genetic Variation in the Bitter Receptors Responsible for Epicatechin Detection Are Associated with BMI in an Elderly Cohort. *Nutrients* **2021**, *13*, 571. [CrossRef] [PubMed]
9. Shakoor, H.; Feehan, J.; Apostolopoulos, V.; Platat, C.; Al Dhaheri, A.S.; Ali, H.I.; Ismail, L.C.; Bosevski, M.; Stojanovska, L. Immunomodulatory Effects of Dietary Polyphenols. *Nutrients* **2021**, *13*, 728. [CrossRef] [PubMed]
10. Simón, J.; Casado-Andrés, M.; Goikoetxea-Usandizaga, N.; Serrano-Maciá, M.; Martínez-Chantar, M.L. Nutraceutical Properties of Polyphenols against Liver Diseases. *Nutrients* **2020**, *12*, 3517. [CrossRef] [PubMed]
11. Vazquez-Cervantes, G.I.; Ortega, D.R.; Blanco Ayala, T.; Pérez de la Cruz, V.; Esquivel, D.F.G.; Salazar, A.; Pineda, B. Redox and Anti-Inflammatory Properties from Hop Components in Beer-Related to Neuroprotection. *Nutrients* **2021**, *13*, 2000. [CrossRef] [PubMed]
12. Gandhi, G.R.; Vasconcelos, A.B.S.; Wu, D.T.; Li, H.B.; Antony, P.J.; Li, H.; Geng, F.; Gurgel, R.Q.; Narain, N.; Gan, R.Y. Citrus Flavonoids as Promising Phytochemicals Targeting Diabetes and Related Complications: A Systematic Review of In Vitro and In Vivo Studies. *Nutrients* **2020**, *12*, 2907. [CrossRef] [PubMed]

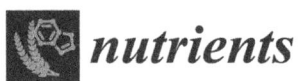

Article

Total Dietary Antioxidant Intake Including Polyphenol Content: Is It Capable to Fight against Increased Oxidants within the Body of Ultra-Endurance Athletes?

Aslı Devrim-Lanpir [1], Pelin Bilgic [2], Tuğba Kocahan [3], Gökhan Deliceoğlu [4], Thomas Rosemann [5] and Beat Knechtle [5,*]

[1] Department of Nutrition and Dietetics, Faculty of Health Sciences, Istanbul Medeniyet University, 34862 Istanbul, Turkey; asli.devrim@medeniyet.edu.tr
[2] Department of Nutrition and Dietetics, Faculty of Health Sciences, Hacettepe University, 06100 Ankara, Turkey; pbilgic@hacettepe.edu.tr
[3] Sport Medicine Physician, Department of Health Services, Sports General Directorship, The Ministry of Youth and Sports, Center of Athlete Training and Health Research, 06100 Ankara, Turkey; tugba.kocahan@sgm.gov.tr
[4] Sport Scientist, Faculty of Sports Science, Kırıkkale University, 71450 Kırıkkale, Turkey; deliceoglugokhan@kku.edu.tr
[5] Institute of Primary Care, University of Zurich, 8091 Zurich, Switzerland; Thomas.rosemann@usz.ch
* Correspondence: beat.knechtle@hispeed.ch; Tel.: +41-(0)-71-226-93-00

Received: 19 May 2020; Accepted: 19 June 2020; Published: 23 June 2020

Abstract: The role of dietary antioxidants on exhaustive exercise-induced oxidative stress has been well investigated. However, the contribution of total dietary antioxidant capacity on exogenous antioxidant defense and exercise performance has commonly been disregarded. The aims of the present investigation were to examine (i) the effects of dietary total antioxidant intake on body antioxidant mechanisms, and (ii) an exhaustive exercise-induced oxidative damage in ultra-endurance athletes. The study included 24 ultra-marathon runners and long-distance triathletes (12 male and 12 female) who underwent an acute exhaustive exercise test (a cycle ergometer (45 min at 65% VO_2max) immediately followed by a treadmill test (75% VO_2max to exhaustion). Oxidative stress-related biomarkers (8-isoprostaglandin F2alpha (8-iso PGF2a), total oxidant status (TOS, total antioxidant status (TAS)) in plasma were collected before and after exercise. Oxidative stress index was calculated to assess the aspect of redox balance. Blood lactate concentrations and heart rate were measured at the 3rd and 6th min after exercise. Dietary antioxidant intake was calculated using the ferric reducing ability of plasma (FRAP) assay. Dietary total antioxidant intake of the subjects was negatively correlated with pre-exercise TOS concentrations (rs = −0.641 in male, and rs = −0.741 in females) and post- vs. pre- (Δ) 8-iso PGF2a levels (rs = −0.702 in male; $p = 0.016$, and rs = −0.682 in females; $p = 0.024$), and positively correlated with Δ TAS concentrations (rs = 0.893 in males; $p = 0.001$, and rs = 0.769 in females; $p = 0.002$) and post- exercise lactate concentrations (rs = 0.795 for males; $p = 0.006$, and rs = 0.642 for females; $p = 0.024$). A positive meaningful ($p = 0.013$) interaction was observed between time at exhaustion and dietary antioxidant intake (rs = 0.692) in males, but not in females. In conclusion, the determination of total dietary antioxidant intake in ultra-endurance athletes may be crucial for gaining a better perspective on body antioxidant defense against exhaustive exercise-induced oxidative stress. However, the effects of dietary antioxidant on exercise performance and recovery rate needs further investigation.

Keywords: ultra-endurance; dietary antioxidants; total antioxidant capacity; exercise intensity; post-exercise recovery; 8-iso prostaglandin F2a

1. Introduction

Ultra-endurance sports such as ultra-marathon races, ultra-cycling, and ultra-triathlon events requires athletes to push their limits, and to perform beyond their capacity for a long period of time [1,2]. It is known that moderate physical activity has quite beneficial effects for the body redox status which is playing a crucial role in exercise adaptation and cell-signaling [3], including a regulatory role in muscle regeneration during muscle damage [4], exercise-induced adaptations of muscle phenotype [5], and activation of the transcriptional factors like sirtuin-1 (SIRT-1) [6]. However, vigorous exercise results in a manifest increase that overwhelms the body antioxidant defenses [5]. It is well-established that exercise-induced oxidative stress caused by prolonged or exhaustive exercise has detrimental effects on skeletal muscles [7], fatigue [8,9], and immune function [10], which could all alter exercise performance.

A lot of research in recent years has focused on exogenous antioxidant supplements' effect on achieving the balance between reactive oxygen species (ROS) and antioxidants in endurance athletes [11–14]. The acute supplementation of the well-known dietary antioxidants such as beta-carotene, vitamin C, vitamin E, selenium, coenzyme Q, thiols, and polyphenols are attracting widespread interest in fighting exercise-induced oxidative stress and enhancing performance [13,15–18]. However, some studies investigating the effects of the supplementations on the body redox status demonstrated that they showed no benefit due to their detrimental effects on decreasing both cell and muscle adaptation against exercise-induced oxidative stress and interfering with the beneficial influences of exercise [19,20]. Furthermore, some studies pointed out that the chronic supplementation may blunt the free radical-induced stress adaptation pathways in exhaustive exercise by interfering with the antioxidant defense against ROS within body systems [19,21,22]. Few studies have addressed that the antioxidant supplementation may be advantageous in athletes where the exogenous antioxidant levels are already depleted [12,23]. Therefore, before a supplementation to athletes should be considered, it is crucial to first determine whether the body antioxidant level is normal, and whether dietary antioxidant intake is needed to assess as well.

Oxidative stress-related research indicated that endogenous antioxidant defense is quite complicated, and is arranged by several antioxidant defense mechanisms affecting the body redox status [12,24–27]. Dietary antioxidants may be crucial for gaining a better perspective on body antioxidant levels. It is well-documented that antioxidant-rich foods provide several bioactive food constituents called phytochemicals that help to eliminate ROS and DNA damage by acting as an inducer of antioxidant defense mechanisms in the body [28,29]. Despite the fact that antioxidant rich-foods such as fresh and dry fruits, vegetables, nuts, and seeds are considered to play a major part in defending exercise-induced oxidative stress [29], studies commonly just focused on dietary micronutrient content disregarding polyphenolic functions, and few researchers have addressed the effects of antioxidant-rich foods on body redox status in athletes [23,30]. Thus, the dietary antioxidant intake effects on endogenous defense mechanisms and exercise performance in ultra-endurance athletes largely remain equivocal.

Numerous oxidative damage biomarkers have been identified during exhaustive or long-period exercise [31], however, the detection of them is mostly limited due to several factors including the lack of sensitivity, the low quantity, the very short half-life, the rapid interaction with antioxidants, the inapplicability of direct detection methods because of the instability, or the need for expensive devices and equipment [32,33]. Therefore, the difficulties in measuring different oxidant molecules, plasma total oxidant status (TOS), and total antioxidant status (TAS) is preferred to define the redox status under certain conditions such as exhaustive performance in athletes [23,34]. In addition to that, since exercise-induced ROS production is well-known to provoke lipid peroxidation, 8-iso prostaglandin F2alpha (8-iso PGF2a) is detected as a stable end product of the arachidonic acid, and defined as a suitable indicator of in vivo lipid peroxidation [35]. Several studies reported a parallel rise in the production of 8-iso PGF2a in plasma or urine, due to the accumulation of lipid peroxidation along with the increase in the intensity of the exercise [34,36–38].

In this study, we aimed to investigate the hormetic role of the dietary antioxidants, and to examine the interaction between the dietary antioxidant intake and the acute exhaustive exercise-induced oxidative stress in ultra-endurance athletes. It was hypothesized (i) that diets rich in antioxidants may increase the body exogenous antioxidant capacity after an exhaustive exercise. Furthermore, we assumed that a high dietary antioxidant consumption may also improve (ii) exercise performance by increasing the time until exhaustion during exercise and (iii) recovery, assessed by post-exercise heart rate and lactate concentrations in ultra-endurance athletes.

2. Materials and Methods

2.1. Study Participants

In total, 12 male (triathletes, $n = 6$; ultra-marathoners, $n = 6$; age 38.5 (31.3–40.0) years; body mass 72.6 (69.6–81.0) kg; body height 179.0 (173.5–184.5) cm; fat mass percentage 12.9 (10.0–16.3)%, fat-free mass 63.8 (60.0–68.3) kg) and 12 female (triathletes, $n = 6$; ultra-marathoners, $n = 6$; age 38.0 ((31.6–44.5) years; body height 162.0 (160.0–166.5) cm; fat mass percentage 19.4 (9.2–12.9)%; fat-free mass 45.5 (42.8–47.9) kg) were recruited from Ancyra Sports Club and local ultra-endurance groups by using study brochures and social media. Inclusion criteria for the study were: age 20–64 years old, being in a good health, training at least 15 h per week, not having any metabolic disease, being a non-smoker, participating at least one ultra-endurance race/event, taking no vitamins, minerals, dietary supplements, antibiotics, and any medication at least during the three months before the study. The lower age of participation was defined by age groups of triathlon and ultra-marathon races. Females with a regular menstrual cycle of physiological length (24–35 days) were included in the study. In addition, females in menopause or using oral contraceptives were excluded from the study. In literature, the influence of menstrual cycle on endurance performance is still controversially discussed. Whilst some studies found no interaction between different menstrual phases and maximal anaerobic performance [39], maximal oxygen consumption, cardiorespiratory variables and blood lactate concentration [40], few studies suggested that some interactions, i.e., VO$_2$max was 2% lower in the luteal phase compared to the early follicular phase, endurance performance and muscle glycogen content were enhanced in the luteal phase. There is no consensus suggesting a specific menstrual phase for use in research on athletic performance. Therefore, to standardize the menstrual phase within subjects [41] and the estrogen effects on body antioxidant capacity by binding estrogen receptors and expand the antioxidant enzyme expressions using intracellular signal pathways [42], and to eliminate the effects of different phases on exercise performance [43], all females performed all exercise tests during mid-follicular phase (low estrogen levels, 7–9 days of the menstrual cycle). Menstrual cycle was calculated starting the first day of their period.

Subjects were informed of all potential risks involved and signed a written informed consent form before participating in the study. The study was performed at the Center of Athlete Training and Health Research of the Ministry of Youth and Sports, and was approved by Hacettepe University Ethics Board and Commission (research ethic project no, KA-180011) and The Ministry of Health (research ethic project no, E182).

2.2. Study Design

Subjects were required to visit the exercise laboratory on two visits. Before the visits, the subjects were informed to attend the laboratory at 8.00 a.m. to 9.00 a.m. after an overnight fast, and to refrain from exhaustive or long-duration exercise on the day preceding the visitations.

At the first visit, anthropometric parameters (body height, body weight, fat mass percentage, fat-free mass) were recorded, maximal oxygen uptake (VO$_2$max) was measured, and a study questionnaire including quantitative food frequency questionnaire was applied to the subjects.

At the second visit, the study exercise test (a cycle ergometer (45 min at 65% VO$_2$max) and immediately followed by a treadmill test (75% VO$_2$max to the exhaustion) was performed, and blood samples were collected immediately before and after the test for analysis of oxidative stress (plasma 8-iso PGF2a) and total oxidant and antioxidant biomarkers, and blood lactate (La⁻) and heart rate were measured before, 3 and 6 min post-exercise to determine exercise performance and post-exercise recovery. Before both the VO_2max test and the study exercise test, subjects were required to consume a standardized breakfast (50 g of carbohydrate, 6 g of protein, 3.5 g of fat) 2 h before the tests.

2.3. Dietary Records Assessment and Dietary Total Antioxidant Capacity Analysis

Dietary intake was determined using a validated quantitative food frequency questionnaire (QFFQ) [44] and 3-day food records. The QFFQ comprised 110 food items, and was used to assess the amount and frequency of total dietary consumption. The QFFQ was applied through face-to-face interviews by a sports dietitian. A photographic Meal and Food Atlas was used to record the quantity and portion size of food items more accurately [45]. The total dietary antioxidant intake was calculated using the intake frequency and total amount of each food item in QFFQ. The Ferric-reducing ability of plasma (FRAP) was calculated for each subject to assess the total antioxidant content of the diet [29]. To determine the dietary FRAP score, the Antioxidant Food Database developed by Carlsen et al. [29], which involves more than 3100 foods, spices, beverages, and herbs, was used. The FRAP assay measures the ability of reduction potential of each food to reduce ferric ($Fe+3$) ions to ferrous ($Fe+2$) ions. The FRAP assay was preferred because the assay does not include glutathione content of foods compared to other assays. This is considered an advantage because glutathione abundant in foods, but it is highly degraded in the human intestine and poorly absorbed in the body. FRAP scores were calculated with the exclusion of coffee in this study, in consistent with literature. Although the main antioxidant content of coffee has reported to be the Maillard products of the coffee which occurs during the roasting process, due to their high molecular weight, the percentage of absorption remains questioned. Therefore, coffee was excluded from total FRAP score to eliminate its effect on obscuring any other interactions between other sources of antioxidants and exercise-induced oxidative stress due to its high antioxidant capacity, in accordance with the literature [46].

An in-depth 24-h dietary recall was collected at the first visit to illustrate how subjects would collect the 3-day food record themselves. Before the second visit, the subjects completed 3-day food records (two working days and one weekend day). The food records data were converted to total daily energy and nutrient intake using the Nutrition Information System Software (BEBIS 6.1) program. When cooked meals were taken into account, the number of vitamins such as ascorbate, folate was adjusted by the software, i.e., the ascorbate was decreased to 50% of the uncooked value. Dietary micronutrient and micronutrient intakes were determined using Recommended Dietary Allowance (RDA) values approved by the National Institutes of Health (NIH) [47].

2.4. Maximal Oxygen uptake (VO_2max) Measurement

Since the study included both ultra-marathon runners and triathletes, and since it has been reported that triathletes who have particularly trained for a triathlon show a similar VO_2max for running and cycling [48], we preferred to measure VO_2max on a treadmill. Before the VO_2max test started, a warm-up of 5 min was performed at 5 km·h⁻¹ and 0% gradient on the treadmill. After 5 min of passive recovery, the incremental running protocol started at 10 km·h⁻¹ and with 0% gradient with the speed increasing by 1 km·h⁻¹ each min until a running speed of 18 km·h⁻¹ was achieved. After reaching and spending 1 min at the speed of 18 km·h⁻¹, whilst the speed was fixed at 18 km·h⁻¹, the gradient was increased by 1% each minute until exhaustion [49]. Heart rate was measured continuously and recorded at intervals of 30 s (Garmin HRM Soft Premium, Olathe, KS, USA). Respiratory parameters were recorded every 30 s (COSMED K5 metabolic cart; COSMED, Rome, Italy). Rating of perceived exertion (RPE) was used to monitor exercise intensity and fatigue during exhaustive exercise. The BORG 6-20 Category Scale was used to measure RPE by asking the subjects how tough they felt during an exercise bout at the end of each stage until volitional exhaustion [50].

VO$_2$max was determined as the highest average of the two highest sequential reading, in the case at least two of the following criteria was observed: (1) Whilst the exercise load increased, VO$_2$ remained stable in the last two stages (range < 2.1 mL·kg^{-1}·min^{-1}), (2) Respiratory exchange ratio (RER) ≥1.10, (3) maximum heart rate (HRmax) >90% of age-predicted HRmax (220-age) and (4) blood lactate concentration ≥8.00 mmol·L^{-1} [51].

2.5. Exercise Protocol

Subjects were initially cycling for 45 min at a submaximal speed (65 ± 5% VO$_2$max), and then immediately followed a running test at 75% VO$_2$max to exhaustion defined as inability to maintain running intensity. The expiration parameters (COSMED K5 metabolic cart; COSMED, Rome, Italy), and heart rate (Garmin HRM Soft Premium, Olathe, KS, USA) were recorded all the exercise period. The exercise test was performed under controlled laboratory conditions (20–25 °C, 40% relative humidity). All athletes were familiarized with cycling on a cycle ergometer and running on a treadmill.

The study protocol was determined based on Montenegro et al. [52], and was slightly changed based on our study aim. The time-to-exhaustion (TTE) exercise protocol was chosen because it has been applied to a similar population, and it has shown a significant decrease in response to exercise intensity [23]. Watson et al. [23] reported that the intensity of TTE exercise under 80% VO$_2$max appeared to have a lower coefficient of variation. According to that, the exercise intensity of the study was arranged at 75% VO$_2$max to exhaustion. The protocol ended with verbal approval by athletes, stating that they could not maintain the exercise intensity. The total running time was recorded.

2.6. Exercise Performance Measurement

Exercise time-to-exhaustion and post-exercise recovery of blood lactate and heart rate parameters were determined as exercise performance measurements.

2.7. Plasma Total Oxidant Status (TOS) and Plasma Total Antioxidant Status (TAS) Analysis

Two 18 mL venous blood parameters were collected into EDTA coated tubes immediately before and after the study exercise protocol. Plasma pellets were obtained by centrifugation at 3000× g for 10 min at 4 °C. Plasma total oxidant status was analyzed using an automated method (Total Oxidant Status Kit, Rel Assay® Diagnostics, Ankara, Turkey). The method is based on the oxidation of Fe^{+3} to Fe^{+2} in the presence of reactive oxidants in the acidic medium. The TOS results were expressed in μmoL H$_2$O$_2$ equivalent/L (μmoL H$_2$O$_2$ eq/L). Plasma total antioxidant status was measured using the colorimetric test system (Total Antioxidant Status Kit, Rel Assay® Diagnostics, Ankara, Turkey). The calibration of reaction was performed using Trolox (a water-soluble analogue of vitamin E, 6-hydroxy-2.5.7.8-tetramethylchroman-2-carboxylic acid), and the total antioxidant status was expressed as μmoL Trolox equivalent/L (μmoL Trolox eq/L).

Oxidative Stress Index (OSI) Calculation

Plasma TOS to TAS ratio was defined as the oxidative stress index (OSI) [53]. Before calculation, the TAS unit expressed in μmoL has to be converted to mmol, and calculated by the following formula;
OSI (arbitrary unit) = TOS (μmoL H$_2$O$_2$ equivalent/l)/TAS (mmol Trolox equivalent/l).

2.8. Plasma 8-isoprostaglandin F2alpha (8-iso PGF2a) Analysis

To assess the exercise-induced oxidative stress, 8-iso PGF2a level in plasma was measured using a competitive enzyme-linked immunosorbent assay kit (Elabscience® Biotechnology Co., Ltd., Houston TX, USA) (sensitivity: 9.38 pg/mL, detection range from 15.63 to 1000 pg/mL).

2.9. Lactate Analysis

To our knowledge, there is no certain suggestion to determine lactate clearance after exhaustive exercise, and its measurement 2 or 3 min after exercise is generally preferred in literature. In addition, Gass et al. [54] conducted a study to determine blood lactate concentration following a maximal exercise in trained athletes and stated that peak lactate values after maximal exertion was reached 6 min after exercise. Therefore, we preferred to measure the blood lactate concentration at the end of each 3 min and after exercise at 3 and 6 min to measure how diet in rich antioxidants effects on post-exercise lactate removal, especially at the peak lactate concentration time as it was practiced by Oh et al. [55] similarly in determining the removal of lactate after high-intensity exercise, and by Di Masi et al. [56] in comparing blood lactate clearance performed during cycling in water immersion and during cycling on land after a similar exercise bout. Blood lactate levels were measured using a validated portable blood lactate analyzer (Lactate plus, Nova Biomedical, Waltham, MA, USA). The quality control solutions provided by the manufacturer were used prior to testing, and a blood sample of 0.7 µL was required to assess the lactate concentration in capillary blood.

2.10. Statistical Analysis

Statistical analysis was performed using IBM SPSS Statistics Software for Windows version 23.0 (IBM Corporation, Armonk, New York, NY, USA). Sample size was calculated by assuming that 8-iso PGF2a levels would increase 70% after exhaustive exercise (Mrakic-Sposta et al.) [37,57], a total of 24 subjects (12 males, 12 females) were required. Prior to analysis, data were tested for normality using the Kolmogorov- Smirnov test, and were found to be non-normally distributed. Therefore, all data were reported as median and interquartile range. The Wilcoxon rank test was used to compare pre- and post-exercise plasma parameters. Effect size (d) for non-parametric tests was calculated using the following formula: $r = z/\sqrt{N}$ [58]. r is referred to as d, z is referred to as z value of Wilcoxon rank tests, N is referred to as the total number of subjects. To determine effect sizes; $d < 0.2$ was classified as a small effect, d between 0.2 and 0.5 was considered as a medium effect, and $d > 0.8$ was considered as a large effect. The Spearman's rho correlation coefficient was performed to measure the strength of an interaction between dietary antioxidant capacity (calculated FRAP score), and pre- and post-exercise changes of plasma oxidative stress, total oxidant and antioxidant parameters, post-exercise changes of heart rate (3rd HR–6th HR), lactate (3rd La$^-$–6th La$^-$), and TTE exercise, adjusted for years of training and average training to prevent their mixing effects on the outcome variables. All data were set at the 5% level ($p < 0.05$).

3. Results

3.1. Subjects

Basic characteristics and dietary intake based on sex of subjects are displayed in Table 1. No difference was observed according to their body weight (per kg) from carbohydrate ($p = 0.085$) and protein ($p = 0.124$) between sexes. The intakes met or exceeded the RDA values with the exception of vitamin E (94.4% of the requirement was met in females), vitamin A (81.0% of the requirement was met in males, and 72.1% of the requirement was met in females), and selenium (95.0% of the requirement was met in females).

Table 1. Basic characteristics and dietary intake of subjects, median (Interquartile range).

Parameter	Males ($n = 12$)	Females ($n = 12$)
Age (y)	38.5 (31.3–40.0)	38.0 ((31.6–44.5)
Height (cm)	179.0 (173.5–184.5)	162.0 (160.0–166.5) *
Body mass (kg)	72.6 (69.6–81.0)	56.5 (53.5–59.0) *
Fat mass percentage (%)	12.9 (10.0–16.3)	19.4 (9.2–12.9) *
Fat-free mass (kg)	63.8 (60.0–68.3)	45.5 (42.8–47.9) *

Table 1. Cont.

Parameter	Males (n = 12)	Females (n = 12)
Maximum oxygen consumption (VO_2 max), mL·min^{-1}·kg^{-1}	60.7 (52.7–65.1)	51.0 (48.7–52.2) *
Baseline training (h·week^{-1})	16.3 (15.0–17.6)	16.4 (15.5–17.0)
Years in ultra-endurance sports (y)	6.0 (2.75–20.0)	10.5 (4.0–20.0)
Dietary intake per day	**%RDA ** **	**%RDA ** **
Energy (kcal)	2571.8 (2057.4–3355.5)	1871.7 (1589.7–2020.0) *
Carbohydrate (%)	36.1 (33.2–41.5)	34.0 (29.6–35.9)
Carbohydrate (g^{-1}·kg^{-1}·d)	3.4 (2.3–3.8)	2.7 (2.1–3.2)
Protein (%)	19.9 (16.7–21.8)	16.3 (14.8–18.2) *
Protein (g^{-1}·kg^{-1}·d)	1.6 (1.3–2.2)	1.3 (1.2–1.3)
Fat (%)	43.8 (40.9–49.9)	49.8 (48.9–52.9) *
Omega 3 (g)	2.9 (2.4–4.1)	2.6 (1.9–3.6)
Omega 6 (g)	25.4 (19.1–32.0)	20.0 (14.6–24.5)
Vitamin C (mg)	145.6 (84.9–186.1) 161.7	98.9 (68.0–121.3) 136.7
Vitamin E (mg)	28.7 (20.8–31.7) 143.6	18.9 (12.5–25.2) * 94.4
Vitamin A (RAE)	729.2 (592.1–815.9) 81.0	505.0 (403.5–915.0) 72.1
Selenium (μg)	52.2 (43.4–65.0) 95.0	57.5 (45.2–62.1) 104.5
Zinc (mg)	14.8 (13.5–20.8) 134.5	10.6 (10.1–11.7) * 132.0

* $p < 0.05$; ** % RDA represents the percentage of median micronutrient intakes of subjects compared to the recommended dietary allowance (RDA).

3.2. Dietary Antioxidant Intake

The amount of dietary antioxidant intake for total and each food group is presented in Figure 1. Including with the contribution of coffee, the coffee comprised 38.5% and 44.6% of total FRAP scores in males and females, respectively. Due to coffee's possible effects on any obscure interactions between other antioxidant sources of FRAP and exercise performance, the total antioxidant intake was assessed excluding the coffee. Foods were grouped as vegetables, fresh fruits, dry fruits, cereals, legumes, nuts and seeds, dairy, meats, eggs, and beverages. No statistical difference was found with regard to the antioxidant capacity for each food group between sexes (sum of FRAP; 16.6 (14.8–22.8) mmol/day and 17.2 (14.1–23.6) mmol/day, males and females respectively) ($p = 0.908$).

3.3. Changes in Plasma Oxidative Stress Biomarkers after Exercise Testing

Table 2 summarizes the role of acute exhaustive exercise on changes of plasma oxidative stress biomarkers. All oxidant and antioxidant biomarkers indicated a significant effect of the exhaustive exercise. Plasma 8-iso PGF2a levels increased up to 444.6 (410.6–482.3) pg/mL from 230.7 (217.9–305.0) pg/mL in males ($d = 0.60$, $p = 0.003$), and up to 458.01 (447.2–556.0) pg/mL from 223.8 (214.2–268.3) pg/mL in females ($d = 0.60$, $p = 0.003$) and the calculated oxidative stress index increased up to 0.4 (0.3–0.4) from 0.3 (0.3–0.4) in males ($d = 0.63$, $p = 0.002$), and up to 0.3 (0.3–0.4) from 0.3 (0.2–0.3) in females ($d = 0.63$, $p = 0.003$) after exercise. The significant increase was also found for total antioxidant parameters (median changes in plasma TAS levels; 13.6 % for males ($d = 0.62$; $p = 0.002$) and 12.0 % for females ($d = 0.63$; $p = 0.002$)). The calculated oxidative stress index suggested an increase after exercise (median changes in OSI; 27.5 % for males ($d = 0.5$, $p = 0.002$) and 20.7 % for females ($d = 0.6$, $p = 0.003$)).

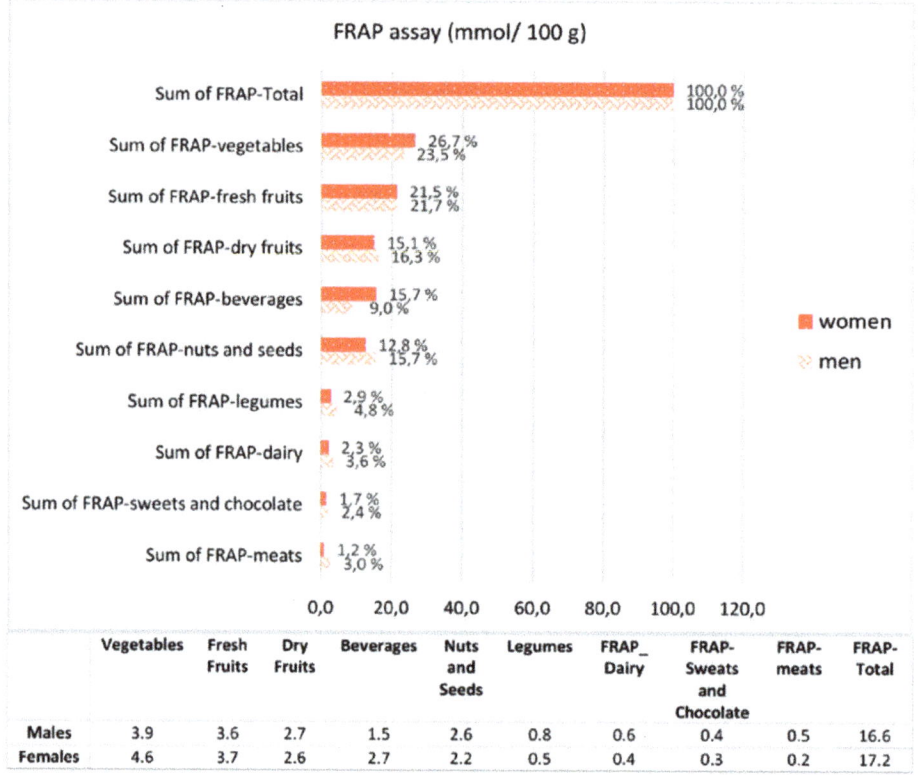

Figure 1. The contribution of foods and beverages to dietary total antioxidant intake according to FRAP assay [27].

Table 2. Plasma oxidative stress parameters before and after the exercise protocol.

Plasma Parameters		Pre-Exercise	Post-Exercise	Δ (Post- vs. Pre-)	Effect Size (d)	Change (%; Range)	p
TOS [a] (µmol H$_2$O$_2$eq/L)	Men	3.9 (3.6–4.5)	5.0 (4.8–7.3)	1.1 (0.5–2.9)	0.50	30.3 (11.0–84.0)	0.015 *
	Women	3.4 (3.2–4.1)	5.0 (4.6–5.6)	1.7 (0.6–2.3)	0.59	48.2 (18.0–65.4)	0.004 *
TAS [b] (µmol Trolox equivalent/L)	Men	1.6 (1.5–1.6)	1.8 (1.7–1.8)	0.2 (0.2–0.3)	0.62	13.6 (11.1–16.1)	0.002 *
	Women	1.4 (1.3–1.5)	1.6 (1.5–1.7)	0.2 (0.1–0.2)	0.63	12.0 (9.5–15.9)	0.002 *
OSI [c]	Men	0.3 (0.3–0.4)	0.4 (0.3 0.4)	0.1 (0.1–0.1)	0.63	27.5 (19.7–40.1)	0.002 *
	Women	0.3 (0.2–0.3)	0.3 (0.3– 0.4)	0.1 (0.0–0.1)	0.60	20.7 (14.1–36.2)	0.003 *
8-iso PGF2α (pg/mL)	Men	230.7 (217.9–305.0)	444.6 (410.6–482.3)	193.5 (171.0–228.0)	0.60	80.5 (58.7–112.6)	0.003 *
	Women	223.8 (214.2–268.3)	458.0 (447.2–556.0)	219.6 (179.0–290.7)	0.60	99.1 (58.6–143.4)	0.003 *

Concentrations are expressed as median (interquartile range). [a] TOS: total oxidant capacity (plasma); [b] TAS: total antioxidant capacity; [c] OSI: oxidative stress index.

3.4. Dietary Antioxidants and Exercise Performance

Table 3 represents the interaction between total dietary antioxidant capacity and both plasma exercise-induced redox status and oxidative stress biomarkers. The years of training and average training time were adjusted to eliminate their confounding effects on the results. Dietary antioxidant intake was negatively correlated to pre-exercise TOS concentrations (rs = −0.641 for males; $p = 0.025$, and rs = −0.741 for females; $p = 0.006$) and Δ(post- vs. pre-) 8-isoPGF2a concentrations (rs = −0.702 for males; $p = 0.016$, and rs = −0.682 for females; $p = 0.024$). A positive correlation between ΔTAS concentrations was observed (rs = 0.893 for males, and rs = 0.769 for females; $p = 0.001$ and $p = 0.002$ respectively).

Table 3. Correlations of pre- and post- exercise plasma biomarkers related to oxidative stress with dietary antioxidant intake, adjusted for years of training, and average training.

		Dietary Antioxidant Intake (FRAP-mmol/day)			
		Males ($n = 12$)		Females ($n = 12$)	
		r	p	r	p
TOS[a] (μmol H_2O_2eq/L)	Pre	−0.641	0.025 *	−0.741	0.006 **
	Post	0.147	0.648	−0.077	0.812
	Δ(Post- vs. Pre-)	0.343	0.216	−0.497	0.101
TAS[b] (μmol Trolox equivalent/L)	Pre	0.225	0.483	0.077	0.812
	Post	0.514	0.087	0.417	0.178
	Δ(Post- vs. Pre-)	0.893	0.001 **	0.769	0.002 **
OSI[c] (arbitrary unit)	Pre	0.320	0.311	−0.451	0.141
	Post	0.056	0.863	−0.077	0.811
	Δ(Post- vs. Pre-)	−0.409	0.187	0.266	0.404
8-isoPGF2a (pg/mL)	Pre	−0.417	0.201	−0.373	0.259
	Post	−0.573	0.066	0.055	0.873
	Δ(Post- vs. Pre-)	−0.702	0.016 *	−0.682	0.024 *
Time-to-exhaustion (min)		0.692	0.013 *	−0.028	0.931
Lactate (mmol/L)	Δ(Post- 3rd La⁻–6th La⁻)	0.795	0.006 **	0.642	0.024 *
Heart rate (HR) (bpm)	Δ(Post- 3rd La⁻–6th La⁻)	0.246	0.440	0.074	0.819
RPE[d]	Post	−0.525	0.079	−0.022	0.945

Spearman's rho correlation. * $p < 0.05$. ** $p < 0.001$; [a] TOS: total oxidant capacity (plasma); [b] TAS: total antioxidant capacity; [c] OSI: oxidative stress index [d] RPE: rating of perceived exertion.

The difference between ΔTOS concentrations was not significantly related to FRAP scores ($p = 0.216$ for males, and $p = 0.101$ for females). The median running time was 26.7 (26.0–28.1) min in males and 26.5 (25.6–27.2) min in female subjects. A positive meaningful ($p = 0.013$) interaction was observed between TTE exercise (rs = 0.692) for males. The median lactate concentration 3 and 6 min after exercise was 12.2 (10.9–13.5) mmol/L and 10.40 (9.5–11.9) mmol/L in males and 10.2 (9.3–11.2) mmol/L and 10.1 (8.6–10.4) mmol/L in females, respectively, and pointed out that the high intensity of the exercise protocol applied in the study. The post-exercise Δlactate concentrations (rs = 0.795 for male athletes, and rs = 0.642 for females; $p = 0.006$ and $p = 0.024$, respectively) were positively correlated to dietary FRAP score. The median heart rate 3 and 6 min after exercise was 146.0 (135.5–153.8) and 132.5 (127.3–147.8) bpm in males and 141.0 (133.3–154.8) and 132.0 (123.3–147.5) bpm in females. No significant relationship was observed between post-exercise Δheart rate values and dietary antioxidant intake ($p = 0.440$ for males and $p = 0.819$). The median of RPE was 19.0 (18.3–20.0) in males and 19.00 (18.3–19.0) in females and indicated that the applied exercise test was perceived as quite exhausting by the subjects. RPE scores were not significantly related to dietary antioxidant intake ($p = 0.079$ for males and $p = 0.945$ for females).

4. Discussion

The main purpose of the present study was to investigate the effects of dietary antioxidant capacity on exhaustive exercise-induced oxidative stress and total oxidant/antioxidant status in ultra-endurance athletes. The main findings were that total dietary antioxidant capacity had a significant influence on body antioxidant defense against acute exhaustive exercise-induced oxidative stress. A diet high in antioxidants was positively related to blood lactate removal after exercise for both sexes, and running time to exhaustion just in males. However, no significant interaction was observed between dietary antioxidants and post-exercise HR recovery. Therefore, the hypothesis that consuming an antioxidant-rich diet would increase the body exogenous antioxidant defenses developed against extreme endurance exercise has been confirmed, but its effects on exercise performance and recovery remained uncertain.

In the present study, the dietary micronutrient analysis indicated that subjects mainly met or exceeded the daily recommended intake except for vitamin E for females and vitamin A for both sexes. Although the consumption of vitamin E and A seemed not problematic and the subjects mostly met the RDA [47], it should be taken into account that the RDA values are designed for non-athletic populations, and athletic populations may require more than a sedentary population, as demonstrated in literature [59]. Considering total dietary antioxidant intake calculated with FRAP, the median dietary antioxidant content was observed 16.6 (14.8–22.8) mmol/day in males and 17.2 (14.1–23.6) mmol/day for females. Carlsen et al. [29] provided no cut-off point for the FRAP score to determine total dietary antioxidant content high in antioxidants. However, Koivisto et al. [60] performed a randomized control placebo trial in elite endurance athletes to investigate the effects of dietary antioxidant intervention during a 3-week altitude training camp on improvement of oxygen-carrying capacity and exercise performance. The total antioxidant concentration of dietary intervention was calculated using the FRAP assay. The FRAP score of 22.2 mmol/day was defined as a diet high in antioxidant, and 2.8 mmol/day was defined as a low antioxidant diet. Comparing with their research [60], the subjects in the present study consumed a moderate-to-high dietary antioxidant diet. Thus, taking together with total dietary antioxidant and micronutrient intake, the subjects' diet may meet the requirements to defense against exhaustive exercise-induced ROS.

In this study, we investigated the role of dietary antioxidants and polyphenolic content on oxidative stress, since research on oxidative stress often ignored its potential impact on oxidative metabolism and performance. Several dietary strategies were applied to diminish or protect against the exercise-induced oxidative damage that caused accumulation of excessive oxygen species, and had an adverse effect on muscle damage, contractile function, lipid peroxidation [34,61]. However, the studies were predominantly carried out by applying antioxidant supplementation, and the effects on oxidative stress remained controversial. Antioxidant micronutrients such as vitamins A, C, E, D, the B vitamins, zinc, beta carotene, and selenium have been commonly studied based on their antioxidant properties [11,13–15,28]. Mastaloudis et al. [14] performed a randomized control placebo trial in runners to investigate the effects of supplementation with 300 IU vitamin E and 1000 mg vitamin C for 6 weeks prior to a 50 km ultra-marathon. Plasma F2-prostanes were elevated just in the placebo group after the ultra-marathon, but inflammation biomarkers (Interleukin-6, C-reactive protein, tumor necrosis alpha) were increased regardless of treatment or placebo. The results pointed out that an antioxidant supplementation protects against exercise-induced oxidative stress, but not against inflammation after an ultra-marathon. McAnulty et al. [62] assessed the effects of vitamin E supplementation with 800 IU for two months prior to a triathlon race (a 2.4-mile ocean swim, a 112-mile bike race and a 26.2-mile run) on plasma homocysteine and oxidative stress biomarkers in triathletes. Cortisol was increased regardless of the treatment, and plasma F2-isoprostanes was significantly increased in the treatment group (181%) compared to the placebo group (97%) suggesting that a prolonged vitamin E supplementation exhibited pro-oxidant characteristics in triathletes during exhaustive exercise. Since the antioxidant supplementation may cause a detrimental effect on body redox metabolism, and research on the effects of dietary antioxidants on exercise performance revealed that antioxidant supplementation has only influenced exercise performance on athletes with clinically nutrient deficiencies [23], the need for understanding the crucial role of dietary antioxidant consumption comes into prominence.

The acute exhaustive exercise increased ROS production and plasma oxidative stress (change in 8-iso PGF2a levels; 80.5% for males, and 99.1% for females) and total oxidant biomarkers (change in TOS levels; 30.3% for males and 48.2% for females) were significantly increased after the exercise. Research on oxidative stress and performance suggested that an increase in 8-iso PGF2a served as a more reliable indicator to determine lipid peroxidation [23,34]. The increase of both plasma 8-iso PGF2a and TOS (as a biomarker of oxidative stress) and the oxidative stress index (as an indicator of increased oxidative status) found in this study are consistent with existing literature [34,37,38,53]. As commonly demonstrated, both exhaustive exercise and a long period of exercise are highly associated with a remarkable accumulation of oxidative radicals beyond the body's limits to defense ROS [35]. Therefore, a detailed insight into the body's antioxidant defense under exhaustive exercise becomes of the utmost importance.

The findings of a meaningful increase of plasma TAS (as a biomarker of antioxidant capacity) after exhaustive exercise test was in contrast to earlier studies [23,63]. A potential explanation for the observed results could be attributed to the body antioxidant defense capacity which was thought to improve with both training and adaptation to exercise [64]. The average years of training of the subjects were 6.0 (2.8–20.0) years for males, and 10.5 (4.0–20.0) years for females suggesting that the longer periods in performance could be an effective factor for the adaptation of the body towards oxidative stress.

It has been reported that a dietary intervention has a significant influence on the exercise-induced F2-isoprostanes concentrations [23]. In line with existing literature, a meaningful negative interaction was found between dietary antioxidant consumption and Δ8-iso PGF2a concentrations indicating that changes in oxidative stress after exercise arises depending of the dietary antioxidant capacity. Furthermore, a meaningful negative interaction between TOS at rest and dietary antioxidant intake (calculated using FRAP assay) was found. These results indicated that antioxidant-rich diet consumption may have a paramount effect on body antioxidant defense.

In the present study, no significant relationship was observed between plasma TAS at rest and diet FRAP scores. Plasma total antioxidant concentration at rest may not be a good predictor to determine the body antioxidant capacity because of its disregarding potential to consider individual antioxidant tissue stores and differences in mobilization ability of the stores in the plasma [34]. Therefore, the determination of the interaction between exercise-induced plasma TAS changes and FRAP scores could be a better choice to interpret the effects of dietary antioxidant intake on exercise-altered antioxidant mechanism of subjects. A positive relationship between exercise-induced changes of total plasma antioxidant capacity and FRAP scores also suggested that these ultra-endurance athletes consumed antioxidant-rich diets which could improve a better antioxidant defense against oxidative damage after exhaustive exercise.

In this study, a time-to-exhaustion exercise protocol was preferred because its effects on oxidative stress have already been confirmed in other studies, and treadmill-based TTE could be classified as a reliable research tool to determine both the endurance performance and the relative exercise intensity in trained athletes [23]. It is well-known that oxidative damage is increasing in line with both exercise duration and exercise intensity [8]. In addition to that, blood lactate concentration and heart rate scores monitored after exercise are also other indicators of exercise performance and post-exercise recovery, and commonly used in clinical practice [65–67]. It is well reported that lactate production gradually increases in line with exercise intensity during exhaustive exercise, and blood lactate clearance rate is a good predictor for the rate of post-exercise recovery [68,69]. Considering all the information related to both exercise performance and post-exercise recovery, a meaningful interaction was observed between dietary antioxidant capacity and TTE and Δlactate concentrations in males. Dietary antioxidant capacity was positively related to Δlactate concentrations in female subjects, but not related to lactate concentrations 3 and 6 min after exercise. All the results addressed that dietary antioxidant intake may affect exercise performance and post-exercise recovery in males. However, the same interaction cannot be confirmed for females when only considering lactate concentrations.

Our findings showed no significant interaction between the FRAP and RPE scores. RPE has been identified as a common indicator to describe how hard an exercise task is during exercise, and has been defined in terms of its strong interaction between exercise intensity [70,71]. Doherty and Smith [71] conducted a meta-analysis related to the role of caffeine on exercise capacity. In their study, the caffeine-mediated improvement of exercise capacity was assessed based on the reduced RPE levels after exercise. A similar interaction between RPE and performance was demonstrated in the study, in which the influence of nitrate and caffeine consumption on exercise performance was examined [72]. The possible explanation why no interaction was detected in our results was that the self-perceived fatigue during exercise was almost similar in all subjects (median 19 for both sexes) and therefore not related to dietary antioxidant consumption.

A limitation of the study was that ultra-endurance athletes compete under more extreme conditions compared to the study exercise protocol. However, we preferred a TTE protocol immediately after a 45 min cycle ergometer exercise with a submaximal speed to push the body's limits, and thus to increase the exercise-induced oxidative stress in subjects. In addition, lactate accumulation concentrations, RPE and HR scores after exercise indicated the strenuousness of the exercise protocol. Future studies may be performed in a competitive ultra-marathon or a triathlon race to ensure more reliable conditions to assess the relationship between the dietary antioxidant intake and its effects on both the body redox balance and exercise performance. On the other hand, the main strength of our study was that this is the first study conducted to calculate total dietary antioxidant content by FRAP assay in ultra-endurance athletes. Furthermore, the determination of the all dietary records and analyses was applied by a qualified sports dietitian. This study provides the framework for future studies to consider the substantial role of dietary antioxidant capacity on both performance and exercise-induced oxidative damage. In future research on exercise-induced oxidative stress, the dietary records should also be investigated to provide more insight into its influence on oxidative balance in ultra-endurance athletes.

5. Conclusions

In conclusion, exhaustive exercise attenuated oxidative stress and altered redox balance in ultra-endurance athletes. We confirmed that total dietary antioxidant capacity had a significant role to assess the exogenous antioxidant defense of the body, therefore a diet rich in antioxidants may provide a better oxidative balance after an exhaustive exercise. Dietary antioxidant intake including antioxidant and polyphenolic content may positively improve both exercise performance and post-exercise recovery, however further work is needed. Our results are encouraging and should be validated in a larger cohort of ultra-endurance athletes.

Author Contributions: Conceptualization, A.D.-L., P.B., G.D., T.K., T.R., and B.K., formal analysis, A.D.-L., investigation, A.D.-L., G.D., and T.K., resources A.D.-L. and T.K., writing-original draft preparation, A.D.-L., T.R., and B.K., writing—review and editing, A.D.-L., P.B., T.R., and B.K., visualization, A.D.-L., P.B., G.D., T.K., T.R., and B.K., supervision, P.B. and B.K. All authors have read and agreed to the published version of the manuscript.

Funding: The study received no external funding.

Acknowledgments: The study was supported by The Ministry of Youth and Sports of Turkey. The authors would like to thank Erkan Tortu, Ebru Aslanoglu, Aslıhan Nefes, Didem Gençal, Mefaret Tekin, Eylem Orhan Aksüt, Salih Sarı, and Bahar Sevgen for their help in collecting data and supports.

Conflicts of Interest: The authors declare no conflict of interest.

References

1. Laursen, P.B. Long distance triathlon: Demands, preparation and performance. *J. Hum. Sport Exerc.* **2011**, *6*, 247–263. [CrossRef]
2. Knechtle, B.; Nikolaidis, P.T. Physiology and pathophysiology in ultra-marathon running. *Front. Physiol.* **2018**, *9*, 634–667. [CrossRef]
3. Sachdev, S.; Davies, K.J.A. Production, detection, and adaptive responses to free radicals in exercise. *Free Radic. Biol. Med.* **2008**, *44*, 215–223. [CrossRef] [PubMed]
4. Teixeira, V.H.; Valente, H.F.; Casal, S.I.; Marques, A.F.; Moreira, P.A. Antioxidants do not prevent postexercise peroxidation and may delay muscle recovery. *Med. Sci. Sports Exerc.* **2009**, *41*, 1752–1760. [CrossRef] [PubMed]
5. Nocella, C.; Cammisotto, V.; Pigozzi, F.; Borrione, P.; Fossati, C.; D'amico, A.; Cangemi, R.; Peruzzi, M.; Gobbi, G.; Ettorre, E.; et al. Impairment between oxidant and antioxidant systems: Short- and Long-Term implications for athletes' health. *Nutrients* **2019**, *11*, 1353. [CrossRef] [PubMed]
6. Liu, H.W.; Kao, H.H.; Wu, C.H. Exercise training upregulates SIRT1 to attenuate inflammation and metabolic dysfunction in kidney and liver of diabetic db/db mice. *Nutr. Metab.* **2019**, *16*. [CrossRef]

7. Pyne, D.B. Exercise-induced muscle damage and inflammation: A review. *Aust. J. Sci. Med. Sport* **1994**, *26*, 49–58. [PubMed]
8. Powers, S.K.; Jackson, M.J. Exercise-induced oxidative stress: Cellular mechanisms and impact on muscle force production. *Physiol. Rev.* **2008**, *88*, 1243–1276. [CrossRef]
9. Barclay, J.K.; Hansel, M. Free radicals may contribute to oxidative skeletal muscle fatigue. *Can. J. Physiol. Pharm.* **1991**, *69*, 279–284. [CrossRef]
10. Reichhold, S.; Neubauer, O.; Bulmer, A.C.; Knasmü, S.; Wagner, K.-H. Endurance exercise and DNA stability: Is there a link to duration and intensity? *Mutat. Res.* **2009**, *682*, 28–38. [CrossRef] [PubMed]
11. Alessio, H.M.; Goldfarb, A.H.; Cao, G. Exercise-induced oxidative stress before and after vitamin C supplementation. *Int. J. Sport Nutr. Exerc. Metab.* **1997**, *7*, 1–9. [CrossRef] [PubMed]
12. McLeay, Y.; Stannard, S.; Houltham, S.; Starck, C. Dietary thiols in exercise: Oxidative stress defence, exercise performance, and adaptation. *J. Int. Soc. Sports Nutr.* **2017**, *14*, 12. [CrossRef] [PubMed]
13. Thompson, D.; Williams, C.; McGregor, S.J.; Nicholas, C.W.; McArdle, F.; Jackson, M.J.; Powell, J.R. Prolonged vitamin C supplementation and recovery from demanding exercise. *Int. J. Sport Nutr.* **2001**, *11*, 466–481. [CrossRef] [PubMed]
14. Mastaloudis, A.; Morrow, J.D.; Hopkins, D.W.; Devaraj, S.; Traber, M.G. Antioxidant supplementation prevents exercise-induced lipid peroxidation, but not inflammation, in ultramarathon runners. *Free Radic. Biol. Med.* **2004**, *36*, 1329–1341. [CrossRef]
15. Gauche, E.; Lepers, R.; Rabita, G.; Leveque, J.M.; Bishop, D.; Brisswalter, J.; Hausswirth, C. Vitamin and mineral supplementation and neuromuscular recovery after a running race. *Med. Sci. Sports Exerc.* **2006**, *38*, 2110–2117. [CrossRef]
16. Vitale, K.C.; Hueglin, S.; Broad, E. Tart Cherry Juice in Athletes. *Curr. Sports Med. Rep.* **2017**, *16*, 230–239. [CrossRef]
17. McAnulty, S.R.; McAnulty, L.S.; Nieman, D.C.; Dumke, C.L.; Morrow, J.D.; Utter, A.C.; Henson, D.A.; Proulx, W.R.; George, G.L. Consumption of blueberry polyphenols reduces exercise-induced oxidative stress compared to vitamin C. *Nutr. Res.* **2004**, *24*, 209–221. [CrossRef]
18. Gaeini, A.A.; Rahnama, N.; Hamedinia, M.R. Effects of vitamin E supplementation on oxidative stress at rest and after exercise to exhaustion in athletic students. *J. Sport. Med. Phys. Fit.* **2006**, *46*, 458–461.
19. Peternelj, T.T.; Coombes, J.S. Antioxidant supplementation during exercise training: Beneficial or detrimental? *Sport. Med.* **2011**, *41*, 1043–1069. [CrossRef]
20. Draeger, C.L.; Naves, A.; Marques, N.; Baptistella, A.B.; Carnauba, R.A.; Paschoal, V.; Nicastro, H. Controversies of antioxidant vitamins supplementation in exercise: Ergogenic or ergolytic effects in humans? *J. Int. Soc. Sports Nutr.* **2014**, *11*, 4. [CrossRef]
21. Michailidis, Y.; Karagounis, L.G.; Terzis, G.; Jamurtas, A.Z.; Spengos, K.; Tsoukas, D.; Chatzinikolaou, A.; Mandalidis, D.; Stefanetti, R.J.; Papassotiriou, I.; et al. Thiol-based antioxidant supplementation alters human skeletal muscle signaling and attenuates its inflammatory response and recovery after intense eccentric exercise. *Am. J. Clin. Nutr.* **2013**, *98*, 233–245. [CrossRef] [PubMed]
22. Petersen, A.C.; McKenna, M.J.; Medved, I.; Murphy, K.T.; Brown, M.J.; Della Gatta, P.; Cameron-Smith, D. Infusion with the antioxidant N-acetylcysteine attenuates early adaptive responses to exercise in human skeletal muscle. *Acta Physiol.* **2012**, *204*, 382–392. [CrossRef] [PubMed]
23. Watson, T.A.; Callister, R.; Taylor, R.D.; Sibbritt, D.W.; Macdonald-Wicks, L.K.; Garg, M.L. Antioxidant restriction and oxidative stress in short-duration exhaustive exercise. *Med. Sci. Sports Exerc.* **2005**, *37*, 63–71. [CrossRef] [PubMed]
24. Radak, Z.; Taylor, A.W.; Ohno, H.; Goto, S. Adaptation to exercise-induced oxidative stress: From muscle to brain. *Exerc. Immunol. Rev.* **2001**, *7*, 90–107.
25. Margaritis, I.; Rousseau, A.S. Does physical exercise modify antioxidant requirements? *Nutr. Res. Rev.* **2008**, *21*, 3–12. [CrossRef]
26. He, F.; Li, J.; Liu, Z.; Chuang, C.-C.; Yang, W.; Zuo, L. Redox Mechanism of Reactive Oxygen Species in Exercise. *Front. Physiol.* **2016**, *7*, 486. [CrossRef]
27. Radak, Z.; Zhao, Z.; Koltai, E.; Ohno, H.; Atalay, M. Oxygen consumption and usage during physical exercise: The balance between oxidative stress and ROS-dependent adaptive signaling. *Antioxid. Redox Signal.* **2013**, *18*, 1208–1246. [CrossRef]

28. Yavari, A.; Javadi, M.; Mirmiran, P.; Bahadoran, Z. Exercise-Induced Oxidative Stress and Dietary Antioxidants. *Asian J. Sport. Med.* **2015**, *6*, 24898. [CrossRef]
29. Carlsen, M.H.; Halvorsen, B.L.; Holte, K.; Bøhn, S.K.; Dragland, S.; Sampson, L.; Willey, C.; Senoo, H.; Umezono, Y.; Sanada, C.; et al. The total antioxidant content of more than 3100 foods, beverages, spices, herbs and supplements used worldwide. *Nutr. J.* **2010**, *9*, 3. [CrossRef]
30. Schneider, C.D.; Bock, P.M.; Becker, G.F.; Moreira, J.C.F.; Bello-Klein, A.; Oliveira, A.R. Comparison of the effects of two antioxidant diets on oxidative stress markers in triathletes. *Biol. Sport* **2018**, *35*, 181–189. [CrossRef]
31. Lee, E.C.; Fragala, M.S.; Kavouras, S.A.; Queen, R.M.; Pryor, J.L.; Casa, D.J. Biomarkers in sports and exercise: Tracking health, performance, and recovery in athletes. *J. Strength Cond. Res.* **2017**, *31*, 2920–2937. [CrossRef] [PubMed]
32. Katerji, M.; Filippova, M. Duerksen-Hughes Penelope Approaches and Methods to Measure Oxidative Stress in Clinical Samples: Research Applications in the Cancer Field. *Oxid. Med. Cell. Longev.* **2019**, 1–29. [CrossRef] [PubMed]
33. Kurutas, E.B. The importance of antioxidants which play the role in cellular response against oxidative/nitrosative stress: Current state. *Nutr. J.* **2016**, *15*, 71–93. [CrossRef] [PubMed]
34. Vezzoli, A.; Dellanoce, C.; Mrakic-Sposta, S.; Montorsi, M.; Moretti, S.; Tonini, A.; Pratali, L.; Accinni, R. Oxidative Stress Assessment in Response to Ultraendurance Exercise: Thiols Redox Status and ROS Production according to Duration of a Competitive Race. *Oxid. Med. Cell. Longev.* **2016**, *2016*, 1–13. [CrossRef]
35. Mastaloudis, A.; Leonard, S.W.; Traber, M.G. Oxidative stress in athletes during extreme endurance exercise. *Free Radic. Biol. Med.* **2001**, *31*, 911–922. [CrossRef]
36. Nieman, D.C.; Henson, D.A.; Mcanulty, S.R.; Mcanulty, L.; Swick, N.S.; Utter, A.C.; Vinci, D.M.; Opiela, S.J.; Morrow, J.D.; Mcan-Ulty, S.R.; et al. Influence of vitamin C supplementation on oxidative and immune changes after an ultramarathon. *J. Appl. Physiol.* **1970**, *92*. [CrossRef]
37. Mrakic-Sposta, S.; Gussoni, M.; Moretti, S.; Pratali, L.; Giardini, G.; Tacchini, P.; Dellanoce, C.; Tonacci, A.; Mastorci, F.; Borghini, A.; et al. Effects of Mountain Ultra-Marathon Running on ROS Production and Oxidative Damage by Micro-Invasive Analytic Techniques. *PLoS ONE* **2015**, *10*, e0141780. [CrossRef]
38. Kennedy, G.; Spence, V.A.; McLaren, M.; Hill, A.; Underwood, C.; Belch, J.J.F. Oxidative stress levels are raised in chronic fatigue syndrome and are associated with clinical symptoms. *Free Radic. Biol. Med.* **2005**, *39*, 584–589. [CrossRef]
39. Janse, D.E.; Jonge, X.; Thompson, B.; Han, A. Methodological Recommendations for Menstrual Cycle Research in Sports and Exercise. *Med. Sci. Sports Exerc.* **2019**, *51*, 2610–2617. [CrossRef]
40. Smekal, G.; Von Duvillard, S.P.; Frigo, P.; Tegelhofer, T.; Pokan, R.; Hofmann, P.; Tschan, H.; Baron, R.; Wonisch, M.; Renezeder, K.; et al. Menstrual cycle: No effect on exercise cardiorespiratory variables or blood lactate concentration. *Med. Sci. Sports Exerc.* **2007**, *39*, 1098–1106. [CrossRef]
41. Joyce, K.M.; Stewart, S.H. Standardization of Menstrual Cycle Dataor the Analysis of Intensive Longitudinal Data. In *Menstrual Cycle*; IntechOpen Limited: London, UK, 2019.
42. Borrás, C.; Gambini, J.; López-Grueso, R.; Pallardó, F.V.; Viña, J. Direct antioxidant and protective effect of estradiol on isolated mitochondria. *Biochim. Biophys. Acta* **2010**, *1802*, 205–211. [CrossRef] [PubMed]
43. Oosthuyse, T.; Bosch, A.N. The effect of the menstrual cycle on exercise metabolism: Implications for exercise performance in eumenorrhoeic women. *Sport. Med.* **2010**, *40*, 207–227. [CrossRef] [PubMed]
44. Marventano, S.; Mistretta, A.; Platania, A.; Galvano, F.; Grosso, G. Reliability and relative validity of a food frequency questionnaire for Italian adults living in Sicily, Southern Italy. *Int. J. Food Sci. Nutr.* **2016**, *67*, 857–864. [CrossRef] [PubMed]
45. Rakicioglu, N.; Acar Tek, N.; Ayaz, A.; Pekcan, G. *Photographic Atlas of Food and Meal Portion Sizes*; Ata Publications: Ankara, Turkey, 2012; ISBN 978-9944-5508-0-2.
46. Mancini, F.R.; Affret, A.; Dow, C.; Balkau, B.; Bonnet, F.; Boutron-Ruault, M.C.; Fagherazzi, G. Dietary antioxidant capacity and risk of type 2 diabetes in the large prospective E3N-EPIC cohort. *Diabetologia* **2018**, *61*, 308–316. [CrossRef]
47. Institute of Medicine; Food and Nutrition Board. Nutrient Recommendations: Dietary Reference Intakes (DRI). Available online: https://ods.od.nih.gov/Health_Information/Dietary_Reference_Intakes.aspx (accessed on 25 April 2020).

48. Hue, O.; Le Gallais, D.; Chollet, D.; Préfaut, C. Ventilatory threshold and maximal oxygen uptake in present triathletes. *Can. J. Appl. Physiol.* **2000**, *25*, 102–113. [CrossRef]
49. Shing, C.M.; Peake, J.M.; Lim, C.L.; Briskey, D.; Walsh, N.P.; Fortes, M.B.; Ahuja, K.D.K.; Vitetta, L. Effects of probiotics supplementation on gastrointestinal permeability, inflammation and exercise performance in the heat. *Eur. J. Appl. Physiol.* **2014**, *114*, 93–103. [CrossRef]
50. Borg, G. Psychophysical bases of perceived exertion. *Med. Sci. Sports Exerc.* **1982**, *14*, 377–381. [CrossRef]
51. Howley, E.; Bassett, D.; Welch, G. Criteria for maximal oxygen uptake: Review and commentary. *Med. Sci. Sports Exerc.* **1995**, *27*, 1292–1300. [CrossRef]
52. Montenegro, C.F.; Kwong, D.A.; Minow, Z.A.; Davis, B.A.; Lozada, C.F.; Casazza, G.A. Betalain-rich supplementation improves exercise performance and recovery in competitive triathletes. *Appl. Physiol. Nutr. Metab.* **2017**, *42*, 166–172. [CrossRef]
53. Erel, O. A new automated colorimetric method for measuring total oxidant status. *Clin. Biochem.* **2005**, *38*, 1103–1111. [CrossRef]
54. Gass, G.C.; Rogers, S.; Mitchell, R. Blood lactate concentration following maximum exercise in trained subjects. *Br. J. Sports Med.* **1981**, *15*, 172–176. [CrossRef] [PubMed]
55. Oh, S.-L.; Chang, H.; Kim, H.-J.; Kim, Y.-A.; Kim, D.-S.; Ho, S.-H.; Kim, S.-H.; Song, W. Effect of HX108-CS supplementation on exercise capacity and lactate accumulation after high-intensity exercise. *J. Int. Soc. Sports Nutr.* **2013**, *10*, 1–21. [CrossRef] [PubMed]
56. Di Masi, F.; De Souza Vale, R.G.; Dantas, E.H.M.; Barreto, A.C.L.; Novaes, J.D.S.; Reis, V.M. Is blood lactate removal during water immersed cycling faster than during cycling on land? *J. Sport. Sci. Med.* **2007**, *6*, 188–192.
57. Viechtbauer, W.; Smits, L.; Kotz, D.; Budé, L.; Spigt, M.; Serroyen, J.; Crutzen, R. A simple formula for the calculation of sample size in pilot studies. *J. Clin. Epidemiol.* **2015**, *68*, 1375–1379. [CrossRef] [PubMed]
58. Cohen, J. *Statistical Power Analysis for the Behavioral Sciences*, 2nd ed.; Lawrence Erlbaum Associates Publishers: Hillsdale, NJ, USA, 1988.
59. Volpe, S.L. Micronutrient Requirements for Athletes. *Clin. Sports Med.* **2007**, *26*, 119–130. [CrossRef] [PubMed]
60. Koivisto, A.E.; Olsen, T.; Paur, I.; Paulsen, G.; Bastani, N.E.; Garthe, I.; Raastad, T.; Matthews, J.; Blomhoff, R.; Bøhn, S.K. Effects of antioxidant-rich foods on altitude-induced oxidative stress and inflammation in elite endurance athletes: A randomized controlled trial. *PLoS ONE* **2019**, *14*, e0217895. [CrossRef]
61. Skenderi, K.P.; Tsironi, M.; Lazaropoulou, C.; Anastasiou, C.A.; Matalas, A.-L.; Kanavaki, I.; Thalmann, M.; Goussetis, E.; Papassotiriou, I.; Chrousos, G.P. Changes in free radical generation and antioxidant capacity during ultramarathon foot race. *Eur. J. Clin. Invest.* **2008**, *38*, 159–165. [CrossRef]
62. McAnulty, S.R.; McAnulty, L.S.; Nieman, D.C.; Morrow, J.D.; Shooter, L.A.; Holmes, S.; Heward, C.; Henson, D.A. Effect of alpha-tocopherol supplementation on plasma homocysteine and oxidative stress in highly trained athletes before and after exhaustive exercise. *J. Nutr. Biochem.* **2005**, *16*, 530–537. [CrossRef]
63. Briviba, K.; Watzl, B.; Nickel, K.; Kulling, S.; Bös, K.; Haertel, S.; Rechkemmer, G.; Bub, A. A half-marathon and a marathon run induce oxidative DNA damage, reduce antioxidant capacity to protect DNA against damage and modify immune function in hobby runners. *Redox Rep.* **2005**, *10*, 325–331. [CrossRef]
64. Kawamura, T.; Muraoka, I. Exercise-induced oxidative stress and the effects of antioxidant intake from a physiological viewpoint. *Antioxidants* **2018**, *7*, 119. [CrossRef]
65. Zhang, Y.; Xun, P.; Wang, R.; Mao, L.; He, K. Can Magnesium Enhance Exercise Performance? *Nutrients* **2017**, *9*, 946. [CrossRef] [PubMed]
66. González-Parra, G.; Mora, R.; Hoeger, B. Maximal oxygen consumption in national elite triathletes that train in high altitude. *J. Hum. Sport Exerc.* **2013**, *8*. [CrossRef]
67. Daniels, J.; Daniels, N. Running economy of elite male and elite female runners. *Med. Sci. Sports Exerc.* **1992**, *24*, 483–489. [CrossRef]
68. Devlin, J.; Paton, B.; Poole, L.; Sun, W.; Ferguson, C.; Wilson, J.; Kemi, O.J. Blood lactate clearance after maximal exercise depends on active recovery intensity. *J. Sports Med. Phys. Fitness* **2014**, *54*, 271–278. [PubMed]
69. Moxnes, J.F.; Sandbakk, Ø. The kinetics of lactate production and removal during whole-body exercise. *Theor. Biol. Med. Model.* **2012**, *9*, 1–14. [CrossRef] [PubMed]

70. Eston, R. Use of ratings of perceived exertion in sports. *Int. J. Sports Physiol. Perform.* **2012**, *7*, 175–182. [CrossRef] [PubMed]
71. Doherty, M.; Smith, P.M. Effects of caffeine ingestion on rating of perceived exertion during and after exercise: A meta-analysis. *Scand. J. Med. Sci. Sport.* **2005**, *15*, 69–78. [CrossRef]
72. Handzlik, M.K.; Gleeson, M. Likely Additive Ergogenic Effects of Combined Preexercise Dietary Nitrate and Caffeine Ingestion in Trained Cyclists. *ISRN Nutr.* **2013**, *2013*. [CrossRef]

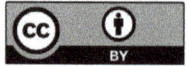

© 2020 by the authors. Licensee MDPI, Basel, Switzerland. This article is an open access article distributed under the terms and conditions of the Creative Commons Attribution (CC BY) license (http://creativecommons.org/licenses/by/4.0/).

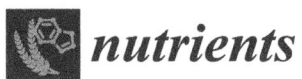

Review

Citrus Flavonoids as Promising Phytochemicals Targeting Diabetes and Related Complications: A Systematic Review of In Vitro and In Vivo Studies

Gopalsamy Rajiv Gandhi [1,2,3], Alan Bruno Silva Vasconcelos [4], Ding-Tao Wu [5], Hua-Bin Li [6], Poovathumkal James Antony [7], Hang Li [1,2], Fang Geng [8], Ricardo Queiroz Gurgel [3], Narendra Narain [9] and Ren-You Gan [1,2,8,*]

[1] Research Center for Plants and Human Health, Institute of Urban Agriculture, Chinese Academy of Agricultural Sciences (CAAS), Chengdu 600103, China; egarajiv@gmail.com (G.R.G.); tiantsai@sina.com (H.L.)
[2] Chengdu National Agricultural Science and Technology Center, Chengdu 600103, China
[3] Postgraduate Program of Health Sciences (PPGCS), Federal University of Sergipe (UFS), Prof. João Cardoso Nascimento Campus, Aracaju, Sergipe 49060-108, Brazil; ricardoqgurgel@gmail.com
[4] Postgraduate Program of Physiological Sciences (PROCFIS), Federal University of Sergipe (UFS), Campus São Cristóvão, São Cristóvão, Sergipe 49100-000, Brazil; abs.vasconcelos@gmail.com
[5] Institute of Food Processing and Safety, College of Food Science, Sichuan Agricultural University, Ya'an 625014, China; DT_Wu@sicau.edu.cn
[6] Guangdong Provincial Key Laboratory of Food, Nutrition and Health, Department of Nutrition, School of Public Health, Sun Yat-sen University, Guangzhou 510080, China; lihuabin@mail.sysu.edu.cn
[7] Department of Microbiology, St. Xavier's College, Kathmandu 44600, Nepal; jamesantonysj@gmail.com
[8] Key Laboratory of Coarse Cereal Processing (Ministry of Agriculture and Rural Affairs), School of Food and Biological Engineering, Chengdu University, Chengdu 610106, China; gengfang@cdu.edu.cn
[9] Laboratory of Flavor and Chromatographic Analysis, Federal University of Sergipe, Campus São Cristóvão, São Cristóvão, Sergipe 49.100-000, Brazil; narendra.narain@gmail.com
* Correspondence: ganrenyou@caas.cn or ganrenyou@yahoo.com; Tel.: +86-28-8020-3193

Received: 25 August 2020; Accepted: 19 September 2020; Published: 23 September 2020

Abstract: The consumption of plant-based food is important for health promotion, especially concerning the prevention and management of chronic diseases. Flavonoids are the main bioactive compounds in citrus fruits, with multiple beneficial effects, especially antidiabetic effects. We systematically review the potential antidiabetic action and molecular mechanisms of citrus flavonoids based on in vitro and in vivo studies. A search of the PubMed, EMBASE, Scopus, and Web of Science Core Collection databases for articles published since 2010 was carried out using the keywords citrus, flavonoid, and diabetes. All articles identified were analyzed, and data were extracted using a standardized form. The search identified 38 articles, which reported that 19 citrus flavonoids, including 8-prenylnaringenin, cosmosiin, didymin, diosmin, hesperetin, hesperidin, isosiennsetin, naringenin, naringin, neohesperidin, nobiletin, poncirin, quercetin, rhoifolin, rutin, sineesytin, sudachitin, tangeretin, and xanthohumol, have antidiabetic potential. These flavonoids regulated biomarkers of glycemic control, lipid profiles, renal function, hepatic enzymes, and antioxidant enzymes, and modulated signaling pathways related to glucose uptake and insulin sensitivity that are involved in the pathogenesis of diabetes and its related complications. Citrus flavonoids, therefore, are promising antidiabetic candidates, while their antidiabetic effects remain to be verified in forthcoming human studies.

Keywords: citrus; diabetes; flavonoids; inflammation; polyphenols

1. Introduction

The genus Citrus covers a large diversity of trees and shrubs, containing 16 species (according to Swingle's classification) or 156 species (according to Tanaka's classification), and is native to subtropical and tropical regions of Asia (from India to North China) and Oceania (Queensland and Australia) [1]. The high phenotypic and genetic variability of the Citrus genus is explained by the sexual compatibility between the Citrus species, allowing natural hybridization, and the long history of human intervention by interspecific hybridization to obtain more useful varieties of the plants [2]. The resulting hybrids are often considered as novel species, in spite of their ability to cross with each other [3]. Additionally, spontaneous natural mutations also increase the diversity of citrus varieties [4].

Citrus fruits are produced and consumed all over the world and represent an annual production of 100 million tons, with 60 million tons being consumed locally, 10 million tons exported, and 30 million tons used in industrial production [5]. The market is dominated by the production of oranges, lemons, limes, pomelos, grapefruit, mandarins, and their hybrids. However, there has recently been increasing consumption of uncommon citrus hybrids, such as yuzu, kaffir lime, blood oranges, and kumquats. The first identification of flavonoids in the Citrus genus dates back to the late nineteenth century when hesperidin was discovered by pioneering biochemistry work [6]. Since then, 44 flavonoids naturally presenting in citrus have been described [7]. Flavonoids are present in diverse citrus fruits, such as bergamots, grapefruits, lemons, limes, mandarins, oranges, and pomelos [8]. Citrus flavonoids include flavones, flavanones, flavonols, isoflavones, anthocyanidins, and flavanols [7]. Some of them are characteristic compounds of the genus, especially polymethoxyflavones (PMFs), while others may selectively present in certain varieties.

Diabetes mellitus is a chronic disease causing 4.2 million deaths and an additional economic burden of 760 million US dollars in health expenditure around the globe in 2019 [9]. According to the latest diabetic data provided by the International Diabetic Federation (IDF), about 463 million adults aged between 20 and 79 years have diabetes, most of them living in low- and middle-income countries, and this is estimated to rise to 700 million by 2045 [9]. The disease is characterized by multiple serious health complications such as nephropathy, neuropathy, and retinopathy that can damage internal organs, particularly the pancreas, heart, liver, adipose tissue, and the kidneys, requiring comprehensive health care and management. It has also become the leading cause of various chronic metabolic diseases [10]. It occurs as a consequence of the irregular catabolism and anabolism of carbohydrates, lipids, and proteins, due to insulin resistance or hypoinsulinism [11]. Abnormal glycemic regulation may increase micro- and macro-vascular diseases, and impair vascular homeostasis. Furthermore, it is suggested that diabetic subjects have an increased risk of physical and cognitive disability, cancer, tuberculosis, and depression [12–15]). Although it is a multifactorial disease, some studies suggest that oxidative stress due to extreme hyperglycemia plays a pivotal role in the initiation of various pathological conditions, such as inflammation and atherosclerosis [15,16].

Many flavonoids derived from citrus fruits have been reported to reduce oxidative stress, improve glucose tolerance and insulin sensitivity, modulate lipid metabolism and adipocyte differentiation, suppress inflammation and apoptosis, and improve endothelial dysfunction [8,17–22], which indicates their potential antidiabetic effect. In order to highlight the antidiabetic potential of citrus flavonoids, we carried out a systematic review to provide related evidence in vitro and in vivo based on the PRISMA (Preferred Reporting Items for Systematic Reviews and Meta-Analyses) guidelines [23]. The article search was conducted in March 2020, and the survey covered articles published since 2010. The search was performed in four databases, including PubMed, EMBASE, Scopus and the Web of Science Core Collection, using the keywords "flavonoid", "citrus", and "diabetes".

The initial search found 1213 articles in the databases (PubMed: 465, EMBASE: 369, Scopus: 247, and Web of Science: 132). The inclusion criteria were in vitro and in vivo studies of citrus flavonoids, articles in English, and published between 2010 and March 2020. The exclusion criteria were articles not in English, human studies, reviews, letters, commentaries, editorials, and case reports. Following the application of the inclusion and exclusion criteria, and after discarding any duplication, we collected

38 articles that contained studies discussing the pharmacological activity of 19 flavonoids of the genus Citrus in relation to diabetes. The flowchart of study selection for this systematic review is provided in Figure 1. This review paper mainly summarizes the antidiabetic potential of the main citrus flavonoids based on in vitro and in vivo studies, and discusses related mechanisms of action of citrus flavonoids.

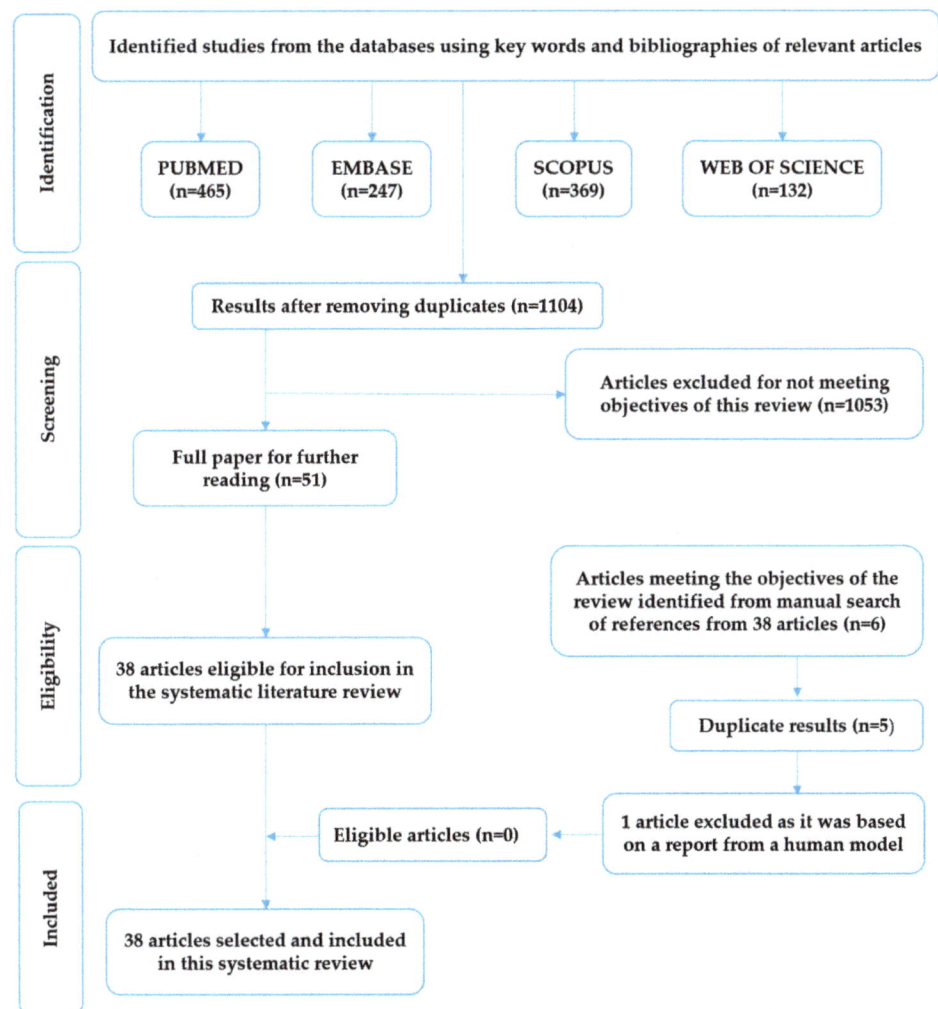

Figure 1. The flowchart of study selection for this systematic review.

2. Main Citrus Flavonoids with Antidiabetic Effects

The 19 citrus flavonoids discussed are presented in Figure 2. The following section summarizes the main antidiabetic flavonoids, discussing their antidiabetic effects and related mechanisms based on in vitro (Table 1) and in vivo (Table 2) studies.

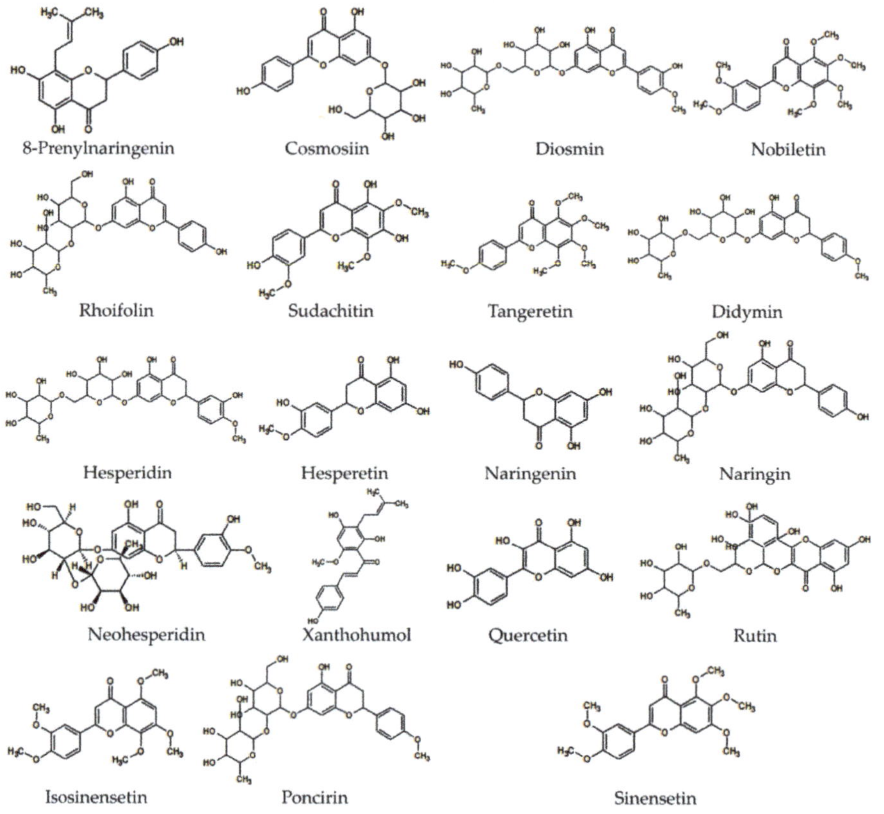

Figure 2. The 19 main citrus flavonoids with antidiabetic effects summarized from 38 articles.

2.1. 8-Prenylnaringenin

8-prenylnaringenin is a prenylflavonoid, more specifically, a xanthohumol metabolite, found in the Citrus genus of plants belonging to the Rutaceae family [24] and exclusively available in nominal concentrations in citrus fruits such as oranges, lemons, grapefruits, and tangerines. Prenylflavonoids are a sub-class of the flavonoid group that represents a group of secondary metabolites derived from 2-phenylchromen-4-one and present a prenyl group attached to the flavone nucleus. Findings from previous studies reported that 8-prenylnaringenin had a protective effect on menopausal and post-menopausal symptoms, as well as exhibiting anticancer activities by the induction of autophagy or by modulating the cell cycle and suppressing the growth of tumor cells when tested in different types of in vitro experimental model systems [25]. It reduced oxidative stress, inflammatory processes, and the secretions of angiogenic factors. It also acted on vascularization processes, such as angiogenesis [26].

In an animal model (C57Bl/6 mice) of type 2 diabetes mellitus induced by a high-fat diet (HFD), Luís et al. showed that 8-prenylnaringenin normalized the expression of Galectin-3 (Gal3), a protein overexpressed during the diabetic state, and was strongly associated with oxidative stress in the liver and kidneys of diabetic mice. In addition, it reduced 3-nitrotyrosine (a marker of cell damage), inflammation, and nitric oxide (NO) production, and promoted the production of glycation end products (AGEs) [27]. Increased levels of AGEs in response to diabetic inflammation have been reported to play a role in tissue stiffness, increased blood pressure, heart failure, and endothelial dysfunction [28]. This polyphenol may, therefore, be a potential therapeutic agent against diabetes mellitus.

2.2. Cosmosiin

Cosmosiin, also known as apigetrin or apigenin-7-O-glucoside, is a glycosyloxyflavone with the molecular formula of $C_{21}H_{20}O_{10}$, that is, apigenin substituted by a beta-D-glucopyranosyl moiety at position 7 via a glycosidic linkage. It is found in a variety of citrus plant species, such as *Citrus grandis* (L.) Osbeck (*red wendun*) and *Citrus aurantium* Linn. of the family Rutaceae. Recently, cosmosiin and its derivatives have been suggested as diabetic therapies [29]. The antidiabetic effect of cosmosiin was reported by Rao et al. in their in vitro study using 3T3-L1 adipocyte cells. Cosmosiin exerted its protective effects through promoting adiponectin secretion, resulting in increased phosphorylation of the insulin receptor-β (IR-β). In addition, it had a positive effect on glucose transporter 4 (GLUT4) translocation [30]. Therefore, these results suggest that cosmosiin has insulin-like activity, which plays a vital role in stimulating glucose uptake into muscles and adipocytes, suggesting that this flavonoid could be beneficial for the management of type 2 diabetes mellitus and related complications.

2.3. Diosmin

Diosmin (3′,5,7-trihydroxy-4′-methoxyflavone-7-ramnoglucoside) is a flavone found in citrus fruits and the leaves of oranges and lemons. This flavone has some important biological activities, such as antioxidant, anti-inflammatory, and anti-apoptotic effects [31]. Diosmin was isolated for the first time in 1925 from *Scrophularia nodosa* Linn. (a perennial herbaceous plant from the family Scrophulariaceae) and used for the first time in 1969 as a therapeutic agent for inflammatory disorders. Currently, it is a medication mainly used for the treatment of diseases, such as chronic venous insufficiency and hemorrhoids [32]. The effect of diosmin on lipid metabolism was evaluated using an animal model of streptozotocin (STZ)-induced diabetes [33]. Interestingly, it was shown to attenuate biochemical markers, such as fasting plasma glucose concentrations, glycosylated hemoglobin (HbA1c), and C-reactive protein (CRP). In addition, it decreased the levels of plasma lipids, including triglycerides (TG), free fatty acids, phospholipids, low-density lipoprotein cholesterol (LDL-C), and very low-density lipoprotein cholesterol (VLDL-C), and decreased high-density lipoprotein cholesterol (HDL-C). Besides, the activity of 3-hydroxy-3-methyl-glutaril-CoA reductase (HMG-CoA reductase), an important enzyme of the metabolic pathway that produces cholesterol, was enhanced in the liver and kidneys of diabetic rats but was inhibited by diosmin treatment. Finally, the activities of the lipoprotein lipase (LPL) and lecithin cholesterol acyl transferase (LCAT) enzymes were also altered by diabetes and normalized by diosmin.

Jain, Bansal, Dalvi, Upganlawar, and Somani [34] showed protective effects of diosmin against biochemical, behavioral, and oxidative stress parameters related to diabetic neuropathy in type 2 diabetic rats fed with an HFD. Diosmin also increased the threshold of nociception in thermal hyperalgesia and tail-flick tests, and improved motor capacity in diabetic rats. In addition, this flavonoid demonstrated a protective effect against oxidative stress, reducing markers of lipid peroxidation (malondialdehyde (MDA) and NO) levels. It also increased the activity of antioxidant enzymes, such as superoxide dismutase (SOD) and reduced glutathione (GSH), suggesting that it may help prevent the early development of diabetic neuropathy in rats.

Hsu, Lin, Cheng, and Wu [35] concluded that diosmin has a beneficial effect through the activation of the imidazoline I-2 receptor (I-2R) and opioid secretion. Diosmin induced β-endorphin-like immunoreactivity secretion in isolated adrenal glands in vitro via calcium-dependent reactions, which evidenced its utility as an antidiabetic drug via inducing opioid secretion. In addition, diosmin attenuated increased plasma glucose concentrations and increased hepatic glycogen levels in diabetic rats. It also activated the I-2R to promote metabolic homeostasis, resulting in reduced blood glucose and lipids in diabetic rats. It is worth mentioning that the administration of diosmin did not produce changes in body weight, food intake, or plasma insulin levels.

Furthermore, diosmin has been reported to have therapeutic potential for behavioral parameters, such as the antinociceptive response and locomotor activity, as well as for the regulation of nociceptive biomarkers linked to the neuropathy caused by diabetes [34]. Taken together, it is suggested that diosmin can attenuate primary effects of diabetes, such as disturbances in plasma glucose and lipoproteins, by modulating key enzymes that regulate glucose metabolism and antioxidant activity.

2.4. Nobiletin

Nobiletin, chemically known as 5,6,7,8,3′,4′-hexamethoxyflavone, is a dietary flavone with the empirical formula $C_{21}H_{22}O_8$ and the molecular weight 402.39. It is found in the peel of various citrus fruits, such as oranges and tangerines [36]. Like other bioflavonoids, nobiletin has shown potential medicinal properties in several pathologies and their associated causes, such as preventing type 2 diabetes [37], protecting against bone mineral density loss [38], treating cancer [39], and lowering blood cholesterol [40]. Studies have suggested that this flavone may be an effective therapeutic molecule for the treatment of metabolic syndromes, such as cardiovascular disease, abdominal obesity, and increased blood pressure.

Mulvihill et al. [41] evaluated its effect on lipoprotein secretion in cultured human hepatoma cells (HepG2) and a mouse model of dyslipidemia and atherosclerosis accompanying insulin resistance. The in vitro results showed that the administration of nobiletin dose-dependently reduced the secretion of apolipoprotein B100-containing lipoproteins, which represents an important risk factor for cardiovascular diseases. This effect happened through the activation of a mitogen-activated protein kinase/extracellular signal-regulated kinase (MAPK/ERK) pathway. MAPK/ERK activation by nobiletin decreased the mRNA expression of microsomal triglyceride transfer protein (MTP), diacylglycerol O-acyltransferase (DGAT)-1, and DGAT2, while it increased hepatic low-density lipoprotein (LDL) receptor (LDLR) mRNA expression. However, the authors found no evidence of nobiletin modulating the tyrosine phosphorylation of the insulin receptor (IR) or the insulin receptor substrate 1 (IRS-1). In addition, TG synthesis and TG mass were significantly lowered in nobiletin-treated cells, with the increase in the mRNA expression of carnitine palmitoyltransferase I α (CPT1-α) and peroxisome proliferator-activated receptor gamma coactivator 1-alpha (PGC1-α). Most of the favorable results observed in the abovementioned in vitro experiment were comparable with the in vivo results, in which nobiletin prevented diet-induced weight gain and reduced dyslipidemia in HFD-fed diabetic mice. The in vivo studies on nobiletin significantly decreased plasma lipids levels (TG and total cholesterol (TC)), reduced the very low-density lipoprotein-total triglyceride (VLDL-TG) secretion rate, and normalized elevated plasma non-esterified fatty acid (NEFA) and glycerol, in addition to reducing TG in both the liver and intestines in HFD-fed obese diabetic mice. In contrast with the in vitro results, nobiletin did not affect the hepatic expression of MTP or DGAT1/2. Nobiletin-treated HFD-fed obese diabetic mice also increased the expression of CPT1-α and PGC1-α, and the rates of fatty acid oxidation. Glucose tolerance tests conducted in the HFD-fed obese diabetic mice revealed that nobiletin normalized the impaired high-fat-diet-induced glucose tolerance, while significantly diminishing hyperinsulinemia and improving insulin sensitivity. Moreover, diet-induced obesity and adipocyte hypertrophy were inhibited in nobiletin-treated HFD-fed obese diabetic mice. It prevented dyslipidemia and hepatic steatosis, and improved metabolic parameters, leading to the prevention of atherosclerosis and a dramatic reduction in the lesions within the aortic sinus compared with the high-fat-diet-fed mice that were not treated with nobiletin.

Onda, Horike, Suzuki, and Hirano [42] added some important evidence from an in vitro study, which showed that nobiletin affected glucose uptake in insulin target cells such as adipocytes, using adipocyte cell lines (murine 3T3-F442 preadipocytes). Nobiletin treatment increased the uptake of [3H]-deoxyglucose in differentiated adipocytes in the presence of insulin. The influence on increased glucose uptake in the adipocytes was associated with several signaling cascade inhibitors that are recognized to promote pathways for glucose incorporation. The results showed that the phosphoinositide 3-kinases (PI3K), protein kinase B (Akt), and the protein kinase A (PKA) pathways were involved in the increase in glucose uptake. These in vitro results encourage further in vivo studies to analyze the antidiabetic action of this polymethoxyflavonoid and its molecular mechanism involved in enhancing glucose uptake via the PI3K/Akt signaling pathway in the insulin target tissues.

To elucidate the antidiabetic mechanism of nobiletin in adipocytes, Kanda et al. [43] conducted a study using 3T3-L1 preadipocyte cells in which nobiletin suppressed lipid accumulation in 3T3-L1 adipocytes, suggesting that nobiletin inhibited adipogenesis in 3T3-L1 cells when the adipocyte differentiation was induced by insulin, 3-isobutyl-1-methylxanthine (IBMX), and dexamethasone (DEX). Regarding the mechanism of action involved in this response, nobiletin did not affect the protein expression of peroxisome proliferator-activated receptor gamma (PPARγ)1 in 3T3-L1 cells; however, it significantly suppressed PPARγ2 protein expression, an important marker in adipogenesis. The transcripts of PPARγ2 and adipocyte protein 2 (aP2), two target genes of PPARγ, were significantly down-regulated by nobiletin treatment. In addition, it suppressed CCAAT-enhancer-binding protein beta (C/EBPβ) expression, suggesting that nobiletin may inhibit adipocyte differentiation by down-regulating PPARγ2 gene expression via decreasing C/EBPβ expression. Finally, nobiletin reduced the phosphorylation of the cAMP-response element-binding protein (CREB) and strongly improved the phosphorylation of the signal transducer and activator of transcription 5 (STAT5), suggesting that a suppressive effect of nobiletin on adipocyte differentiation was involved due to the enhanced activation of STAT5 by the regulation of PPARγ activity.

Furthermore, Parkar, Bhatt, and Addepalli [44] hypothesized that nobiletin, due to its metalloproteinase (MMP)-2- and MMP-9-inhibitory and antioxidant potential, could ameliorate the cardiovascular dysfunction in diabetes. In an animal model of STZ-induced diabetes, nobiletin treatment reduced the mean arterial pressure in the diabetic rats in comparison to vehicle-treated rats. Heart rate fell rapidly and dramatically after the administration of STZ; however, nobiletin increased the heart rate and kept the condition normal. Additionally, in connection to other cardiac parameters, nobiletin reduced MMP-2 and MMP-9 enzymatic activities in the heart, improved the cardiac hypertrophy index, attenuated the deterioration in the morphology of cardiomyocytes, and reduced diabetes-induced myocardial fibrosis in the rats. Nobiletin also showed antioxidant effects by improving myocardial SOD and catalase activity and decreasing MDA levels. Moreover, nobiletin ameliorated vascular reactivity and collagen levels in the aortae of rats.

Zhang et al. [45] also investigated the therapeutic effect of nobiletin on STZ-induced diabetic cardiomyopathy in mice. Echocardiography and hemodynamic measurements showed a protective effect on cardiac function in nobiletin-treated mice. Nobiletin treatment significantly attenuated the mRNA expression of nicotinamide-adenine dinucleotide phosphate-reduced (NADPH) oxidase isoforms (p67phox, p22phox, and p91phox), suggesting its potential antioxidant effect. Nobiletin improved SOD1 activity and decreased MDA levels in cardiac tissue, reinforcing the positive influence on oxidative-stress-related disorders. These effects were also accompanied by anti-inflammatory responses, such as the modulation of the mRNA expression of pro-inflammatory cytokines (tumor necrosis factor-alpha (TNF-α) and interleukin (IL)-6) in diabetic myocardium treated with nobiletin. In addition, the authors highlighted the fact that nobiletin treatment did not produce any significant effect on blood glucose levels. However, the treatment decreased the expression of transforming growth factor (TGF)-β1, connective tissue growth factor (CTGF), fibronectin, and collagen Iα, and also reduced cardiac fibrosis in the nobiletin-treated mice. Nobiletin also reduced phosphor-kappaB-α (IκB-α) expression, with the subsequent inhibition of phosphor-p65 activity. These results indicate that the treatment with nobiletin mitigated cardiac dysfunction and interstitial fibrosis, which may be due to its constructive action on the suppression of the c-Jun N-terminal kinase (JNK), P38, and nuclear factor kappa B (NF-κB) signaling pathways.

A recent study tested the hypothesis that nobiletin provides metabolic protection against the phosphorylation of AMP-activated protein kinase (AMPK) and acetyl-CoA carboxylase (ACC) in three different mouse models; mice deficient in hepatic AMPK (*Ampkβ1-/-*), mice incapable of the inhibitory phosphorylation of ACC (*AccDKI*), and mice with adipocyte-specific AMPK deficiency (*iβ1β2AKO*) [46]. Nobiletin was able to activate (increase the phosphorylation of) AMPK in human hepatocarcinoma HepG2 cells in the presence of high glucose. Additionally, ACC phosphorylation, which was suppressed by hyperglycemia, was reversed through nobiletin treatment. In vitro nobiletin-treated cells had reduced lipogenesis and increased fatty acid oxidation independent of AMPK. In summary, the results of this study showed that nobiletin treatment attenuated obesity, hepatic steatosis, dyslipidemia, and insulin resistance, and protected metabolism in three mouse models independently of AMPK activation. The authors also emphasized the potential therapeutic convenience of this citrus flavonoid nobiletin, specifically in the management of metabolic syndromes such as diabetes and obesity, and further in-depth studies are warranted to investigate the primary mechanism of action that influences insulin sensitivity.

Nobiletin has, therefore, been shown to have potent antidiabetic, anti-obesity, and hypolipidemic effects by modulating several physiological pathways. In addition, it acted as an immunomodulatory molecule, attenuating inflammatory and oxidative stress markers, which are linked to the various diabetic complications. This evidence reinforces the therapeutic potential of nobiletin for diabetes in in vitro experimental systems and animal models, which should be further verified in humans.

2.5. Rhoifolin

Rhoifolin, with the molecular formula $C_{27}H_{30}O_{14}$, is one of the most common flavonoids and is used extensively in preclinical investigations to explore its pharmacological effects in a wide range of chronic diseases including diabetes and obesity. It is found in several citrus fruits such as bitter oranges, grapefruits, lemons, and unripe grapes [47,48]. Previous studies found that rhoifolin influenced several biological activities, with antioxidant [49], anti-inflammatory [50], hepatoprotective [51], and anticancer potential [52].

Rhoifolin was also isolated from *Citrus grandis* (L.) Osbeck leaves, and its insulin-mimetic action was reported by Rao et al. in an in vitro study using differentiated 3T3-L1 adipocytes cells. It was found to act via promoting adiponectin secretion, the phosphorylation of IR-β, and GLUT4 translocation, which are considered to be critically involved in diabetic complications [30]. The action of rhoifolin against these genes may provide novel targets for combating insulin-resistance-associated diseases.

Table 1. The main characteristics of in vitro studies using citrus flavonoids for the management of diabetes mellitus.

Flavonoids	Class	Concentrations and Duration of the Treatment	In Vitro Models	Effects and Molecular Mechanisms	Ref.
Nobiletin	Flavone	1, 2.5, 5, 10, and 20 µM; 24 h	HepG2 cells (human hepatoma cells)	Nobiletin activated mitogen-activated protein kinase-extracellular signal-related kinase (MAPK/ERK), resulting in the marked inhibition of apolipoprotein B100 secretion. It neither induced the phosphorylation of the insulin receptor (IR) or insulin receptor substrate-1(IRS-1) tyrosine nor triggered lipogenesis associated with insulin resistance.	[41]
Rhoifolin and cosmosiin from Citrus grandis (L.) Osbeck leaves	Flavone	Rhoifolin: 0.001–5 µM; cosmosiin: 1–20 µM; 24 h	3T3-L1 adipocyte cells	Rhoifolin and cosmosiin exerted antidiabetic effects by promoting adiponectin secretion, the tyrosine phosphorylation of IR-β, and glucose transporter 4 (GLUT4) translocation. These bioactive molecules may help in insulin resistance-related treatment for diabetic complications.	[30]
Tangeretin and nobiletin	Flavone	5–50 mM; 24 h	3T3-F442A preadipocytes	Tangeretin and nobiletin induced increased glucose uptake in murine adipocytes, suggesting that the action was mediated by phosphatidylinositol 3-kinase (PI3K) as well as protein kinase B (Akt) and protein kinase A (PKA)/cAMP-response element-binding protein (CREB) signaling-dependent pathways.	[42]
Flavonoids from Citrus aurantium Linn. include naringin, esperidin, poncirin, sosiensetin, sineesytin, nobiletin, and tangeretin	Flavone and flavanone	0, 10, and 50 µg/mL; 0–6 days	3T3-L1 preadipocytes	C. aurantium containing flavonoids decreased the expression of key adipocyte differentiation regulators, including CCAAT-enhancer binding protein family (C/EBPβ and C/EBPα) and peroxisome proliferator-activated receptor gamma (PPARγ); it reduced adipogenesis and the accumulation of cytoplasmic lipid droplets during differentiation in 3T3-L1 cells.	[53]
Nobiletin	Flavone	0, 1, 10, and 100 µM; 7 days	3T3-L1 preadipocytes	Nobiletin suppressed the differentiation of 3T3-L1 preadipocytes into adipocytes by down-regulating the expression of the gene coding for PPARγ2. In addition, nobiletin reduced the phosphorylation of CREB and strongly improved the phosphorylation of signal transducer and activation of transcription (STAT)5.	[43]
Sudachitin	Flavone	30 mmol/L; 48 h	Primary myoblasts	Sudachitin increased mitochondrial biogenesis and improved mitochondrial function, leading to an improvement in lipid and glucose metabolism mediated via the sirtuin (Sirt) 1-AMP-activated protein kinase (AMPK)-peroxisome proliferator-activated receptor gamma coactivator-1- alpha (PGC-1α) pathway.	[54]
Naringenin	Flavanone	0, 10, and 50 µM; 3 h	RAW 264 (macrophages) cells and 3T3-L1 adipocytes	Naringenin inhibited the monocyte chemoattractant protein-1 (MCP-1)'s mRNA expression and secretion in the adipocytes in a dose-dependent manner. It also prevented the MCP-1 production stimulated by the interaction between the adipocytes and the infiltrated macrophages.	[55]
Hesperidin and naringin	Flavanone	0.25, 0.5, 1, and 2 mg/mL; 1 and 24 h	Pancreatic islets	Hesperidin and naringin increased the production and the release of insulin from the islet cells and decreased the intestinal glucose absorption.	[56]
Quercetin	Flavanol	10 and 100 mM; 24 h	L6 myotubes	Quercetin activated the adenosine monophosphate kinase (AMPK)-P38 MAPK pathway and up-regulated glucose transporter type 4 (GLUT4)/AKT mRNA expression to induce glucose uptake in skeletal muscle cell lines.	[57]
Diosmin	Flavone	0.01–1 µmol/L; 24 h	Transfected imidazoline receptor (I-R) gene in CHO-K1 cells (Chinese hamster ovary cell)	Diosmin enhanced calcium influx in I-R gene-transfected CHO-K1 cells. Diosmin effectively activated the I-R gene via inducing opioid secretion, showing utility as an antidiabetic drug.	[35]

Table 1. Cont.

Flavonoids	Class	Concentrations and Duration of the Treatment	In Vitro Models	Effects and Molecular Mechanisms	Ref.
Hesperidin	Flavanone	12.5, 25, and 50 μmol/L; 6 h	RGC-5 cells (retinal ganglial cells)	Hesperidin protected against a high level of glucose-induced cell apoptosis by down-regulating caspase-9, caspase-3, and Bax/Bcl-2. Furthermore, it significantly inhibited the phosphorylation of c-Jun N-terminal kinases (JNK) and activated p38 MAPK in high glucose-fed RGC-5 cells.	[58]
Hesperidin and hesperetin	Flavanone	40, 80, 120, 160, and 200 μM; 24 h	Rat liver cells	Flavonoids hesperidin and hesperetin inhibited the activities of two gluconeogenesis enzymes, alanine aminotransferase (ALT) and aspartate aminotransferase (AST), indicating their effectiveness in treating AST and ALT-mediated metabolic disorders, including in diabetes mellitus.	[59]
Tangeretin	Flavone	0, 2.5, 5, and 10 μM; 24 h	Human glomerular mesangial cells (MCs)	Tangeretin very effectively inhibited high glucose (HG)-induced cell proliferation, oxidative stress, and extracellular matrix (ECM) expression in the human glomerular mesangial cells (MCs) via inactivating the extracellular signal-regulated kinase (ERK) signaling pathway. It also displayed therapeutic potential in the management of diabetic nephropathy.	[60]
Didymin	Flavanone	10 and 20 μM; 6 and 24 h	Human umbilical vein endothelial cells (HUVECs)	Didymin protected against high glucose (HG)-induced human umbilical vein endothelial cells by modulating the expression of intercellular adhesion molecule (ICAM)-1 and vascular cell adhesion protein (VCAM)-1, and regulating nuclear factor kappa B (NF-κB)-mediated inflammatory cytokines and chemokines. Didymin prevented HG-induced endothelial dysfunction and death via antioxidative and anti-inflammatory activities.	[61]
Didymin	Flavanone	10–30 μM; 15 and 30 min, 1 and 24 h, 28 days	HepG2 (human hepatocarcinoma) cell line	Didymin inhibited α-glucosidase, activated the insulin-signaling pathway, and improved insulin sensitivity. It showed potent inhibitory activity against the key enzymes involved in diabetes mellitus, including protein tyrosine phosphatase 1B (PTP1B), α-glucosidase, advanced glycation end products (AGEs), and aldose reductase (AR).	[62]
Naringenin	Flavanone	0.01–1 μM; 1 and 24 h	NSC34 (mouse neuroblastoma and embryonic spinal cord motor neurons) cell line	Naringenin suppressed neuronal apoptosis and enhanced antioxidant protective effects in methylglyoxal (MG)-treated NSC34 cells. It prevented MC-induced hyperglycemia-related neurotoxicity via regulating insulin-like growth factor 1 receptor (IGF-1R)-mediated signaling.	[63]
Naringenin	Flavanone	0, 1, 10, and 50 μM; 30 min, 3 and 6 h	3T3-L1 (adipocytes) and RAW264 (macrophages) cells	Naringenin inhibited monocyte chemotactic protein (MCP)-3 expression in 3T3-L1 adipocytes and a coculture of 3T3-L1 adipocytes and RAW264 macrophages. It did not affect the expression of macrophage inflammatory protein-2 (MIP-2), a key chemokine for neutrophil migration and activation, in macrophages or a coculture of adipocytes and macrophages.	[64]
Nobiletin	Flavone	10 μM; 1 and 4 h	HepG2 (human hepatocarcinoma) cell line	Nobiletin increased pAMPK in HepG2 incubated with high glucose content, in which the phosphorylation of AMPK was suppressed, which was comparable to the action carried out by the reference standards (resveratrol and metformin).	[46]

2.6. Sudachitin

Sudachitin (5,7,4′-trihydroxy-6,8,3′-trimethoxyflavone), also known as menthocubanone, is a polymethoxylated flavone originally found in the skin of *Citrus sudachi* Hort. fruit. Sudachitin belongs to the class of organic compounds known as 8-O-methylated flavonoids and has been detected commonly in citrus fruits, such as mandarin oranges and bitter oranges [65]. It exhibits diverse biological activities, such as the suppression of inflammatory bone destruction [66], induction of apoptosis in human keratinocyte HaCaT cells [67], enhancement of antigen-specific cellular and humoral immune responses [68], and inhibition of matrix metalloproteinase (MMP)-1 and MMP-3 production in TNF-α-stimulated human periodontal ligament cells [69].

The effects of sudachitin on glucose, lipid, and energy metabolism in an HFD experimental obesity model using C57BL/6J mice and diabetic *db/db* mice fed a normal diet were investigated by Tsutsumi et al. [54], and it was found that sudachitin reduced the weight gain in the HFD mice without changing the food intake. It also ameliorated the elevated adipose tissue mass, increased subcutaneous fat deposits, and elevated visceral fat composition, and normalized adipocyte size and function. In addition, it reduced hyperinsulinemia and hyperglycemia, improved glucose tolerance, ameliorated plasma leptin levels, decreased visceral fat content, increased plasma adiponectin levels, and improved insulin sensitivity. A possible explanation for these effects could be the ability of sudachitin to modulate metabolism-related genes, such as by modulating the mRNA expression of GLUT4 and transcripts of uncoupling protein 1 and 3 (UCP1 and UCP3) in white adipose tissue and the liver, which were significantly increased in the white adipose tissue of the diabetic animals. Besides, it was able to decrease the levels of the mRNA transcripts encoding FAS ligand, ACC1, and ACC2 in the liver. Tsutsumi et al. also reported that sudachitin promoted energy expenditure by activating the sirtuin (Sirt)1–PGC1α pathway, increased basal muscle skeletal adenosine triphosphate (ATP) contents, and increased mitochondrial citrate synthase activity. Sudachitin also improved insulin sensitivity and reduced fasting blood glucose and TG levels in diabetic *db/db* mice. Finally, an important in vitro study carried out by Tsutsumi et al. showed that sudachitin influenced the mitochondrial biogenesis by activating vital signaling pathways in myocytes, increasing the expression of genes such as nuclear respiratory factor 1 and 2 (NRF1 and NRF2) and mitochondrial transcription factor A (mtTFA). Sudachitin treatment increased the mitochondrial number and activity. Therefore, these observations indicate that sudachitin has good potential for managing obesity and diabetes and its associated complications.

2.7. Tangeretin

Tangeretin is an O-polymethoxylated flavone with methoxy groups at positions 5, 6, 7, 8, and 4′, and is found in tangerines and orange peel. It performs a number of biologically beneficial activities and has antioxidant, anti-inflammatory, antitumor, hepatoprotective, and neuroprotective potential [70]. The properties of this flavonoid with respect to diabetes and its associated comorbidities have also been widely studied. Regarding the antidiabetic effects of tangeretin, in vitro evidence confirmed that it increased glucose uptake in differentiated 3T3-F442 adipocytes, even in the presence of insulin. In addition, results showed that 3T3-F442 adipocyte glucose uptake by the PI3K, Akt, and PKA pathways was increased following treatment with this polymethoxyflavonoid [42].

Sundaram, Shanthi, and Sachdanandam [71] evaluated the antihyperglycemic potential of tangeretin regarding the activities of key enzymes linked with carbohydrate and glycogen metabolism in diabetic rats. Tangeretin treatment reduced blood glucose to near-normal levels, increased hemoglobin (Hb), and decreased hemoglobin (Hb)A1c levels, besides reversing the obese body weight and liver weight changes induced by diabetes. In addition, tangeretin normalized the activities of key hepatic enzymes and reinstated the levels of glycogen and the activities of glycogen synthase and glycogen phosphorylase. Histopathological analysis showed a significant increase in the regeneration of pancreatic β-cells in the islets of Langerhans in tangeretin-treated diabetic rats compared with those in the non-treated diabetic animals.

Furthermore, Sundaram, Shanthi, and Sachdanandam [72] used a diabetic animal model to gain more therapeutic information on the mechanism of the action regarding the antioxidant, anti-inflammatory, and cardio-protective effectiveness of tangeretin. The oral administration of tangeretin reversed the body weight and heart weight changes by its insulinotropic action. Tangeretin administrated to the diabetic rats attenuated and normalized the lipid profiles in the plasma and cardiac tissues. These effects were mediated through the modification of the activities of key enzymes (LCAT, LPL, and HMG-CoA reductase) of lipid metabolism in the liver and increased GLUT4 expression in the heart tissues of diabetic rats. Moreover, tangeretin administration in diabetic rats decreased the levels of lipid peroxidation by increasing the activities of antioxidant enzymes (SOD, catalase (CAT), glutathione peroxidase (GPx), and glutathione reductase (GR)). It also caused a significant reduction in both inflammatory cytokines (TNF-α and IL-6) and cardiac marker enzymes (aspartate aminotransferase (AST), lactate dehydrogenase (LDH), and creatine phosphokinase (CPK)) in the plasma and heart tissues. Additionally, tangeretin treatment markedly decreased the nuclear translocation of NF-κB and TNF-α according to immunostaining in cardiac tissues. In summary, the results suggest that tangeretin treatment plays a beneficial role in regulating diabetes and its associated cardiovascular risk.

Chen, Ma, Sun, and Zhu [60] elucidated the effects of tangeretin on high glucose-induced oxidative stress and extracellular matrix (ECM) accumulation in human glomerular mesangial cells (HGMCs) and discovered the underlying mechanisms. The important inflammatory factor TGF-β1's expression induced by high glucose was efficiently suppressed in tangeretin-treated cells. The citrus molecule suppressed reactive oxygen species (ROS) and MDA production, while it increased SOD activity. In addition, high glucose treatment greatly increased the expression of fibronectin and collagen IV in HGMCs, which was then reversed by tangeretin treatment. The extracellular signal-regulated kinase (ERK) pathway plays an important role in the development of diabetic nephropathy, and this study concluded that tangeretin can modulate ERK signaling through preventing the activation of the ERK signaling pathway in high glucose-stimulated mast cells (MCs). These results highlighted tangeretin as a curative agent in the management of diabetic nephropathy, the leading cause of morbidity and mortality resulting in end-stage renal disease.

Therefore, tangeretin has a promising role in research into diabetic therapy, since its effects appear to be consistent and reliable in diabetic preclinical studies. Its major effects include attenuating biochemical parameters related to diabetic conditions, modulating key enzymes of lipid and glycolytic metabolism, attenuating inflammation and oxidative-stress-signaling markers, and exhibiting protective effects on the heart and liver tissues, which are considered to be vital in diabetic metabolic disorders.

2.8. Didymin

Didymin ((S)-5,7-dihydroxy-4′-methoxyflavanone-7-β-rutinoside) is an oral bioactive citrus flavonoid-O-glycoside belonging to a flavanone class found in several citrus fruits, such as oranges, lemons, grapefruits, and mandarins [73]. Although it has great antioxidant potential, didymin is mainly mentioned in the literature in relation to its potent anticancer capacity, having an antiproliferative effect and preventing the growth of cancer cells [74–76]. The effects of didymin against endothelial dysfunction, a pathological process involved in atherogenesis, were described by Shukla, Sonowal, Saxena, and Ramana [61], who demonstrated the role of this flavanone in inhibiting the apoptosis of human umbilical vein endothelial cells induced by high glucose, via modulating oxidative stress signals, leading to the generation of ROS as well as the activation of caspase-3 and Erk1/2 and regulation of the Bcl2 protein. Moreover, didymin also alleviated high glucose-induced endothelial dysfunction by preventing monocyte adhesion to endothelial cells, restoring endothelial nitric oxide synthase (eNOS) and NO levels, reducing the levels of several inflammatory cytokines, such as TNF-α, interferon gamma (INF-γ), IL-1β, IL-2, and IL-6. Thus, these results demonstrated that it could be developed as a natural therapeutic agent against hyperglycemia-induced endothelial dysfunction and mortality.

Ali et al. [62] evaluated the antidiabetic potential of didymin and the molecular mechanisms underlying its effects in the insulin-resistant HepG2 cell line. In vitro experiments showed that didymin inhibited human recombinant aldose reductase (HRAR), rat lens aldose reductase (RLAR), α-glucosidase, and AGE formation. It also activated the insulin-signaling pathway and resulted in improved insulin sensitivity. Together, these physiological effects led to a potent antidiabetic effect. Regarding the molecular mechanisms related to these effects, didymin reduced the expression of protein tyrosine phosphatase (PTP1B) and increased the phosphorylation of IRS-1, PI3K, glycogen synthase kinase 3β (GSK3β), and Akt, besides reducing two key enzymes, leading to diminished hepatic glucose production in insulin-resistant HepG2 cells. Molecular docking studies indicated that didymin possessed high affinity and tight binding capacity for the active sites of HRAR, RLAR, PTP1B, and α-glucosidase. Additionally, didymin showed important vascular effects through the activation of molecular pathways that result in glycemic control, highlighting the great therapeutic potential for diabetes and diabetes-associated complications. Thus, further clinical trials are warranted to investigate the use of didymin as a potential lead candidate to protect against metabolic disorders targeting various organs.

2.9. Hesperidin

Hesperidin is a flavanone glycoside commonly found in citrus fruits such as oranges, tangerines, lemons, and grapefruits, and is one of the most important non-essential nutrients for human beings [77]. Its name originated from the word "hesperidium", which denotes fruits derived from citrus trees. The consumption of hesperidin appears to influence blood pressure and improve antioxidant status in humans [78]. This citrus flavanone is a widely used dietary supplement, alone or in combination with other bioflavonoids, for the treatment or prevention of disturbances in the vascular system (reducing capillary permeability) and as an anti-inflammatory, antioxidant, or anticarcinogenic herbal medicine [79,80]. The majority of the medicinal properties of this bioflavonoid have been attributed to its ability to modulate pro-inflammatory cytokines, such as TNF-α, IL-1β, and IL-6, and reduce inflammation and oxidative stress in biological systems, as demonstrated in different animal models of inflammatory reactions [81].

One of the most common chronic diseases that can be treated with this flavonoid is diabetes, as Akiyama et al. [82] reported. The authors used an animal model of STZ-induced diabetes to assess the effect of hesperidin on biochemical markers, glucose-regulating enzymes, and parameters of bone loss in marginal type 1 diabetic rats. Hesperidin reduced blood glucose and serum insulin and normalized the enzymatic activities of glucose-6-phosphatase (G6Pase), glucokinase (GK), and other hepatic enzymes important in glycemic control. In addition, Mahmoud et al. [83] showed that hesperidin treatment could attenuate hyperglycemia-mediated oxidative stress and suppress the production of pro-inflammatory cytokines, such as TNF-α and IL-6, in HFD/STZ-induced type 2 diabetic rats. These results corroborate those of El-Marasy et al. [84], who reported that the oral administration of hesperidin reduced blood glucose, decreased levels of MDA and IL-6, and increased GSH and brain-derived neurotropic factor (BDNF) levels in the brains of rats with diabetes. Hesperidin also normalized the levels of monoamines in the brain, specifically, norepinephrine and dopamine, and elevated brain levels of serotonin. The results obtained were also reflected in physical and behavioral parameters, since hesperidin reduced the immobility time of rats with diabetes in the forced swimming test.

Visnagri, Kandhare, Chakravarty, Ghosh, and Bodhankar [85] evaluated the effect of hesperidin against diabetic neuropathic pain in rats. Hesperidin treatment inhibited the reduction in motor nerve and sensory nerve conduction velocity induced by diabetes. Impaired neural conduction velocity can affect sensory, nociceptive, and motor responses. However, hesperidin normalized the sensorial responses by attenuating the increased mechanical and thermal hyperalgesia in diabetic rats. This bioflavonoid also attenuated several diabetic biochemical parameters, such as high blood glucose, TC, and serum TG, increased the plasma concentration of insulin, and had positive effects on hemodynamic variables, important in the treatment of diabetes and the associated cardiovascular complications. Finally, hesperidin showed neural-protective effects, accompanied by a reduced infiltration of neutrophils and macrophages in the sciatic nerve and reduced mRNA expression of neural TNF-α and IL-1β, two important pro-inflammatory cytokines involved in the progression of diabetes. In addition, it restored the distortion of the architecture of the sciatic nerve caused by STZ-induced necrosis, edema, and congestion on nerve fibers.

Mahmoud, Ahmed, Ashour, and Abdel-Moneim [56] generated more information regarding the mechanism of action of hesperidin as a natural antidiabetic product using HFD/STZ-induced type 2 diabetic rats and in vitro studies. The oral administration of hesperidin was shown to reduce fasting glucose and attenuate insulin resistance in diabetic rats, and increase the release of insulin in isolated pancreatic islets. In addition, it normalized the activities of metabolic enzymes, such as glucose-6-phosphatase, glycogen phosphorylase, and fructose-1,6-bisphosphatase. This bioflavonoid was also found to increase glucose uptake in isolated pancreatic cells. It has been shown that the antidiabetic effects of hesperidin are mainly due to its capacity to increase the mRNA and protein expression of GLUT4 in adipose tissue, in addition to decreasing intestinal glucose absorption.

Liu, Liou, Hong, and Liu [58] conducted experiments to evaluate the effects and mechanisms of hesperidin on different pathophysiological parameters of diabetic retinopathy using retinal RGC-5 ganglial cells. It is well established that oxidative stress plays an important role in diabetes, and it is characterized by high concentrations of ROS and the lipid peroxidation marker MDA, as well as a reduction in the activity of antioxidant enzymes. The higher levels of intracellular ROS, MDA, and protein carbonyl in RGC-5 cells under high concentrations of glucose were down-regulated by hesperidin, and the reduced activities of SOD, GPx, and catalase (CAT) were recovered. The authors also showed that hesperidin blocked the high glucose-induced elevation of the cell apoptosis regulator Bax and decreased Bcl-2 concentrations in high glucose-exposed RGC-5 cells. It also down-regulated caspase-9 and caspase-3, lowered the Bax/Bcl-2 ratio, and restored mitochondrial function, confirming that cells can be protected by hesperidin from high glucose-induced apoptosis through a mitochondrially mediated pathway. Moreover, this citrus flavone significantly inhibited the phosphorylation of JNK and activated p38 mitogen-activated protein kinases (p38 MAPK), proving its vital effect of protecting cells from ROS injury and cellular death.

According to Zareei, Boojar, and Amanlou [59], alanine aminotransferase (ALT) and AST are two liver pyridoxal phosphate-dependent enzymes involved in gluconeogenesis and amino acid metabolism that catalyze the intermediary reactions of glucose and protein metabolism. The increased activity of these enzymes has been observed in liver metabolic syndrome, atherogenesis, and type I and type II diabetes. In rat liver cells, different concentrations of hesperidin exhibited inhibitory effects against ALT and AST activities; therefore, it can be considered a potential compound for designing a safe and effective agent for the management of diabetes mellitus-associated hepatic injury.

Li, Kandhare, Mukherjee, and Bodhankar [86] conducted several experiments in diabetic animals aiming to evaluate the effectiveness of hesperidin against diabetic foot ulcers induced by injecting STZ followed by excision wounds created on the dorsal surface of the foot. In addition, hesperidin treatment in diabetes-induced rats inhibited weight loss, reduced insulin concentrations, normalized blood glucose, reduced food and water intake, increased SOD and GSH levels, and reduced MDA and NO levels. The results presented by Li, Kandhare, Mukherjee, and Bodhankar also showed that this flavanone exhibited beneficial effects in the treatment of wounds, since it attenuated the morphological changes caused, and reduced the edema and inflammatory infiltration of polymorphonuclear cells, in addition to accelerating angiogenesis and vasculogenesis. These effects can be attributed to the regulatory action of hesperidin on important biomarkers, such as vascular endothelial growth factor c (VEGF-c); angiopoietin-1, the ligand for the tyrosine kinase receptor Tie2 (Ang-1/Tie-2); TGF-β; and Smad-2/3.

In STZ-induced diabetic animals, Dokumacioglu et al. [87] supported some of the previously reported data about this citrus flavonoid hesperidin and added more important molecular findings, which showed that hesperidin significantly decreased serum total cholesterol, TG, LDL C, VLDL C, and MDA levels and increased GSH concentrations but did not change HDL-C levels. Additionally, histological analysis showed that treatment with hesperidin led to an improvement in the degenerated islet cells in diabetic rats. The study also reported a reduction in pro-inflammatory cytokines in diabetic rats. The authors speculated that the control of weight loss in the diabetic rats treated with hesperidin might result from the organized regulation of TNF-α and IL-6 levels in adipose tissue. Studies reported that the increased secretion of TNF-α and IL-6 by subcutaneous fat tissue correlates with obesity and adiposity, and such was also suggested to be associated with the origination of diabetic microvascular complications [88,89].

2.10. Hesperetin

Hesperetin ((S) -2,3-dihydro-5,7-dihydroxy-2- (3-hydroxy-4-methoxyphenyl) -4-benzopyran), an important citrus flavonoid and aglycone form of hesperidin, is a bitter compound mainly found in bitter oranges and lemons [90]. It is interesting to note that hesperetin has a higher bioavailability compared to hesperidin due to the rutinoside moiety attached to the flavonoid, and this seems to contribute to its superior anti-inflammatory and antioxidant properties [91]. Hesperetin is widely studied in several pathological conditions and exhibits neuroprotective effects [92], anticancer properties [93], anti-neuroinflammatory potential [94], antioxidant effects [95], and anti-inflammatory [96] activities, among others.

Zareei, Boojar, and Amanlou [59] investigated and evaluated the effect of hesperetin on the AST and ALT enzymes in the liver of rats and concluded that hesperetin exclusively inhibited ALT and AST activities in diabetes-induced rats. Therefore, their study hypothesized that hesperetin may be a potential compound for designing safe and effective drugs for the management of increased ALT- and AST-related disorders, which are especially found in diabetes. Furthermore, Revathy, Subramani, Sheik Abdullah, and Udaiyar [97] showed that hesperetin exhibited an antihyperglycemic effect by reducing blood glucose and enhancing plasma insulin and glycogen levels in an animal model of STZ-induced diabetes. Hesperetin treatment ameliorated vascular congestion and mononuclear cellular infiltration, and improved hepatic architecture, which was damaged by profound hyperglycemia. Hesperetin also alleviated the abnormality caused by hyperglycemia in pancreatic β-cells, inducing a notable extension of islets, improved staining in pancreatic β-cells, and boosting the number of insulin immune-positive cells of the islets. It also recovered the diabetes-induced damaged kidney tissue by reducing marked tubular necrosis, improving the architecture of the glomerulus and renal cortex, and attenuating interstitial inflammation in rat renal tissues.

Samie, Sedaghat, Baluchnejadmojarad, and Roghani [98] assessed the beneficial effect of hesperetin on diabetes-associated testicular injury in diabetic rats. Like other bioflavonoids, hesperetin was also able to prevent body weight loss, DNA fragmentation, and testicular oxidative stress and/or apoptosis; increase serum testosterone levels; reduce serum glucose, MDA, ROS, and protein carbonyl levels; and prevent caspase 3 activity in diabetic animals. Hesperetin treatment also showed important antioxidant effects by increasing glutathione, mitochondrial membrane potential (mMP), and ferric reducing antioxidant power (FRAP) levels, besides improving the activities of enzymes such as SOD, CAT, and GPx. Finally, hesperetin showed positive effects on testicular function and improved sperm counts, motility, and viability, as well as reducing inflammatory cytokines (TNF-α and IL-17) and preventing damage to the seminiferous tubules in diabetic rats.

Overall, hesperetin exhibits anti-inflammatory and antioxidant effects in diabetes-mediated metabolic disorders. These results suggest that hesperetin specifically modulates biochemical parameters linked to liver enzymes, in addition to protecting the vital organs affected by the deleterious effects of profound hyperglycemia. Thus, further clinical trials should be carried out to verify hesperetin as an important potential treatment against diabetes and related metabolic complications.

Table 2. Description of the main characteristics of animal studies using citrus flavonoids for the management of diabetes mellitus.

Flavonoids	Class	Animal Models	Dose/Route/Duration of the Experiment	Effects and Molecular Mechanisms	Ref.
Hesperidin	Flavanone	Wistar Rats	Hesperidin-containing animal diet (10 g/kg diet); 28 days	Hesperidin attenuated hyperglycemia and hyperlipidemia by decreasing blood glucose and normalizing hepatic glucose-regulating enzyme activities but did not affect bone tissue and bone metabolic parameters in streptozotocin (STZ)-injected marginal diabetic weanling rats.	[82]
Rutin	Flavonol	Wistar Rats	50 mg/kg (*intraperitoneal*); 45 days	Rutin significantly reduced the blood glucose level, improved the lipid profiles, and normalized the activities of hepatic enzymes in STZ-induced diabetic rats. It also regulated hyperglycemia and dyslipidemia, and inhibited the progression of liver and heart dysfunction in STZ-induced diabetic rats.	[99]
Nobiletin	Flavone	C57BL/6 Ldlr-/- Mice	Nobiletin (0.1 or 0.3% mixed in high-fat Western diet); 56 to 182 days	Nobiletin regulated liver biomarkers by increasing hepatic and peripheral insulin sensitivity, improving glucose tolerance, and protecting against the development of atherosclerosis.	[41]
Naringenin	Flavanone	Wistar Rats	10 mg/kg (*intraperitoneal*); 35 days	Naringenin ameliorated aortic reactivity dysfunction in diabetic rats by attenuating lipid peroxidation and oxidative injury via a nitric acid-dependent pathway.	[100]
Hesperidin and naringin	Flavanone	Wistar Rats	50 mg/kg (*oral administration*); 28 and 30 days	Hesperidin and naringin lowered the level of pro-inflammatory cytokine (tumor necrosis factor-alpha (TNF-α) and interleukin (IL)-6) production and enhanced antioxidant defenses in a type 2 diabetes rat model by normalizing the altered blood glucose and antioxidant parameters in the liver.	[83]
Diosmin	Flavone	Wistar Rats	100 mg/kg (*intragastric*); 45 days	Diosmin attenuated lipid abnormalities in the diabetic rats via reducing the plasma and tissue lipids significantly, along with a profound increase in high-density lipoprotein cholesterol (HDL-C) levels.	[33]
Hesperidin	Flavanone	Wistar Rats	25, 50, or 100 mg/kg (*oral administration*); 21 days	Hesperidin reduced hyperglycaemia, decreased malondialdehyde (MDA) and IL-6 levels, and enhanced the brain-derived neurotrophic factor (BDNF) and monoamines in the brain, thereby enabling it to be effective in treating and managing neurogenesis in diabetic rats.	[84]
Naringenin	Flavanone	Wistar Rats	20, 50, and 100 mg/kg (*oral administration*); 56 days	Naringenin restored hyperglycemia, down-regulated superoxide dismutase activity, and reversed chemical and thermal hyperalgesia in the diabetic rats, showing its preventive and therapeutic effectiveness in diabetic neuropathy treatment.	[101]
Diosmin	Flavone	Sprague-Dawley Rats	50 and 100 mg/kg (*oral administration*); 28 days	Diosmin significantly restored the blood glucose levels, antioxidant parameters, and lipid profiles in the diabetic rats. It also improved their thermal hyperalgesia, cold allodynia, and walking function.	[34]
Sudachitin	Flavone	C57BL/6 J and db/db Mice	5 mg/kg (*oral administration*); 84 days	Sudachitin significantly improved dyslipidemia, reduced triglyceride and free fatty acid contents, enhanced glucose tolerance, and reduced insulin resistance in the diabetic mice. β-oxidation of fatty acids was also markedly enhanced via increased mitochondrial biogenesis.	[54]
Tangeretin	Flavone	Wistar Rats	25, 50, and 100 mg/kg (*intragastric*); 30 days	Tangeretin normalized the levels and activities of plasma glucose, insulin, glycosylated hemoglobin, and key enzymes of carbohydrate metabolism in the livers of diabetic rats.	[71]

Table 2. Cont.

Flavonoids	Class	Animal Models	Dose/Route/Duration of the Experiment	Effects and Molecular Mechanisms	Ref.
Hesperidin	Flavanone	Sprague-Dawley Rats	25, 50, and 100 mg/kg (oral administration); 28 days	Hesperidin decreased the levels of STZ-induced hyperglycemia and pro-inflammatory cytokines and increased the nociceptive threshold, motor nerve conduction velocity, sensory nerve conduction velocity, insulin levels, and Na-K-adenosine triphosphate (ATP)ase activity in the diabetic rats.	[85]
Naringenin	Flavanone	C57BL/6J Mice	100 mg/kg (oral administration); 14 days	Naringenin suppressed macrophage infiltration into the adipose tissues of the high-fat diet (HFD)-fed obese mice. It also down-regulated monocyte chemoattractant protein-1 (MCP-1) in the adipose tissues via inhibiting the c-Jun NH2-terminal kinase (JNK) pathway.	[55]
Neohesperidin	Flavanone	KK-Ay and C57BL/6 Mices	50 mg/kg (oral administration); 42 days	Neohesperidin attenuated fasting blood glucose and insulin resistance. The levels of total cholesterol, triglycerides, and leptins were significantly decreased, while the phosphorylation of AMP-activated protein kinase (AMPK) and its target genes was increased in the drug-treated mice. It also significantly decreased the size of epididymal adipocytes in the diabetic mice.	[102]
Hesperidin and naringin	Flavanones	Wistar Rats	50 mg/kg (oral administration); 30 days	Hesperidin and naringin significantly reduced the glucose level, restored the altered parameters of glucose metabolism, and enhanced adipose tissue glucose transporter type 4 (GLUT4) mRNA and protein expression in the diabetic rats.	[36]
Tangeretin	Flavone	Wistar Rats	100 mg/kg (intragastric); 30 days	Tangeretin significantly reduced plasma and cardiac lipid profiles by regulating key lipid metabolic enzymes in the livers of diabetic rats. It also markedly restored the GLUT4 expression, antioxidant enzyme activities, and levels of inflammatory cytokines in the heart tissues of the tangeretin-treated diabetic rats.	[72]
Nobiletin	Flavone	Wistar rats	10 and 25 mg/kg (oral administration); 28 days	Nobiletin substantially ameliorated hemodynamic parameters, oxidative stress, collagen levels, matrix metalloproteinase (MMP)-2 levels, and MMP-9 levels in the diabetic rats. It also markedly attenuated deterioration in the morphology of cardiomyocytes.	[44]
Nobiletin	Flavone	C57BL/6 Mice	50 mg/kg (oral administration); 77 days	Nobiletin significantly decreased the expression of nicotinamide adenine dinucleotide (NADH) oxidase isoforms p67phox, p22phox, and p91phox, and attenuated oxidative stress in diabetic mice. It also ameliorated the development of cardiac dysfunction and interstitial fibrosis by down-regulating the c-Jun N-terminal kinase (JNK), P38, and nuclear factor kappa B NF-κB signaling pathways.	[45]
Diosmin	Flavone	Sprague-Dawley Rats	160 mg/kg (intraperitoneal); 7 days	Diosmin reduced hyperglycemia by enhancing the secretion of β-endorphin from the adrenal glands via imidazoline 1–2 receptor (I-2R) activation, which triggered the opioid receptors to attenuate gluconeogenesis metabolism in the livers of diabetic rats. It decreased the hepatic glycogen content and plasma lipid profiles in STZ-induced diabetic rats. However, it did not adversely affect the body weight, food intake, and plasma insulin level in the diabetic rats.	[35]

Table 2. Cont.

Flavonoids	Class	Animal Models	Dose/Route/Duration of the Experiment	Effects and Molecular Mechanisms	Ref.
Hesperidin and quercetin	Flavanone and flavone	Wistar Rats	100 mg/kg (oral administration); 15 days	Hesperidin and quercetin exerted positive effects on insulin metabolism. They lowered the levels of triglycerides, MDA, TNFα, and IL-6, and restored the level of glutathione (GSH) in experimental diabetic rats induced by STZ.	[87]
Hesperidin	Flavanone	Sprague-Dawley Rats	25, 50, and 100 mg/kg (oral administration); 21 days	Hesperidin ameliorated the increased levels of blood glucose, serum insulin, food intake, and water intake in STZ- induced diabetes. It also had a protective effect on the wound architecture by accelerating angiogenesis and vasculogenesis via the up-regulation of vascular endothelial growth factor c (VEGF-c), Angiopoietin (Ang)-1/Tie-2, transforming growth factor (TGF-β), and small mothers against decapentaplegic (Smad)-2/3 mRNA expression to enhance wound healing in the chronic diabetic foot ulcer condition in the diabetic rats.	[86]
Xanthohumol and 8-prenylnaringenin	Prenylflavonoid	C57Bl/6 Mice	0.1% of flavonoids dissolved in ethanol; 140 days	Xanthohumol and 8-prenylnaringenin have a potent therapeutic effect on diabetic mice, as evidenced by the decreased levels of diabetes-linked biochemical parameters in the liver and kidney. They also decreased the overexpression of galectin-3 (Gal3), which was correlated with oxidative stress in diabetic mice.	[27]
Naringin	Flavanone	Sprague-Dawley Rats	100 mg/kg (oral administration); 28 days	Naringin reduced blood glucose, total cholesterol, triglycerides, and low-density lipoproteins in fructose-fed rats. Naringin restored acetylcholine-mediated vasorelaxation, suggesting its potential influence on fructose-induced metabolic alterations and endothelial dysfunction. Naringin improved serum nitrate/nitrite (NOx), endothelial nitric oxide synthase (eNOS), and phosphorylated eNOS (p-eNOS) protein expression, and preserved endothelium-dependent relaxation in the aortae of the fructose-fed rats.	[103]
Hesperetin	Flavanone	Wistar Rats	40 mg/kg (intragastric); 45 days	Hesperetin reduced the blood glucose level and enhanced the plasma insulin and the hepatic glycogen levels in the STZ-induced diabetic rats. It also restored the altered hepatic glucose metabolic enzymes, lipid profiles, and serum biomarkers, and protected from STZ-mediated structural alterations and functional changes in the liver, kidneys, and pancreatic β-cells of diabetic animals.	[97]
Hesperetin	Flavanone	Wistar Rats	50 mg/kg (oral administration); 46 days	Hesperetin significantly reduced the serum glucose level and improved the serum testosterone level in the STZ-induced diabetic rats. Additionally, it augmented the testicular antioxidant enzymes and attenuated the testicular inflammatory markers, such as TNFα and IL-17, besides preventing the seminiferous tubules' damage in diabetic rats.	[98]
Naringenin	Flavanone	C57BL/6J Mice	100 mg/kg (oral administration); 14 days	Naringenin inhibited neutrophil infiltration into the adipose tissues of the high-fat diet (HFD)-fed mice by reducing the expression of several chemokines, including monocyte chemoattractant protein (MCP)-1 and MCP-3, in the adipose tissues.	[64]
Nobiletin	Flavone	Ldlr−/− and Ampkβ1−/− mice from a C57BL/6J background	0.3% of nobiletin mixed in HFD; 84–126 days	Nobiletin attenuated obesity, hepatic steatosis, dyslipidemia, and insulin resistance, and improved energy utilization in HFD-fed mice. It conferred metabolic protection independently of AMPK activation in the liver and adipose tissues.	[46]

2.11. Naringenin

Naringenin (5,7-dihydroxy-2- (4-hydroxyphenyl) chroman-4-one) is a citrus flavanone mainly found in grapefruits, bergamots, and oranges. Numerous pharmacological activities of naringenin have already been reported in the scientific literature. It is widely used as a dietary supplement in different treatments, often in combination with other herbal preparations. Naringenin (aglycone) and naringin are flavanones that display strong anti-inflammatory and antioxidant activities [104].

Since cardiovascular diseases (CVDs) remain the leading cause of morbidity and mortality in diabetic patients, Fallahi, Roghani, and Moghadami [100] focused their study on investigating the cardiovascular potential of this natural flavonoid in diabetes. More specifically, the authors investigated its aortic reactivity, since increased serum glucose and ROS cause vascular endothelial dysfunction. Naringenin prevented weight loss and lowered the increased plasma glucose concentration in diabetic animals, suggesting its cardioprotective effects. This bioflavonoid exhibited beneficial effects on the cardiovascular system by reducing the maximum contractile response of endothelium-intact rings and improving endothelium-dependent relaxation in response to acetylcholine (ACh). These effects seem to be dependent on modulating the NO pathway, since the pretreatment of endothelium-intact rings with the NOS inhibitor N (G)-nitro-l-arginine methyl ester (L-NAME) significantly attenuated the observed responses in diabetic rats.

Hasanein and Fazeli [101] also investigated the antidiabetic effects of naringenin but with a special focus on its effectiveness in diabetes-induced hyperalgesia and allodynia. Naringenin attenuated chemical and thermal hyperalgesia, as well as allodynia. Since oxidative stress and inflammation are also found in diabetic neuropathy, the study showed that naringenin administration increased the activity of SOD, an endogenous enzyme closely intertwined with oxidative stress during the diabetic condition.

Furthermore, using an HFD-induced obesity animal model (C57BL/6J Mice), Yoshida et al. [55] evaluated the anti-inflammatory effects of naringenin and its mechanism of action. Naringenin did not affect HFD-induced changes in serum biochemical parameters, such as glucose, TC, and TG levels. However, it was able to reduce the mRNA expression of the Mac-2 gene, an important macrophage marker. Reinforcing its anti-inflammatory effect, the administration of naringenin reduced monocyte chemoattractant protein 1 (MCP-1) expression in adipose tissue from HFD-fed mice, and in adipocyte and macrophage co-cultures, which is one of the key chemokines, one of its main roles being to suppress the migration and infiltration of monocytes/macrophages into adipose tissue. In addition, naringenin inhibited HFD-induced JNK phosphorylation but did not interfere in the expression of IκB-α, a member of a family of cellular proteins that function to inhibit the NF-κB transcription factor. In summary, these results suggest that naringenin suppresses macrophage infiltration and can modulate the chemoattraction of inflammatory cells via the regulation of MCP-1 expression in adipocytes via a JNK-dependent pathway in obesity-related metabolic disorders.

Tsuhako, Yoshida, Sugita, and Kurokawa [64] conducted an in vivo experiment with a HFD-induced obese and insulin-resistant animal model, as well as with in vitro assays, using 3T3-L1 (adipocytes) and RAW264 (macrophages) cells to confirm their hypothesis that naringenin has effects on inflammatory cell infiltration into adipose tissue, in addition to being able to modulate vital chemokines and cytokines. The recruitment of immune cells was observed in obese adipose tissue, which contributes to the initiation and progression of obesity-linked diseases, such as insulin resistance and type 2 diabetes mellitus. They showed that naringenin suppressed the neutrophil infiltration into adipose tissue in obese mice. Naringenin also produced an anti-inflammatory response in the adipose tissues in mice by reducing the levels of the chemokines and/or cytokines MCP-1, macrophage inflammatory protein (MIP)-1α, MIP-2, and MCP-3 and causing a noticeable reduction in the pro-inflammatory cytokine IL-6, although TNF-α was not affected. In the in vitro analyses, naringenin significantly reduced MCP-3 expression at the transcriptional and secretion levels in 3T3-L1 adipocytes, as well as in a co-culture of 3T3-L1 adipocytes and RAW264 macrophages. Thus, the authors suggest that naringenin suppresses neutrophil infiltration into adipose tissue via the regulation of vital inflammatory mediators connected to immune-cell functions.

Similar to other citrus flavonoids, naringenin has also been observed to be a potent NF-κB pathway regulator that directly leads to the obstruction of ROS accumulation due to its ability to act as a scavenger of free radicals and up-regulate the activity of both prooxidant and antioxidant enzymes, which is the most remarkable dual property of this flavonoid [55]. In addition, recent findings also point out that naringenin can down-regulate vital chemokines, which have a significant role in the recruitment and infiltration of inflammatory cells into adipose tissue, and stop the advancement of metabolic disorders, such as insulin resistance and type 2 diabetes mellitus.

2.12. Naringin

Naringin is a flavanone-7-O-glycoside located between the flavanone naringenin and the disaccharide neohesperidose. It occurs naturally in citrus fruits, predominantly in grapefruits. Similarly to naringenin, naringin is widely sold as a food supplement because of its cardioprotective, neuroprotective, and immunomodulatory properties [105]. When ingested by humans, naringin is metabolized by naringinase in the liver, so the main product of this metabolism is naringenin, which seems to be responsible, at least in part, for the biological effects attributed to this biomolecule. Naringin showed beneficial effects in acute and chronic models, such as those of diabetic neuropathy [106], pleurisy [107], asthma [108,109], cancer [110], behavioral deficits [111], Alzheimer's disease [112], and chronic fatigue [113], and in experimental models for inflammation and oxidative stress induced by cisplatin [114].

Mahmoud et al. [83] conducted two studies, in 2012 and 2015, to evaluate the antidiabetic potential of naringin. According to the authors, naringin attenuated hyperglycemia-mediated oxidative stress parameters (MDA and NO) and pro-inflammatory cytokine (TNF-α and IL-6) secretion and production in HFD/STZ-induced type 2 diabetic rats. The authors confirmed that the oral administration of naringin normalized the activities of important enzymes in hepatic glycolytic metabolism, such as G6Pase, glycogen phosphorylase, and fructose-1,6-bisphosphatase. In addition, naringin increased the release of insulin from isolated islets in the presence of IL-1β and decreased intestinal glucose absorption. Its antioxidant effects were also verified due to the reduction of NO in isolated pancreatic islets. The mechanism of the action responsible for the effects of naringin may be related to the increased expression of GLUT4 in adipose tissue, which aids in the uptake of free circulating glucose from the blood to peripheral tissues.

Malakul, Pengnet, Kumchoom, and Tunsophon [103] investigated the effect of naringin on fructose-induced endothelial dysfunction in rats and its fundamental mechanisms. Rats that had consumed fructose in drinking water showed significantly increased levels of blood glucose, TC, TG, and LDL C. Consequently, naringin treatment significantly brought these parameters back to near normal. Fructose impaired endothelial function, but vascular smooth muscle function was unaffected by fructose treatment. Interestingly, naringin restored endothelial function in the aortic rings, confirming a vasoprotective effect. In addition, naringin improved serum nitrate/nitrite (NOx), eNOS, and phosphorylated eNOS (p-eNOS) protein expression. Therefore, the authors concluded that the vascular potential of naringin was moderately attributed to improving NO bioavailability, increasing eNOS activity, and obstructing the accumulation of peroxynitrite in the aortae.

In summary, the results of these studies demonstrate the related curative potential of naringin in attenuating oxidative damage and inflammatory cascades. Moreover, it exhibits a unique preserving effect on endothelial dysfunction, an important factor in the development of diabetic complications, especially atherosclerosis and cardiovascular diseases.

2.13. Neohesperidin

Neohesperidin (hesperetin-7-neohesperidoside) is a flavanone glycoside, a weak-polar molecule with a bitter taste, found in various citrus fruits [115]. Neohesperidin, a dihydrochalcone, is a substance mainly obtained from bitter oranges and has unique properties such as masking undesirable flavors and enhancing fruity and citrus flavors, which gives this molecule great value for the food industry and nutraceuticals firms [116]. This flavanone has a wide range of biological activities, including neuroprotective activity [117] and anti-proliferative effects [118]. Recently, neohesperidin was found to inhibit common allergic responses in vivo and in vitro [119], exhibit protective effects in progressive pulmonary fibrosis [120], and show anti-osteoclastic properties, presenting it as a potential anti-catabolic biomolecule for the treatment of osteoporosis [121].

The antidiabetic potential of neohesperidin was investigated by Jia et al. [102], who evaluated the effect of this active compound derived from *Citrus aurantium* Linn. in diabetic KK-Ay mice induced via a formulated diet (6.0% fat, 18% proteins, and 8.0% water). Neohesperidin had no significant effect on the body weight and food intake in the experimental diabetic mice; nevertheless, it increased glucose tolerance and insulin sensitivity and reduced the blood glucose levels affected by diabetic illness. Neohesperidin treatment also significantly reduced total cholesterol and TG, in addition to decreasing ALT, but it did not modulate AST levels, showing its key hypoglycemic and hypolipidemic properties.

Histological studies showed that neohesperidin-treated diabetic mice had a marked reduction in lipid accumulation in the liver and decreased adipocyte size compared with water-treated KK-Ay diabetic mice. Neohesperidin was shown to have hypolipidemic effects via exerting a profound influence on markers, such as the mRNA levels of PPAR-α, PPAR-γ, and their target genes, including stearoyl-CoA desaturase (SCD)-1, carnitine palmitoyltransferase (CPT)-1, adaptor complex (AP)-2, UCP-2, fatty acid synthase (FAS), and acyl-CoA oxidase (ACOX), in liver tissue. The expression of SCD-1 and FAS in diabetic mice was significantly down-regulated by neohesperidin treatment, whereas the expression of ACOX was significantly up-regulated. Finally, neohesperidin treatment resulted in the increased phosphorylation of AMPK. These data demonstrate that neohesperidin may have pronounced potential for the prevention of obesity-linked diabetes mellitus [102].

2.14. Xanthohumol

Xanthohumol or 3'-[3,3-dimethylallyl]-2',4',4-trihydroxy-6'-methoxychalcone, found in citrus plants in the family Rutaceae, is a bioactive antioxidant molecule linked to a wide range of bioactivities, including anticarcinogenic, anti-inflammatory, and antioxidant properties [122,123]. A study included in our survey demonstrated that xanthohumol reduced the expression of Gal3, a protein responsible for multiple complications and diabetic progression in HFD-fed type 2 diabetic C57Bl/6 mice. In addition to reducing Gal3 expression, xanthohumol has also been shown to reduce oxidative stress biomarkers associated with diabetes such as 3-nitrotyrosine and AGEs in the liver and kidneys, validating its remedial effect against this chronic metabolic disease [27].

2.15. Quercetin

This citrus flavonoid is probably one of the most studied flavonol compounds, which may be due to its ubiquitous presence in different citrus plants. It also has many therapeutic properties that include anti-inflammatory, antinociceptive, and anticancer effects. Oranges, mandarins, limes, lemons, sour oranges, and grapefruits are common sources of quercetin [124]. Quercetin is, therefore, considered the most important citrus flavonoids because of its ability to modulate the essential inflammatory mediators that accompany metabolic diseases. This flavonol is one of the most popular citrus flavonoids in the global fruit market, and it is commonly used as a constituent in nutraceuticals and food supplements. A number of products containing this flavonoid have been patented because of its outstanding therapeutic applicability as a disease-fighting antioxidant molecule that can improve the health and well-being of individuals [125].

Dhanya, Arya, Nisha, and Jayamurthy [57] investigated the molecular mechanism of quercetin by screening it in skeletal muscle (L6 myotubes) cells and showed that it improved glucose uptake via regulation of the AMPK pathway. The authors demonstrated that the AMPK pathway has a significant role in 2-NBDG (2-deoxy-2-[(7-nitro-2,1,3-benzoxadiazol-4-yl)amino]-D-glucose) uptake and that this was induced by quercetin. The adenosine monophosphate/adenosine triphosphate ratio (AMP/ATP) is an essential factor for cellular AMPK activation, and quercetin pretreatment caused an increase in both the AMP-to-ATP ratio and the adenosine diphosphate (ADP)-to-ATP ratio, an effect correlated with its activity on mitochondrial membrane depolarization. In addition, quercetin pretreatment in L6 myotubes induced a significant up-regulation of the mRNA levels of both AMPK and its downstream target p38 MAPK. Interestingly, calcium-calmodulin mediated protein kinase (CaMKK), AMPK, and MAPK, the key signaling molecules involved in the AMPK signaling pathway, were up-regulated by quercetin treatment in vitro, reinforcing the evidence of its participation in this vital signaling pathway related to the management of insulin signaling. In addition, quercetin was found to increase GLUT4 expression and translocation in a skeletal muscle cell line. Therefore, quercetin possesses antidiabetic potential via activating multiple therapeutic targets to rectify insulin resistance through bypassing different metabolic pathways.

However, Dokumacioglu et al. [87] have reported some controversial results regarding the effect of quercetin on diabetes. Although quercetin treatment decreased various diabetes-related biochemical parameters, such as TC, TG, LDL C, VLDL C, and MDA, it did not alter the HDL-C level and the GSH concentration. Histological analysis showed that treatment with quercetin led to an increase in the regeneration of β-cells in the pancreatic islets. However, it was also reported that quercetin administration in diabetic animals regulated the levels of pro-inflammatory cytokines, such as TNF-α and IL-6. In addition, quercetin also blocked the weight loss in diabetic rats, which could be the result of quercetin regularizing TNF-α and IL-6 secretion in adipose cells and the consequent decrease in fat tissue.

2.16. Rutin

Rutin (quercetin 3-rutinoside, $C_{27}H_{30}O_{16}$) is a glycosidic flavonoid commonly present in dietary sources. The main citrus fruit sources of rutin are oranges, grapefruits, lemons, and limes. Treatment with rutin was found to exert a great modulatory impact on the secretion of IL-1β, IL-2, IL-4, and IL-6. These are vital immunomodulatory cytokines secreted by the immune cells, and abnormal levels of secretion and their action during inflammation can cause cytokine-mediated organ dysfunction and tissue damage during long-term diseases such as diabetes mellitus, cancer, and rheumatoid arthritis [126]. Its immunomodulatory and anti-inflammatory effects on chronic metabolic disorders characterized by hyperglycemia suggest that rutin may be an excellent biomolecule to use in the treatment of these disorders and their associated complaints.

Fernandes et al. [99] investigated the benefit of rutin treatment for various biochemical alterations in experimental diabetic animals. Rutin reduced blood glucose and improved the lipid profile. In addition, it prevented changes in the activities of ALT, AST, and LDH in the serum, liver, and heart, indicating the protective effect of the molecule against hepatic and cardiac toxicity in diabetic rats. Rutin was also able to decrease hepatic and cardiac levels of TG and elevate the glycogen concentration. It showed hypoglycemic and hypolipidemic effects in diabetic rats and, more importantly, prevented liver and heart damage caused by the uncontrolled accumulation of diabetes-mediated ROS.

Besides the single flavonoid compound mentioned above, the citrus extract, rich in different flavonoids, also shows an antidiabetic effect. A study by Kim et al. [53] investigated the effects of *Citrus aurantium* Linn., which contains major flavonoids including naringin, hesperidin, poncirin, isosiennsetin, sineesytin, nobiletin, and tangeretin, on the inhibition of adipogenesis and adipocyte differentiation in 3T3-L1 cells. The mixed actions of the flavonoids from *C. aurantium* showed anti-adipogenic properties and inhibited the differentiation of 3T3-L1 preadipocytes into adipocytes, in addition to also reducing the amount of lipid droplets, and preventing lipid and triglyceride accumulation. Flavonoid-rich *C. aurantium* was able to modulate the insulin signaling cascade, via the inhibition of Akt activation and GSK3β phosphorylation. Finally, it down-regulated the expression of C/EBPβ and subsequently inhibited the activation of PPARγ and C/EBPα, which are related to lipid accumulation and lipid metabolism. Thus, these results highlight the actions of these vital flavonoids present in *C. aurantium* in improving hyperglycemia and dyslipidemia, while inhibiting the progression of diabetes.

3. Composition of Antidiabetic Citrus Flavonoids in Common Citrus Fruit Sources

Few review reports and original articles concern the composition of some major flavonoids in the genus *Citrus*. In our survey, the majority of the antidiabetic studies reported used citrus flavanones (hesperidin, didymin, naringin, neohesperidin, and poncirin), flavones (rhoifolin, diosmin, and rutin), and polymethoxyflavones (nobiletin, sinesetin, and tangeretin). The flavonoid composition of long-life orange juice comprises hesperidin (76.9 mg/L) and didymin (9.9 mg/L) [127]. The composition of tangerine or mandarin hand-squeezed juice comprised didymin (4.44–9.50 mg/L), hesperidin (123.3–206.7 mg/L), tangeritin (5.99–31.8 mg/L), nobiletin (5.49–28.2 mg/L), and sinensetin (0.30–2.00 mg/L), whereas the peeled fruit of tangerines or mandarins contained higher contents of hesperidin (841–1898 mg/kg) and didymin (45–112 mg/kg) [128]. The flavonoid contents in fresh weight (FW) peels and peel extracts of citrus fruits, such as oranges, clementines, and mandarins, were poncirin (2.49–18.85 mg/g FW), didymin (3.22–13.94 mg/g FW), neohesperidin (3.20–11.67 mg/g FW), hesperidin (83.4–234.1 mg/g FW), naringin (only in mandarin) (19.49 mg/g FW), rhoifolin (4.54–10.39 mg/g FW), diosmin (4.01–18.06 mg/g FW), and rutin (8.16–42.13 mg/g FW) [129].

In addition, Gattuso et al. [130] have reviewed the flavonoid contents in various citrus juices extensively. For example, sweet orange juice contains hesperidin (28.6 mg/100 mL), didymin (1.89 mg/100 mL), poncirin (1.04 mg/100 mL), rhoifolin (0.05 mg/100 mL), diosmin (0.09 mg/100 mL), nobiletin (0.33 mg/100 mL), sinesetin (0.37 mg/100 mL), and tangeretin (0.04 mg/100 mL); clementine juice possess hesperidin (39.9 mg/100 mL), naringin (0.08 mg/100 mL), and diosmin (1.25 mg/100 mL); lemon juice has hesperidin (20.5 mg/100 mL) and diosmin (3.12 mg/100 mL); grapefruit juice contains didymin (0.30 mg/100 mL), hesperidin (0.93 mg/100 mL), naringin (23.0 mg/100 mL), neohesperidin (1.21 mg/100 mL), poncirin (1.26 mg/100 mL), rutin (3.26 mg/100 mL), rhoifolin (0.28 mg/100 mL), nobiletin (0.15 mg/100 mL), tangeretin (0.12 mg/100 mL), hesperetin (0.74 mg/100 mL), naringenin (2.70 mg/100 mL), and quercetin (0.19 mg/100 mL); the juice of a hybrid between lemon and sweet oranges contains naringin (2.23 mg/100 mL), neohesperidin (1.60 mg/100 mL), poncirin (6.41 mg/100 mL), rhoifolin (0.37 mg/100 mL), and diosmin (0.39 mg/100 mL); mandarin orange juice has didymin (1.44 mg/100 mL), hesperidin (24.3 mg/100 mL), nobiletin (0.23 mg/100 mL), sinensetin (1.05 mg/100 mL), and tangeretin (0.26 mg/100 mL); hybrid mandarin orange juice contains hesperidin (0.15 mg/100 mL); and bitter orange juice has naringin (1.97 mg/100 mL), neohesperidin (0.87 mg/100 mL), poncirin (0.73 mg/100 mL), diosmin (0.15 mg/100 mL), nobiletin (0.2 mg/100 mL), and tangeretin (0.08 mg/100 mL).

However, few studies have reported the relationships between the antidiabetic effects and the structure of citrus flavonoids, which should be investigated in the future to elucidate their structure–function relationships.

4. Conclusions

In conclusion, using bioactive molecules from plant dietary sources is a fascinating therapeutic process but requires detailed knowledge of their effects drawn from different types of experimental models when used in the treatment of various syndromes. In this review study, the 19 flavonoids of the Citrus genus surveyed present diverse effects and related molecular mechanisms for the treatment and management of diabetic mellitus and related complications. The related antidiabetic mechanisms of citrus flavonoids are illustrated in Figures 3 and 4. These citrus flavonoids attenuated tissue damage arising from prolonged exposure to elevated glucose levels, mainly by increasing endogenous antioxidants, such as SOD, CAT, and GPx, and reducing the concentration of ROS. Regarding the key molecular mechanisms, citrus flavonoids modulate vital metabolic signaling markers via increasing the expression of IRS-1, PI3K, GSK3β, Akt, and PPARγ, and decreasing the expression of PTP1B. The citrus flavonoids are also involved in activating and increasing the expression of the imidazoline I-2R, opioid secretion, GLUT4, and IR, and they also modulate the expression of eNOS, MCP-1 and 3, NF-κB, the cytokines TNFα and INFγ, IL1β, IL-2, and IL-6. All of these processes result in the attenuation of inflammatory mediators linked to the pathogenesis and progression of diabetic vascular complications by increasing glucose uptake in peripheral tissues. This also has a preventive effect against high glucose-induced cell proliferation.

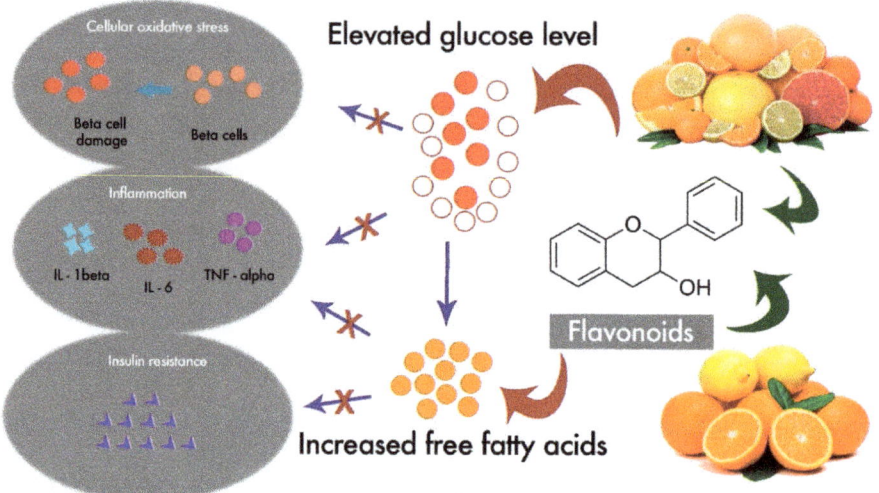

Figure 3. Proposed antidiabetic mechanisms of action of citrus flavonoids. The pictorial representation summarizes the current knowledge that citrus flavonoids could improve the pathogenesis of diabetes and its complications via attenuating cellular oxidative stress, inflammatory markers (interleukin (IL) -1beta, IL-6, tumor necrosis factor (TNF)-alpha), and insulin resistance.

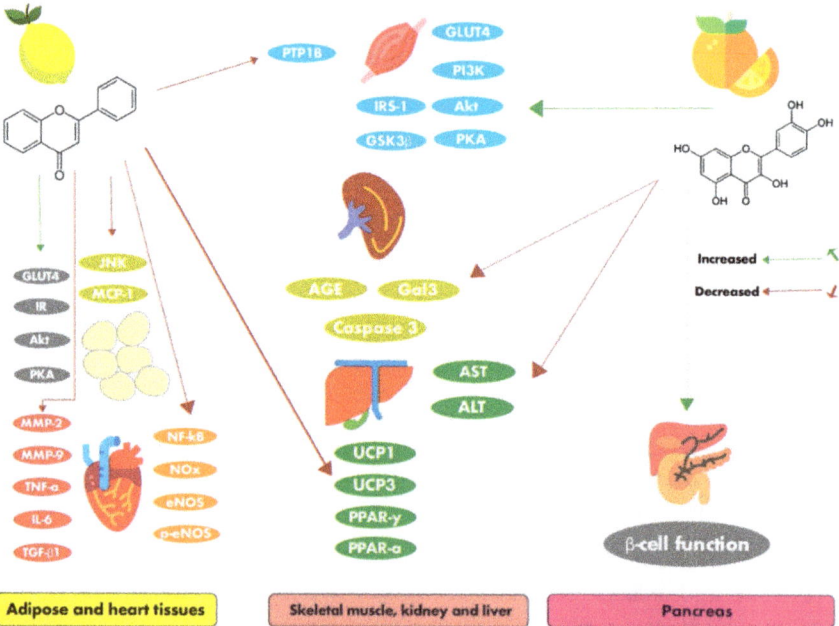

Figure 4. Citrus flavonoids target several molecular markers that are involved in the regulation of blood glucose levels. Citrus flavonoids can increase adipose tissue glucose transporter 4 (GLUT4), insulin receptors (IR), protein kinase B (PKB) or Akt, and protein kinase A (PKA); decrease skeletal

muscle protein tyrosine phosphatase 1B (PTP1B); and up-regulate GLUT4, phosphoinositide 3-kinases (PI3K), insulin receptor substrate (IRS)-1, Akt, PKA, and glycogen synthase kinase 3β (GSK3β) expression in the skeletal muscle tissue. They also improve β-cell function. On the other hand, citrus flavonoid molecules can decrease c-Jun N-terminal kinase (JNK) and monocyte chemoattractant protein (MCP)-1 in the adipose tissue, and down-regulate nuclear factor kappa B (NF-κB), nitrate/nitrite (NOx), endothelial nitric oxide synthase (eNOS), matrix metalloproteinases (MMPs), and inflammatory mediators in the heart tissue. They also reduce the glycation end products (AGEs), Galectin-3 (Gal3), and caspase 3 expression in the kidney and decrease the uncoupling protein (UCP), proliferator-activated receptor (PPAR), aspartate aminotransferase (AST), and alanine aminotransferase (ALT) levels in the liver tissue.

In the future, more detailed research is still required into these compounds, along with the development of various drug delivery vehicles that facilitate their controlled release and increase their absorption, bioavailability, and potency. Conducting human clinical trials is the only fool-proof method for determining the efficacy of citrus flavonoids in humans. Therefore, it is important to undertake human clinical trials based on the current knowledge about these compounds using modern molecular technological tools to identify the mechanisms of action in different pathways and molecular gene expression studies using type 2 diabetes-related genes.

Moreover, easier and cheaper methods to isolate pure compounds should be further explored so that comprehensive studies can be conducted on every potential antidiabetic citrus flavonoid. Emphasis must be given to the citrus flavonoids as safer, novel antidiabetic agents, rather than being overly dependent on synthetic antidiabetic drugs. Accurate scientific information on citrus flavonoids should be collected and distributed as widely as possible through publications and seminars.

Overall, the Citrus species are valuable natural sources of flavonoids and a promising source for future treatments aimed at the prevention and management of diabetes and related complications. To the best of our knowledge, this is the first review that summarizes the effects of major citrus flavonoids on the vital physiological pathways and biochemical parameters related to diabetes. This can contribute to the understanding of their biological profiles in current therapies and assist in the development of future therapies for the treatment of diabetes.

Author Contributions: Conceptualization, G.R.G. and R.-Y.G.; data curation, G.R.G. and H.-B.L.; formal analysis, G.R.G.; funding acquisition, R.-Y.G.; project administration, R.-Y.G.; supervision, R.-Y.G.; writing—original draft, G.R.G. and A.B.S.V.; writing—review and editing, P.J.A., H.-B.L., D.-T.W., H.L., F.G., R.Q.G., N.N., and R.-Y.G. All authors have read and agreed to the published version of the manuscript.

Funding: This study was supported by the Central Public-interest Scientific Institution Basal Research Fund (No. Y2020XK05); Local Financial Funds of the National Agricultural Science and Technology Center, Chengdu (No. NASC2020KR02); and the National Key R & D Program of China (No. 2018YFC1604405).

Conflicts of Interest: The authors declare no conflict of interest.

References

1. Zech-Matterne, V.; Fiorentino, G. *AGRUMED: Archaeology and History of Citrus Fruit in the Mediterranean: Acclimatization, Diversifications, Uses*; Collection du Centre Jean Bérard, Publications du Centre Jean Bérard: Naples, Italy, 2017. [CrossRef]
2. Luro, F.; Gatto, J.; Costantino, G.; Pailly, O. Analysis of genetic diversity in *Citrus*. *Plant Genet. Resour.* **2011**, *9*, 218–221. [CrossRef]
3. Goulet, B.E.; Roda, F.; Hopkins, R. Hybridization in plants: Old ideas, new techniques. *Plant Physiol.* **2017**, *173*, 65–78. [CrossRef] [PubMed]
4. Ollitrault, P.; Navarro, L. Citrus. In *Fruit Breeding*; Badenes, M., Byrne, D., Eds.; Springer: Boston, MA, USA, 2012; Volume 8, pp. 623–662. [CrossRef]
5. Gill, H.; Garg, H. *Citrus Pathology*; IntechOpen: London, UK, 2017. [CrossRef]
6. Man, M.Q.; Yang, B.; Elias, P.M. Benefits of hesperidin for cutaneous functions. *Evid. Based Complement. Alternat. Med.* **2019**, *2019*, 2676307. [CrossRef] [PubMed]

7. Tripoli, E.; Guardia, M.L.; Giammanco, S.; Majo, D.D.; Giammanco, M. Citrus flavonoids: Molecular structure, biological activity and nutritional properties: A review. *Food Chem.* **2007**, *104*, 466–479. [CrossRef]
8. Mahmoud, A.M.; Hernández Bautista, R.J.; Sandhu, M.A.; Hussein, O.E. Beneficial effects of citrus flavonoids on cardiovascular and metabolic health. *Oxid. Med. Cell. Longev.* **2019**, *2019*, 5484138. [CrossRef]
9. Diabetes Atlas 9th edition 2019. Available online: https://www.diabetesatlas.org/en/ (accessed on 25 August 2020).
10. Reach, G.; Pechtner, V.; Gentilella, R.; Corcos, A.; Ceriello, A. Clinical inertia and its impact on treatment intensification in people with type 2 diabetes mellitus. *Diabetes Metab.* **2017**, *43*, 501–511. [CrossRef]
11. Cho, N.H.; Shaw, J.E.; Karuranga, S.; Huang, Y.; da Rocha Fernandes, J.D.; Ohlrogge, A.W.; Malanda, B. IDF Diabetes Atlas: Global estimates of diabetes prevalence for 2017 and projections for 2045. *Diabetes Res. Clin. Pract.* **2018**, *138*, 271–281. [CrossRef]
12. Gray, S.P.; Jandeleit-Dahm, K. The pathobiology of diabetic vascular complications—Cardiovascular and kidney disease. *J. Mol. Med.* **2014**, *92*, 441–452. [CrossRef]
13. Wong, E.; Backholer, K.; Gearon, E.; Harding, J.; Freak-Poli, R.; Stevenson, C.; Peeters, A. Diabetes and risk of physical disability in adults: A systematic review and meta-analysis. *Lancet Diabetes Endocrinol.* **2013**, *1*, 106–114. [CrossRef]
14. Heinonen, S.E.; Genové, G.; Bengtsson, E.; Hübschle, T.; Åkesson, L.; Hiss, K.; Benardeau, A.; Ylä-Herttuala, S.; Jönsson-Rylander, A.-C.; Gomez, M.F. Animal models of diabetic macrovascular complications: Key players in the development of new therapeutic approaches. *J. Diabetes Res.* **2015**, *2015*, 404085. [CrossRef]
15. Zhang, P.; Li, T.; Wu, X.; Nice, E.C.; Huang, C.; Zhang, Y. Oxidative stress and diabetes: Antioxidative strategies. *Front. Med.* **2020**. [CrossRef] [PubMed]
16. Yaribeygi, H.; Sathyapalan, T.; Atkin, S.L.; Sahebkar, A. Molecular mechanisms linking oxidative stress and diabetes mellitus. *Oxid. Med. Cell. Longev.* **2020**, *2020*, 8609213. [CrossRef] [PubMed]
17. Li, C.; Schluesener, H. Health-promoting effects of the citrus flavanone hesperidin. *Crit. Rev. Food Sci. Nutr.* **2017**, *57*, 613–631. [CrossRef] [PubMed]
18. Millar, C.L.; Duclos, Q.; Blesso, C.N. Effects of dietary flavonoids on reverse cholesterol transport, HDL metabolism, and HDL function. *Adv. Nutr.* **2017**, *8*, 226–239. [CrossRef] [PubMed]
19. Rees, A.; Dodd, G.F.; Spencer, J.P.E. The effects of flavonoids on cardiovascular health: A review of human intervention trials and implications for cerebrovascular function. *Nutrients* **2018**, *10*, 1852. [CrossRef]
20. Zaidun, N.H.; Thent, Z.C.; Latiff, A.A. Combating oxidative stress disorders with citrus flavonoid: Naringenin. *Life Sci.* **2018**, *208*, 111–122. [CrossRef]
21. Zhang, X.; Li, X.; Fang, H.; Guo, F.; Li, F.; Chen, A.; Huang, S. Flavonoids as inducers of white adipose tissue browning and thermogenesis: Signalling pathways and molecular triggers. *Nutr. Metab.* **2019**, *16*, 47. [CrossRef]
22. Kopustinskiene, D.M.; Jakstas, V.; Savickas, A.; Bernatoniene, J. Flavonoids as anticancer agents. *Nutrients* **2020**, *12*, 457. [CrossRef]
23. Moher, D.; Liberati, A.; Tetzlaff, J.; Altman, D.G. Preferred reporting items for systematic reviews and meta-analyses: The PRISMA statement. *PLoS Med.* **2009**, *6*, e1000097. [CrossRef]
24. Żołnierczyk, A.K.; Mączka, W.K.; Grabarczyk, M.; Wińska, K.; Woźniak, E.; Anioł, M. Isoxanthohumol—Biologically active hop flavonoid. *Fitoterapia* **2015**, *103*, 71–82. [CrossRef]
25. Štulíková, K.; Karabín, M.; Nešpor, J.; Dostálek, P. Therapeutic perspectives of 8-prenylnaringenin, a potent phytoestrogen from hops. *Molecules* **2018**, *23*, 660. [CrossRef] [PubMed]
26. Negrão, R.; Costa, R.; Duarte, D.; Taveira Gomes, T.; Mendanha, M.; Moura, L.; Vasques, L.; Azevedo, I.; Soares, R. Angiogenesis and inflammation signaling are targets of beer polyphenols on vascular cells. *J. Cell. Biochem.* **2010**, *111*, 1270–1279. [CrossRef] [PubMed]
27. Luís, C.; Costa, R.; Rodrigues, I.; Castela, Â.; Coelho, P.; Guerreiro, S.; Gomes, J.; Reis, C.; Soares, R. Xanthohumol and 8-prenylnaringenin reduce type 2 diabetes-associated oxidative stress by downregulating galectin-3. *Porto Biomed. J.* **2018**, *4*, e23. [CrossRef] [PubMed]
28. Petrie, J.R.; Guzik, T.J.; Touyz, R.M. Diabetes, hypertension and cardiovascular disease: Clinical insights and vascular mechanisms. *Can. J. Cardiol.* **2018**, *34*, 575–584. [CrossRef]
29. Munhoz, A.C.M.; Frode, T.S. Isolated compounds from natural products with potential antidiabetic activity—A systematic review. *Curr. Diabetes Rev.* **2018**, *14*, 36–106. [CrossRef] [PubMed]

30. Rao, Y.K.; Lee, M.J.; Chen, K.; Lee, Y.C.; Wu, W.S.; Tzeng, Y.M. Insulin-mimetic action of rhoifolin and cosmosiin isolated from *Citrus grandis* (L.) Osbeck leaves: Enhanced adiponectin secretion and insulin receptor phosphorylation in 3T3-L1 cells. *Evid. Based Complement. Alternat. Med.* **2011**, *2011*, 624375. [CrossRef]
31. Shalkami, A.S.; Hassan, M.; Bakr, A.G. Anti-inflammatory, antioxidant and anti-apoptotic activity of diosmin in acetic acid-induced ulcerative colitis. *Hum. Exp. Toxicol.* **2018**, *37*, 78–86. [CrossRef]
32. Bogucka-Kocka, A.; Woźniak, M.; Feldo, M.; Kocki, J.; Szewczyk, K. Diosmin—Isolation techniques, determination in plant material and pharmaceutical formulations, and clinical use. *Nat. Prod. Commun.* **2013**, *8*, 1934578X1300800435. [CrossRef]
33. Srinivasan, S.; Pari, L. Antihyperlipidemic effect of diosmin: A citrus flavonoid on lipid metabolism in experimental diabetic rats. *J. Funct. Foods* **2013**, *5*, 484–492. [CrossRef]
34. Jain, D.; Bansal, M.K.; Dalvi, R.; Upganlawar, A.; Somani, R. Protective effect of diosmin against diabetic neuropathy in experimental rats. *J. Integr. Med.* **2014**, *12*, 35–41. [CrossRef]
35. Hsu, C.C.; Lin, M.H.; Cheng, J.T.; Wu, M.C. Diosmin, a citrus nutrient, activates imidazoline receptors to alleviate blood glucose and lipids in type 1-like diabetic rats. *Nutrients* **2017**, *9*, 684. [CrossRef]
36. Huang, H.; Li, L.; Shi, W.; Liu, H.; Yang, J.; Yuan, X.; Wu, L. The multifunctional effects of nobiletin and its metabolites in vivo and in vitro. *Evid. Based Complement. Alternat. Med.* **2016**, *2016*, 2918796. [CrossRef] [PubMed]
37. Lee, Y.-S.; Cha, B.-Y.; Choi, S.-S.; Choi, B.-K.; Yonezawa, T.; Teruya, T.; Nagai, K.; Woo, J.-T. Nobiletin improves obesity and insulin resistance in high-fat diet-induced obese mice. *J. Nutr. Biochem.* **2013**, *24*, 156–162. [CrossRef] [PubMed]
38. Wang, Y.; Xie, J.; Ai, Z.; Su, J. Nobiletin-loaded micelles reduce ovariectomy-induced bone loss by suppressing osteoclastogenesis. *Int. J. Nanomed.* **2019**, *14*, 7839–7849. [CrossRef]
39. Goh, J.X.H.; Tan, L.T.; Goh, J.K.; Chan, K.G.; Pusparajah, P.; Lee, L.H.; Goh, B.H. Nobiletin and derivatives: Functional compounds from citrus fruit peel for colon cancer chemoprevention. *Cancers* **2019**, *11*, 867. [CrossRef]
40. Nohara, K.; Nemkov, T.; D'Alessandro, A.; Yoo, S.H.; Chen, Z. Coordinate regulation of cholesterol and bile acid metabolism by the clock modifier nobiletin in metabolically challenged old mice. *Int. J. Mol. Sci.* **2019**, *20*, 4281. [CrossRef] [PubMed]
41. Mulvihill, E.E.; Assini, J.M.; Lee, J.K.; Allister, E.M.; Sutherland, B.G.; Koppes, J.B.; Sawyez, C.G.; Edwards, J.Y.; Telford, D.E.; Charbonneau, A.; et al. Nobiletin attenuates VLDL overproduction, dyslipidemia, and atherosclerosis in mice with diet-induced insulin resistance. *Diabetes* **2011**, *60*, 1446–1457. [CrossRef] [PubMed]
42. Onda, K.; Horike, N.; Suzuki, T.; Hirano, T. Polymethoxyflavonoids tangeretin and nobiletin increase glucose uptake in murine adipocytes. *Phytother. Res.* **2013**, *27*, 312–316. [CrossRef]
43. Kanda, K.; Nishi, K.; Kadota, A.; Nishimoto, S.; Liu, M.C.; Sugahara, T. Nobiletin suppresses adipocyte differentiation of 3T3-L1 cells by an insulin and IBMX mixture induction. *Biochim. Biophys. Acta* **2012**, *1820*, 461–468. [CrossRef]
44. Parkar, N.A.; Bhatt, L.K.; Addepalli, V. Efficacy of nobiletin, a citrus flavonoid, in the treatment of the cardiovascular dysfunction of diabetes in rats. *Food Funct.* **2016**, *7*, 3121–3129. [CrossRef]
45. Zhang, N.; Yang, Z.; Xiang, S.Z.; Jin, Y.G.; Wei, W.Y.; Bian, Z.Y.; Deng, W.; Tang, Q.Z. Nobiletin attenuates cardiac dysfunction, oxidative stress, and inflammatory in streptozotocin: Induced diabetic cardiomyopathy. *Mol. Cell. Biochem.* **2016**, *417*, 87–96. [CrossRef] [PubMed]
46. Morrow, N.M.; Burke, A.C.; Samsoondar, J.P.; Seigel, K.E.; Wang, A.; Telford, D.E.; Sutherland, B.G.; O'Dwyer, C.; Steinberg, G.R.; Fullerton, M.D.; et al. The citrus flavonoid nobiletin confers protection from metabolic dysregulation in high-fat-fed mice independent of AMPK. *J. Lipid Res.* **2020**, *61*, 387–402. [CrossRef] [PubMed]
47. Refaat, J.; Desoukey, S.Y.; Ramadan, M.A.; Kamel, M.S. Rhoifolin: A review of sources and biological activities. *Int. J. Pharmacogn.* **2015**, *2*, 102–109. [CrossRef]
48. Liao, S.; Song, F.; Feng, W.; Ding, X.; Yao, J.; Song, H.; Liu, Y.; Ma, S.; Wang, Z.; Lin, X.; et al. Rhoifolin ameliorates titanium particle-stimulated osteolysis and attenuates osteoclastogenesis via RANKL-induced NF-κB and MAPK pathways. *J. Cell. Physiol.* **2019**, *234*, 17600–17611. [CrossRef] [PubMed]

49. Phan, V.K.; Nguyen, T.M.; Minh, C.V.; Nguyen, H.K.; Nguyen, H.D.; Nguyen, P.T.; Nguyen, X.C.; Nguyen, H.N.; Nguyen, X.N.; Heyden, Y.V.; et al. Two new C-glucosyl benzoic acids and flavonoids from Mallotus nanus and their antioxidant activity. *Arch. Pharm. Res.* **2010**, *33*, 203–208. [CrossRef] [PubMed]
50. Cheng, L.; Ren, Y.; Lin, D.; Peng, S.; Zhong, B.; Ma, Z. The anti-inflammatory properties of Citrus *wilsonii tanaka* extract in LPS-induced RAW 264.7 and primary mouse bone marrow-derived dendritic cells. *Molecules* **2017**, *22*, 1213. [CrossRef]
51. Sultana, B.; Yaqoob, S.; Zafar, Z.; Bhatti, H.N. Escalation of liver malfunctioning: A step toward Herbal Awareness. *J. Ethnopharmacol.* **2018**, *216*, 104–119. [CrossRef]
52. Koyuncu, I. Evaluation of anticancer, antioxidant activity and phenolic compounds of *Artemisia absinthium* L. Extract. *Cell. Mol. Biol.* **2018**, *64*, 25–34. [CrossRef]
53. Kim, G.S.; Park, H.J.; Woo, J.H.; Kim, M.K.; Koh, P.O.; Min, W.; Ko, Y.G.; Kim, C.H.; Won, C.K.; Cho, J.H. *Citrus aurantium* flavonoids inhibit adipogenesis through the Akt signaling pathway in 3T3-L1 cells. *BMC Complement. Altern. Med.* **2012**, *12*, 31. [CrossRef]
54. Tsutsumi, R.; Yoshida, T.; Nii, Y.; Okahisa, N.; Iwata, S.; Tsukayama, M.; Hashimoto, R.; Taniguchi, Y.; Sakaue, H.; Hosaka, T.; et al. Sudachitin, a polymethoxylated flavone, improves glucose and lipid metabolism by increasing mitochondrial biogenesis in skeletal muscle. *Nutr. Metab.* **2014**, *11*, 32. [CrossRef]
55. Yoshida, H.; Watanabe, H.; Ishida, A.; Watanabe, W.; Narumi, K.; Atsumi, T.; Sugita, C.; Kurokawa, M. Naringenin suppresses macrophage infiltration into adipose tissue in an early phase of high-fat diet-induced obesity. *Biochem. Biophys. Res. Commun.* **2014**, *454*, 95–101. [CrossRef] [PubMed]
56. Mahmoud, A.M.; Ahmed, O.M.; Ashour, M.B.; Abdel-Moneim, A. In vivo and in vitro antidiabetic effects of citrus flavonoids; a study on the mechanism of action. *Int. J. Diabetes Dev. Ctries.* **2015**, *35*, 250–263. [CrossRef]
57. Dhanya, R.; Arya, A.D.; Nisha, P.; Jayamurthy, P. Quercetin, a lead compound against type 2 diabetes ameliorates glucose uptake via AMPK pathway in skeletal muscle cell line. *Front. Pharmacol.* **2017**, *8*, 336. [CrossRef]
58. Liu, W.; Liou, S.S.; Hong, T.Y.; Liu, I.M. Protective effects of hesperidin (citrus flavonone) on high glucose induced oxidative stress and apoptosis in a cellular model for diabetic retinopathy. *Nutrients* **2017**, *9*, 1323. [CrossRef] [PubMed]
59. Zareei, S.; Boojar, M.M.A.; Amanlou, M. Inhibition of liver alanine aminotransferase and aspartate aminotransferase by hesperidin and its aglycone hesperetin: An in vitro and in silico study. *Life Sci.* **2017**, *178*, 49–55. [CrossRef]
60. Chen, F.; Ma, Y.; Sun, Z.; Zhu, X. Tangeretin inhibits high glucose-induced extracellular matrix accumulation in human glomerular mesangial cells. *Biomed. Pharmacother.* **2018**, *102*, 1077–1083. [CrossRef]
61. Shukla, K.; Sonowal, H.; Saxena, A.; Ramana, K.V. Didymin prevents hyperglycemia-induced human umbilical endothelial cells dysfunction and death. *Biochem. Pharmacol.* **2018**, *152*, 1–10. [CrossRef]
62. Ali, M.Y.; Zaib, S.; Rahman, M.M.; Jannat, S.; Iqbal, J.; Park, S.K.; Chang, M.S. Didymin, a dietary citrus flavonoid exhibits anti-diabetic complications and promotes glucose uptake through the activation of PI3K/Akt signaling pathway in insulin-resistant HepG2 cells. *Chem. Biol. Interact.* **2019**, *305*, 180–194. [CrossRef]
63. Tseng, Y.-T.; Hsu, H.-T.; Lee, T.-Y.; Chang, W.-H.; Lo, Y.-C. Naringenin, a dietary flavanone, enhances insulin-like growth factor 1 receptor-mediated antioxidant defense and attenuates methylglyoxal-induced neurite damage and apoptotic death. *Nutr. Neurosci.* **2019**, 1–11. [CrossRef]
64. Tsuhako, R.; Yoshida, H.; Sugita, C.; Kurokawa, M. Naringenin suppresses neutrophil infiltration into adipose tissue in high-fat diet-induced obese mice. *J. Nat. Med.* **2019**, *74*, 229–237. [CrossRef] [PubMed]
65. Nakagawa, H.; Takaishi, Y.; Tanaka, N.; Tsuchiya, K.; Shibata, H.; Higuti, T. Chemical constituents from the peels of *Citrus sudachi*. *J. Nat. Prod.* **2006**, *69*, 1177–1179. [CrossRef] [PubMed]
66. Ohyama, Y.; Ito, J.; Kitano, V.J.; Shimada, J.; Hakeda, Y. The polymethoxy flavonoid sudachitin suppresses inflammatory bone destruction by directly inhibiting osteoclastogenesis due to reduced ROS production and MAPK activation in osteoclast precursors. *PLoS ONE* **2018**, *13*, e0191192. [CrossRef] [PubMed]
67. Abe, S.; Hirose, S.; Nishitani, M.; Yoshida, I.; Tsukayama, M.; Tsuji, A.; Yuasa, K. Citrus peel polymethoxyflavones, sudachitin and nobiletin, induce distinct cellular responses in human keratinocyte HaCaT cells. *Biosci. Biotechnol. Biochem.* **2018**, *82*, 2064–2071. [CrossRef]

68. Mitani, M.; Minatogawa, Y.; Nakamoto, A.; Nakamoto, M.; Shuto, E.; Nii, Y.; Sakai, T. Sudachitin, polymethoxyflavone from *Citrus sudachi*, enhances antigen-specific cellular and humoral immune responses in BALB/c mice. *J. Clin. Biochem. Nutr.* **2019**, *64*, 158–163. [CrossRef] [PubMed]
69. Hosokawa, Y.; Hosokawa, I.; Ozaki, K.; Matsuo, T. Sudachitin inhibits matrix metalloproteinase-1 and -3 production in tumor necrosis factor-α-stimulated human periodontal ligament cells. *Inflammation* **2019**, *42*, 1456–1462. [CrossRef]
70. Ashrafizadeh, M.; Ahmadi, Z.; Mohammadinejad, R.; Afshar, E.G. Tangeretin: A mechanistic review of its pharmacological and therapeutic effects. *J. Basic Clin. Physiol. Pharmacol.* **2020**, *31*, 20190191. [CrossRef]
71. Sundaram, R.; Shanthi, P.; Sachdanandam, P. Effect of tangeretin, a polymethoxylated flavone on glucose metabolism in streptozotocin-induced diabetic rats. *Phytomedicine* **2014**, *21*, 793–799. [CrossRef]
72. Sundaram, R.; Shanthi, P.; Sachdanandam, P. Tangeretin, a polymethoxylated flavone, modulates lipid homeostasis and decreases oxidative stress by inhibiting NF-κB activation and proinflammatory cytokines in cardiac tissue of streptozotocin-induced diabetic rats. *J. Funct. Foods* **2015**, *16*, 315–333. [CrossRef]
73. Yao, Q.; Lin, M.T.; Zhu, Y.D.; Xu, H.L.; Zhao, Y.Z. Recent trends in potential therapeutic applications of the dietary flavonoid didymin. *Molecules* **2018**, *23*, 2547. [CrossRef]
74. Hung, J.Y.; Hsu, Y.L.; Ko, Y.C.; Tsai, Y.M.; Yang, C.J.; Huang, M.S.; Kuo, P.L. Didymin, a dietary flavonoid glycoside from citrus fruits, induces Fas-mediated apoptotic pathway in human non-small-cell lung cancer cells in vitro and in vivo. *Lung Cancer* **2010**, *68*, 366–374. [CrossRef]
75. Singhal, J.; Nagaprashantha, L.D.; Vatsyayan, R.; Awasthi, S.; Singhal, S.S. Didymin induces apoptosis by inhibiting N-Myc and upregulating RKIP in neuroblastoma. *Cancer Prev. Res.* **2012**, *5*, 473–483. [CrossRef] [PubMed]
76. Wei, J.; Huang, Q.; Bai, F.; Lin, J.; Nie, J.; Lu, S.; Lu, C.; Huang, R.; Lu, Z.; Lin, X. Didymin induces apoptosis through mitochondrial dysfunction and up-regulation of RKIP in human hepatoma cells. *Chem. Biol. Interact.* **2017**, *261*, 118–126. [CrossRef] [PubMed]
77. Peterson, J.J.; Beecher, G.R.; Bhagwat, S.A.; Dwyer, J.T.; Gebhardt, S.E.; Haytowitz, D.B.; Holden, J.M. Flavanones in grapefruit, lemons, and limes: A compilation and review of the data from the analytical literature. *J. Food Compos. Anal.* **2006**, *19*, S74–S80. [CrossRef]
78. Rangel-Huerta, O.D.; Aguilera, C.M.; Martin, M.V.; Soto, M.J.; Rico, M.C.; Vallejo, F.; Tomas-Barberan, F.; Perez-de-la-Cruz, A.J.; Gil, A.; Mesa, M.D. Normal or high polyphenol concentration in orange juice affects antioxidant activity, blood pressure, and body weight in obese or overweight adults. *J. Nutr.* **2015**, *145*, 1808–1816. [CrossRef]
79. Nandakumar, N.; Balasubramanian, M.P. Hesperidin a citrus bioflavonoid modulates hepatic biotransformation enzymes and enhances intrinsic antioxidants in experimental breast cancer rats challenged with 7, 12-dimethylbenz (a) anthracene. *J. Exp. Ther. Oncol.* **2012**, *9*, 321–335.
80. Mahmoud, A.M.; Mohammed, H.M.; Khadrawy, S.M.; Galaly, S.R. Hesperidin protects against chemically induced hepatocarcinogenesis via modulation of Nrf2/ARE/HO-1, PPARγ and TGF-β1/Smad3 signaling, and amelioration of oxidative stress and inflammation. *Chem. Biol. Interact.* **2017**, *277*, 146–158. [CrossRef]
81. Carballo-Villalobos, A.I.; González-Trujano, M.E.; Alvarado-Vázquez, N.; López-Muñoz, F.J. Pro-inflammatory cytokines involvement in the hesperidin antihyperalgesic effects at peripheral and central levels in a neuropathic pain model. *Inflammopharmacology* **2017**, *25*, 265–269. [CrossRef]
82. Akiyama, S.; Katsumata, S.; Suzuki, K.; Ishimi, Y.; Wu, J.; Uehara, M. Dietary hesperidin exerts hypoglycemic and hypolipidemic effects in streptozotocin-induced marginal type 1 diabetic rats. *J. Clin. Biochem. Nutr.* **2010**, *46*, 87–92. [CrossRef]
83. Mahmoud, A.M.; Ashour, M.B.; Abdel-Moneim, A.; Ahmed, O.M. Hesperidin and naringin attenuate hyperglycemia-mediated oxidative stress and proinflammatory cytokine production in high fat fed/streptozotocin-induced type 2 diabetic rats. *J. Diabetes Complicat.* **2012**, *26*, 483–490. [CrossRef]
84. El-Marasy, S.A.; Abdallah, H.M.; El-Shenawy, S.M.; El-Khatib, A.S.; El-Shabrawy, O.A.; Kenawy, S.A. Anti-depressant effect of hesperidin in diabetic rats. *Can. J. Physiol. Pharmacol.* **2014**, *92*, 945–952. [CrossRef]
85. Visnagri, A.; Kandhare, A.D.; Chakravarty, S.; Ghosh, P.; Bodhankar, S.L. Hesperidin, a flavanoglycone attenuates experimental diabetic neuropathy via modulation of cellular and biochemical marker to improve nerve functions. *Pharm. Biol.* **2014**, *52*, 814–828. [CrossRef] [PubMed]

86. Li, W.; Kandhare, A.D.; Mukherjee, A.A.; Bodhankar, S.L. Hesperidin, a plant flavonoid accelerated the cutaneous wound healing in streptozotocin-induced diabetic rats: Role of TGF-ß/Smads and Ang-1/Tie-2 signaling pathways. *EXCLI J.* **2018**, *17*, 399–419. [CrossRef] [PubMed]
87. Dokumacioglu, E.; Iskender, H.; Sen, T.M.; Ince, I.; Dokumacioglu, A.; Kanbay, Y.; Erbas, E.; Saral, S. The effects of hesperidin and quercetin on serum tumor necrosis factor-alpha and interleukin-6 levels in streptozotocin-induced diabetes model. *Pharmacogn. Mag.* **2018**, *14*, 167–173. [CrossRef] [PubMed]
88. Tilg, H.; Hotamisligil, G.S. Nonalcoholic fatty liver disease: Cytokine-adipokine interplay and regulation of insulin resistance. *Gastroenterology* **2006**, *131*, 934–945. [CrossRef] [PubMed]
89. Mehta, S.; Farmer, J.A. Obesity and inflammation: A new look at an old problem. *Curr. Atheroscler. Rep.* **2007**, *9*, 134–138. [CrossRef]
90. Somerset, S.M.; Johannot, L. Dietary flavonoid sources in Australian adults. *Nutr. Cancer* **2008**, *60*, 442–449. [CrossRef]
91. Furtado, A.F.; Nunes, M.A.; Ribeiro, M.H. Hesperidinase encapsulation towards hesperitin production targeting improved bioavailability. *J. Mol. Recognit.* **2012**, *25*, 595–603. [CrossRef]
92. Paramita, P.; Sethu, S.N.; Subhapradha, N.; Ragavan, V.; Ilangovan, R.; Balakrishnan, A.; Srinivasan, N.; Murugesan, R.; Moorthi, A. Neuro-protective effects of nano-formulated hesperetin in a traumatic brain injury model of *Danio rerio*. *Drug Chem. Toxicol.* **2020**, 1–8. [CrossRef]
93. Kottaiswamy, A.; Kizhakeyil, A.; Padmanaban, A.; Bushra, F.; Vijay, V.R.; Lee, P.S.; Verma, N.K.; Kalaiselvan, P.; Samuel, S. The citrus flavanone hesperetin induces apoptosis in CTCL cells via STAT3/Notch1/NFκB-mediated signaling axis. *Anticancer Agents Med. Chem.* **2020**. [CrossRef]
94. Jo, S.H.; Kim, M.E.; Cho, J.H.; Lee, Y.; Lee, J.; Park, Y.D.; Lee, J.S. Hesperetin inhibits neuroinflammation on microglia by suppressing inflammatory cytokines and MAPK pathways. *Arch. Pharm. Res.* **2019**, *42*, 695–703. [CrossRef]
95. Kim, W.J.; Lee, S.E.; Park, Y.G.; Jeong, S.G.; Kim, E.Y.; Park, S.P. Antioxidant hesperetin improves the quality of porcine oocytes during aging *in vitro*. *Mol. Reprod. Dev.* **2019**, *86*, 32–41. [CrossRef]
96. Chen, X.; Wei, W.; Li, Y.; Huang, J.; Ci, X. Hesperetin relieves cisplatin-induced acute kidney injury by mitigating oxidative stress, inflammation and apoptosis. *Chem. Biol. Interact.* **2019**, *308*, 269–278. [CrossRef] [PubMed]
97. Jayaraman, R.; Subramani, S.; Sheik Abdullah, S.H.; Udaiyar, M. Antihyperglycemic effect of hesperetin, a citrus flavonoid, extenuates hyperglycemia and exploring the potential role in antioxidant and antihyperlipidemic in streptozotocin-induced diabetic rats. *Biomed. Pharmacother.* **2018**, *97*, 98–106. [CrossRef] [PubMed]
98. Samie, A.; Sedaghat, R.; Baluchnejadmojarad, T.; Roghani, M. Hesperetin, a citrus flavonoid, attenuates testicular damage in diabetic rats via inhibition of oxidative stress, inflammation, and apoptosis. *Life Sci.* **2018**, *210*, 132–139. [CrossRef]
99. Fernandes, A.A.; Novelli, E.L.; Okoshi, K.; Okoshi, M.P.; Di Muzio, B.P.; Guimarães, J.F.; Fernandes Junior, A. Influence of rutin treatment on biochemical alterations in experimental diabetes. *Biomed. Pharmacother.* **2010**, *64*, 214–219. [CrossRef] [PubMed]
100. Fallahi, F.; Roghani, M.; Moghadami, S. Citrus flavonoid naringenin improves aortic reactivity in streptozotocin-diabetic rats. *Indian J. Pharmacol.* **2012**, *44*, 382–386. [CrossRef]
101. Hasanein, P.; Fazeli, F. Role of naringenin in protection against diabetic hyperalgesia and tactile allodynia in male Wistar rats. *J. Physiol. Biochem.* **2014**, *70*, 997–1006. [CrossRef]
102. Jia, S.; Hu, Y.; Zhang, W.; Zhao, X.; Chen, Y.; Sun, C.; Li, X.; Chen, K. Hypoglycemic and hypolipidemic effects of neohesperidin derived from *Citrus aurantium* L. in diabetic KK-A(y) mice. *Food Funct.* **2015**, *6*, 878–886. [CrossRef]
103. Malakul, W.; Pengnet, S.; Kumchoom, C.; Tunsophon, S. Naringin ameliorates endothelial dysfunction in fructose-fed rats. *Exp. Ther. Med.* **2018**, *15*, 3140–3146. [CrossRef]
104. Alam, M.A.; Subhan, N.; Rahman, M.M.; Uddin, S.J.; Reza, H.M.; Sarker, S.D. Effect of citrus flavonoids, naringin and naringenin, on metabolic syndrome and their mechanisms of action. *Adv. Nutr.* **2014**, *5*, 404–417. [CrossRef]
105. Chen, R.; Qi, Q.L.; Wang, M.T.; Li, Q.Y. Therapeutic potential of naringin: An overview. *Pharm. Biol.* **2016**, *54*, 3203–3210. [CrossRef] [PubMed]

106. Kandhare, A.D.; Raygude, K.S.; Ghosh, P.; Ghule, A.E.; Bodhankar, S.L. Neuroprotective effect of naringin by modulation of endogenous biomarkers in streptozotocin induced painful diabetic neuropathy. *Fitoterapia* **2012**, *83*, 650–659. [CrossRef] [PubMed]
107. Ahmad, S.F.; Attia, S.M.; Bakheet, S.A.; Zoheir, K.M.A.; Ansari, M.A.; Korashy, H.M.; Abdel-Hamied, H.E.; Ashour, A.E.; Abd-Allah, A.R.A. Naringin attenuates the development of carrageenan-induced acute lung inflammation through inhibition of NF-κb, STAT3 and pro-inflammatory mediators and enhancement of IκBα and anti-inflammatory cytokines. *Inflammation* **2015**, *38*, 846–857. [CrossRef] [PubMed]
108. Jiao, H.Y.; Su, W.W.; Li, P.B.; Liao, Y.; Zhou, Q.; Zhu, N.; He, L. Therapeutic effects of naringin in a guinea pig model of ovalbumin-induced cough-variant asthma. *Pulm. Pharmacol. Ther.* **2015**, *33*, 59–65. [CrossRef]
109. Xiong, G.; Liu, S.; Gao, J.; Wang, S. Naringin protects ovalbumin-induced airway inflammation in a mouse model of asthma. *Inflammation* **2016**, *39*, 891–899. [CrossRef]
110. Zhang, Y.S.; Li, Y.; Wang, Y.; Sun, S.Y.; Jiang, T.; Li, C.; Cui, S.X.; Qu, X.J. Naringin, a natural dietary compound, prevents intestinal tumorigenesis in Apc (Min/+) mouse model. *J. Cancer Res. Clin. Oncol.* **2016**, *142*, 913–925. [CrossRef]
111. Kwatra, M.; Jangra, A.; Mishra, M.; Sharma, Y.; Ahmed, S.; Ghosh, P.; Kumar, V.; Vohora, D.; Khanam, R. Naringin and sertraline ameliorate doxorubicin-induced behavioral deficits through modulation of serotonin level and mitochondrial complexes protection pathway in rat hippocampus. *Neurochem. Res.* **2016**, *41*, 2352–2366. [CrossRef]
112. Sachdeva, A.K.; Kuhad, A.; Chopra, K. Naringin ameliorates memory deficits in experimental paradigm of Alzheimer's disease by attenuating mitochondrial dysfunction. *Pharmacol. Biochem. Behav.* **2014**, *127*, 101–110. [CrossRef] [PubMed]
113. Vij, G.; Gupta, A.; Chopra, K. Modulation of antigen-induced chronic fatigue in mouse model of water immersion stress by naringin, a polyphenolic antioxidant. *Fundam. Clin. Pharmacol.* **2009**, *23*, 331–337. [CrossRef]
114. Chtourou, Y.; Aouey, B.; Kebieche, M.; Fetoui, H. Protective role of naringin against cisplatin induced oxidative stress, inflammatory response and apoptosis in rat striatum via suppressing ROS-mediated NF-κB and P53 signaling pathways. *Chem. Biol. Interact.* **2015**, *239*, 76–86. [CrossRef]
115. Zhang, J.; Sun, C.; Yan, Y.; Chen, Q.; Luo, F.; Zhu, X.; Li, X.; Chen, K. Purification of naringin and neohesperidin from Huyou (*Citrus* changshanensis) fruit and their effects on glucose consumption in human HepG2 cells. *Food Chem.* **2012**, *135*, 1471–1478. [CrossRef] [PubMed]
116. Gong, N.; Zhang, B.; Yang, D.; Gao, Z.; Du, G.; Lu, Y. Development of new reference material neohesperidin for quality control of dietary supplements. *J. Sci. Food Agric.* **2015**, *95*, 1885–1891. [CrossRef] [PubMed]
117. Hwang, S.-L.; Yen, G.-C. Neuroprotective effects of the citrus flavanones against H2 O2 -induced cytotoxicity in PC12 cells. *J. Agric. Food Chem.* **2008**, *56*, 859–864. [CrossRef] [PubMed]
118. Bellocco, E.; Barreca, D.; Laganà, G.; Leuzzi, U.; Tellone, E.; Ficarra, S.; Kotyk, A.; Galtieri, A. Influence of l-rhamnosyl-d-glucosyl derivatives on properties and biological interaction of flavonoids. *Mol. Cell. Biochem.* **2009**, *321*, 165–171. [CrossRef]
119. Zhao, T.; Hu, S.; Ma, P.; Che, D.; Liu, R.; Zhang, Y.; Wang, J.; Li, C.; Ding, Y.; Fu, J.; et al. Neohesperidin suppresses IgE-mediated anaphylactic reactions and mast cell activation via Lyn-PLC-Ca$^{(2+)}$ pathway. *Phytother. Res.* **2019**, *33*, 2034–2043. [CrossRef] [PubMed]
120. Guo, J.; Fang, Y.; Jiang, F.; Li, L.; Zhou, H.; Xu, X.; Ning, W. Neohesperidin inhibits TGF-β1/Smad3 signaling and alleviates bleomycin-induced pulmonary fibrosis in mice. *Eur. J. Pharmacol.* **2019**, *864*, 172712. [CrossRef]
121. Tan, Z.; Cheng, J.; Liu, Q.; Zhou, L.; Kenny, J.; Wang, T.; Lin, X.; Yuan, J.; Quinn, J.M.W.; Tickner, J.; et al. Neohesperidin suppresses osteoclast differentiation, bone resorption and ovariectomised-induced osteoporosis in mice. *Mol. Cell. Endocrinol.* **2017**, *439*, 369–378. [CrossRef]
122. Jiang, C.H.; Sun, T.L.; Xiang, D.X.; Wei, S.S.; Li, W.Q. Anticancer activity and mechanism of xanthohumol: A prenylated flavonoid from hops (*Humulus lupulus* L.). *Front. Pharmacol.* **2018**, *9*, 530. [CrossRef]
123. Li, F.; Yao, Y.; Huang, H.; Hao, H.; Ying, M. Xanthohumol attenuates cisplatin-induced nephrotoxicity through inhibiting NF-κB and activating Nrf2 signaling pathways. *Int. Immunopharmacol.* **2018**, *61*, 277–282. [CrossRef]
124. Wang, S.; Yang, C.; Tu, H.; Zhou, J.; Liu, X.; Cheng, Y.; Luo, J.; Deng, X.; Zhang, H.; Xu, J. Characterization and metabolic diversity of flavonoids in *Citrus* species. *Sci. Rep.* **2017**, *7*, 10549. [CrossRef]

125. Sharma, A.; Sharma, P.; Singh Tuli, H.; Sharma, A.K. Phytochemical and Pharmacological Properties of Flavonols. In *eLS*; John Wiley & Sons: Chichester, UK, 2018; pp. 1–12. [CrossRef]
126. Gautam, R.; Singh, M.; Gautam, S.; Rawat, J.K.; Saraf, S.A.; Kaithwas, G. Rutin attenuates intestinal toxicity induced by Methotrexate linked with anti-oxidative and anti-inflammatory effects. *BMC Complement. Altern. Med.* **2016**, *16*, 99. [CrossRef] [PubMed]
127. Klimczak, I.; Małecka, M.; Szlachta, M.; Gliszczyńska-Świgło, A. Effect of storage on the content of polyphenols, vitamin C and the antioxidant activity of orange juices. *J. Food Compos. Anal.* **2007**, *20*, 313–322. [CrossRef]
128. Stuetz, W.; Prapamontol, T.; Hongsibsong, S.; Biesalski, H. Polymethoxylated flavones, flavanone glycosides, carotenoids, and antioxidants in different cultivation types of tangerines (*Citrus reticulata* Blanco cv. Sainampueng) from Northern Thailand. *J. Agric. Food Chem.* **2010**, *58*, 6069–6074. [CrossRef] [PubMed]
129. Ramful, D.; Bahorun, T.; Bourdon, E.; Tarnus, E.; Aruoma, O.I. Bioactive phenolics and antioxidant propensity of flavedo extracts of Mauritian citrus fruits: Potential prophylactic ingredients for functional foods application. *Toxicology* **2010**, *278*, 75–87. [CrossRef] [PubMed]
130. Gattuso, G.; Barreca, D.; Gargiulli, C.; Leuzzi, U.; Caristi, C. Flavonoid composition of citrus juices. *Molecules* **2007**, *12*, 1641–1673. [CrossRef]

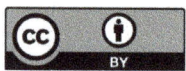

© 2020 by the authors. Licensee MDPI, Basel, Switzerland. This article is an open access article distributed under the terms and conditions of the Creative Commons Attribution (CC BY) license (http://creativecommons.org/licenses/by/4.0/).

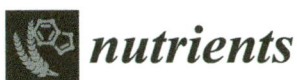

Article

Inula britannica Inhibits Adipogenesis of 3T3-L1 Preadipocytes via Modulation of Mitotic Clonal Expansion Involving ERK 1/2 and Akt Signaling Pathways

Hyung-Seok Yu, Won-Ju Kim, Won-Young Bae, Na-Kyoung Lee and Hyun-Dong Paik *

Department of Food Science and Biotechnology of Animal Resources, Konkuk University, Seoul 05029, Korea; hyungseok_yu@naver.com (H.-S.Y.); jootopaz22@naver.com (W.-J.K.); won5483101@naver.com (W.-Y.B.); lnk11@konkuk.ac.kr (N.-K.L.)
* Correspondence: hdpaik@konkuk.ac.kr; Tel.: +82-2-2049-6011

Received: 1 September 2020; Accepted: 1 October 2020; Published: 3 October 2020

Abstract: The flower of *Inula britannica* contains various phenolic compounds with prophylactic properties. This study aimed to determine the anti-adipogenic effect of an *I. britannica* flower aqueous extract (IAE) and its underlying mechanisms in the 3T3-L1 preadipocytes and to identify the phenolic compounds in the extract. Treatment with IAE inhibited the adipogenesis of 3T3-L1 preadipocytes by showing a dose-dependently suppressed intracellular lipid accumulation and significantly mitigated expression levels of lipogenesis- and adipogenesis-associated biomarkers including transcription factors. IAE exerted an anti-adipogenic effect through the modulation of the early phases of adipogenesis including mitotic clonal expansion (MCE). Treatment with IAE inhibited MCE by arresting the cell cycle at the G0/G1 phase and suppressing the activation of MCE-related transcription factors. Furthermore, IAE inhibited adipogenesis by regulating the extracellular signal-regulated kinase 1/2 and Akt signaling pathways. Protocatechuic acid, chlorogenic acid, kaempferol-3-*O*-glucoside, and 6-methoxyluteolin, which are reported to exhibit anti-adipogenic properties, were detected in IAE. Therefore, modulation of early phases of adipogenesis, especially MCE, is a key mechanism underlying the anti-adipogenic activity of IAE. In summary, the anti-obesity effects of IAE can be attributed to its phenolic compounds, and hence, IAE can be used for the development of anti-obesity products.

Keywords: *Inula britannica*; anti-obesity; adipogenesis; lipogenesis; mitotic clonal expansion; ERK 1/2 signaling pathways; Akt signaling pathways

1. Introduction

Adipose tissue is crucially involved in various biological functions such as energy homeostasis, hormonal regulation, and metabolism by secreting the hormones, growth factors, and adipokines as well as function as an energy reservoir [1,2]. However, a chronic imbalance between the intake and consumption of energy promotes the aberrant growth of adipose tissue accompanying hyperplasia and/or hypertrophy of the adipocytes, consequently resulting in the development of obesity [3]. Obesity is a growing socioeconomic health concern as it is pathologically associated with development of the various degenerative disease such as type-2 diabetes mellitus, hypertension, dyslipidemia, and cardiovascular disease [4]. According to recent reports of the Centers for Disease Control and Prevention, prevalence of obesity in the United States of America has been increased over the past decade and it was estimated that approximately 20% of children and 40% of adults were obese in 2017–2018 [5]. Additionally, the increasing prevalence of obesity has led to an annual increase in extra medical expenditure for obesity and obesity-associated disorders as a socioeconomic burden [6].

Hence, considerable funds have been invested in the development of therapeutic strategies for obesity. Major strategies to mitigate the disease include decreasing appetite, enhancing energy expenditure, and inhibiting lipogenesis [7].

Adipogenesis, which is a multi-step process of adipocyte formation, involves commitment of pluripotent mesenchymal stem cells into preadipocytes and the differentiation of preadipocytes into mature adipocytes. The 3T3-L1 cell line, which is derived from the murine preadipocyte, is a well-established model for studying adipogenesis and can be differentiated into mature adipocytes under experimental conditions [8,9]. Adipogenesis in the 3T3-L1 preadipocytes comprises an early phase, an intermediate phase, and a terminal phase of differentiation. During adipogenesis, the preadipocytes are first growth-arrested, thereafter treated with hormonal inducers to initiate the early phases of differentiation, which includes synchronous re-entry into the cell cycle and mitotic clonal expansion (MCE). Subsequently, the cell cycle is terminated to undergo terminal phases of differentiation, which is associated with sequential changes in gene expression [10–12]. The MCE is a prerequisite for the differentiation of 3T3-L1 preadipocytes, underscoring the correlation between the cell cycle regulation and the differentiation in this adipogenesis model system [13,14]. Additionally, the activation of extracellular signal-regulated kinase (ERK) 1/2 and Akt signaling cascades is responsible for the MCE, as these signaling pathways mediate cell survival and cell cycle progression, consequently promoting adipogenesis [15,16].

Adipogenesis is modulated by multiple transcription factors such as signal transducer and activator of transcription-3 (STAT3), CCAAT/enhancer-binding proteins (C/EBPs), and peroxisome proliferator-activator receptor (PPAR)-γ [17]. During the early phase of differentiation, STAT3 and C/EBP-β are expressed in response to hormonal stimulation, continuously acquiring the DNA-binding activity to undergo MCE, and finally triggering the activation of C/EBP-α and PPAR-γ, the major transcription factors in terminal differentiation. The activation of C/EBP-α and PPAR-γ leads to the termination of MCE and modulation of the expression of genes involved in the differentiated phenotype [18]. In the adipocytes, de novo lipogenesis is markedly increased during terminal differentiation due to the upregulated expression of triacylglycerol-associated enzymes such as fatty acid-binding protein (FABP) 4, fatty acid synthase (FAS), perilipin, and stearoyl-CoA desaturase (SCD)-1. Particularly, perilipin is involved in the storage of lipids by coating lipid droplets and preventing lipolysis. This results in the accumulation of intracellular lipids, which promotes the expansion of the adipose tissue [7,12,14].

In response to increasing awareness of personal health, dietary polyphenols are garnering interest in the prevention and improvement of various disorders as an alternative medicine based on their biological functionalities [19]. Nutritional, clinical, and epidemiological studies have supported the evidence that appropriate dosage of dietary phenolic compounds improves human health by decreasing the risk and preventing the development of degenerative disorders with reduced adverse effects [20,21]. Medicinal herbs are an abundant source of diverse dietary polyphenols exhibiting prophylactic properties and therapeutic efficacy in various diseases including inflammatory- and obesity-associated disorders [19,22]. *Inula britannica* is a flowering wild plant distributed in eastern Asia and is used for medicinal purposes based on traditional applications. The flower of *I. britannica* exhibits neuroprotective, antimicrobial, anti-tumor, and anti-inflammatory properties [19,23,24], which are potentially attributable to its bio-active compounds such as flavonoids, sesquiterpene lactones, and polysaccharides [25–28]. For example, polysaccharides derived from the flower of *I. britannica* demonstrated hypoglycemic and anti-hyperlipidemic properties in an alloxan-induced diabetic mouse model [29]. However, the effects of *I. britannica* on adipogenesis and the underlying molecular mechanism have not been examined. Therefore, this study aimed to determine the anti-adipogenic effect of aqueous extract of *I. britannica* flower and its underlying mechanisms in the 3T3-L1 preadipocytes and to identify the phenolic compounds in the extract.

2. Materials and Methods

2.1. Chemicals and Reagents

Dulbecco's modified Eagle's medium (DMEM), water, trypsin-EDTA solution, phosphate-buffered saline (PBS), and antibiotics solution (penicillin, 10,000 U/mL; streptomycin, 10,000 µg/mL) were purchased from Hyclone Laboratories, Inc. (South Logan, UT, USA). Newborn calf serum (NCS), fetal bovine serum (FBS), and 0.4% trypan blue solution were purchased from Life Technologies (Carlsbad, CA, USA). Halt^{TM} protease and phosphatase inhibitor cocktails and reagents for quantitative real-time polymerase chain reaction (qRT-PCR) were purchased from Thermo Scientific Pierce (Waltham, MA, USA). Equipment and reagents for western blotting analysis were purchased from Bio-Rad (Hercules, CA, USA). The anti-FAS, anti-perilipin, anti-SCD-1, anti-FABP4, anti-adiponectin, anti-PPAR-γ, anti-C/EBP-α, anti-cyclin-dependent kinase (CDK)-4, anti-p27^{KIP1}, anti-p-mitogen-activated protein kinase kinase (MEK) (Ser217/221), anti-ERK, anti-p-ERK (Thr202/Tyr204), anti-Akt, anti-p-Akt (Ser473), anti-mammalian target of rapamycin (mTOR), anti-p-mTOR (Ser2448), anti-p70S6K, anti-p-p70S6K (Ser371), anti-p-glycogen synthase kinase (GSK)-3β (Ser21/9), anti-p-cdc2 (Tyr15), and anti-p-STAT3 (Tyr705) primary antibodies and horseradish peroxidase (HRP)-conjugated secondary antibodies were purchased from Cell Signaling Technology, Inc. (Beverly, MA, USA). The other primary antibodies were purchased from Santa Cruz Biotechnology (Santa Cruz, CA, USA). Other chemicals including 3-isobutyl-1-methylxanthine (IBMX), dexamethasone (DEX), and insulin solution were purchased from Sigma-Aldrich (St. Louis, MO, USA).

2.2. Sample Preparation

The *I. britannica* flower aqueous extract (IAE) was prepared as previously described with minor modifications [24]. Briefly, commercially purchased dried flowers of *I. britannica* (Herb Kingdom Agriculture, Namwon, Korea) were pulverized and subjected to aqueous extraction (1:10; *I. britannica* powder:distilled water; w/v) for 72 h at 60 °C. The extract was filtered through a 0.45-µm filter, lyophilized, and stored at −20 °C until further use. The IAE was filtered through a 0.2-µm filter before use in subsequent experiments.

2.3. Cell Culture and Adipocyte Differentiation

The 3T3-L1 preadipocytes (American Type Culture Collection, Rockville, MD, USA) were cultured and maintained in growth medium (DMEM supplemented with 10% NCS and 1% antibiotic solution) at 5% CO_2 and 37 °C in a humidified atmosphere. The differentiation of preadipocytes was performed as described previously [7]. Briefly, two-day-post-confluent 3T3-L1 preadipocytes (designated as day 0) were induced to differentiate by replacing the growth medium with the differentiation medium (MDI) comprising DMEM supplemented with 10% FBS, 1% antibiotics solution, adipogenic hormonal cocktail (0.5 mM IBMX, 1 µM DEX, and 5 µg/mL insulin). The cells were incubated for 48 h (day 0–2) and the culture medium was replenished with DMEM containing 10% FBS, 1% antibiotics solution, and 5 µg/mL insulin once every two days until day 8. During differentiation, the cells were treated with different concentrations (0–200 µg/mL) of IAE for periods indicated in the figure captions. To examine the mechanism underlying the anti-adipogenic effect of IAE, the cells were treated with 10 µM of specific inhibitors (U0126, ERK 1/2 inhibitor; LY294002, Akt inhibitor) for 1 h prior to MDI treatment. The undifferentiated and differentiated cells were defined as negative control groups and positive control groups, respectively.

2.4. Oil Red O Staining and Intracellular Triglyceride Quantification

The 3T3-L1 preadipocytes were plated in 60 mm cell culture dishes (1.0×10^5 cells/dish) and differentiated into mature adipocytes as described in Section 2.3. The cells were rinsed twice with PBS and fixed with 4% neutral paraformaldehyde for 1 h at 4 °C. After washing with PBS, cells were maintained in 60% isopropyl alcohol for 5 min. The intracellular lipid droplets were stained with filtered (0.45 μm) 0.3% Oil Red O solution (w/v, in 60% isopropyl alcohol) for 1 h. Following the aspiration of residual Oil Red O solution, cells were rinsed five times with PBS. The images were acquired using a Nikon Eclipse E400-microscope/camera (Nikon, Tokyo, Japan). The Oil Red O dye was eluted with 100% isopropyl alcohol, and the absorbance was measured at 500 nm. The concentrations of intracellular triglycerides were assessed using a commercial kit (BioVision, Milpitas, CA, USA).

2.5. Cell Viability

Cell viability was assessed with 3-(4,5-dimethylthiazol-2-yl)-2,5-diphenyltetrazolium bromide (MTT) assay [30]. The cells plated in 24-well culture plates (2.0×10^4 cells/well) were cultured in the growth medium for 48 h. The culture medium was replenished with the growth medium containing different concentrations of IAE and incubated for 48 h. The cells were then treated with MTT solution (dissolved in growth medium) at a final concentration of 0.5 mg/mL. Following the removal of the supernatant, the formazan deposits were dissolved in 1 mL of dimethyl sulfoxide. The absorbance was measured at 570 nm. Cell viability was represented as a percentage relative to that in the control groups. The effect of IAE on the cell viability of mature adipocytes was examined on day 8.

2.6. Immunoblotting

Western blotting analysis was performed as described previously with a minor modification [31]. The 3T3-L1 preadipocytes plated in 60 mm culture dishes (1.0×10^5 cells/dish) were incubated and differentiated for various intervals in the presence of different concentrations of IAE. The cells were rinsed thrice with ice-cold PBS and lysed using a Pro-prep protein extraction buffer (iNtRON Biotechnology, Gyeonggi-do, Korea) supplemented with protease and phosphatase inhibitor cocktails. The lysates were sonicated (1 Amp; pulse-on, 5 s; pulse-off, 5 s) for 25 s in an ice-bath and centrifuged ($15,000 \times g$, 30 min, 4 °C). The protein concentration in the supernatant was determined using the DC^{TM} Protein Assay Kit (Bio-Rad). Equal amounts (25–40 μg) of cellular proteins were subjected to sodium dodecyl sulfate-polyacrylamide gel electrophoresis. The resolved proteins were transferred onto a polyvinyl difluoride membrane. The membrane was blocked with 5% skim milk and probed with the primary antibodies. Furthermore, the membrane was incubated with the HRP-conjugated secondary antibodies. The protein bands were detected using x-ray blue films and the enhanced chemiluminescence detection kit (Bio-Rad). The density of each protein band was measured using the ImageJ software (National Institutes of Health, Bethesda, MD, USA).

2.7. qRT-PCR

The qRT-PCR analysis was performed as described previously [31]. The 3T3-L1 preadipocytes seeded in 6-well culture plates (5×10^4 cells/well) were differentiated until day 8, as described in Section 2.3. The cells were rinsed thrice with ice-cold PBS and subjected to RNA extraction using the commercial RNeasy Kit (Qiagen, Hilden, Germany). An equal amount (1 μg) of total RNA was reverse-transcribed to complementary DNA using a RevertAid^{TM} first-strand cDNA synthesis kit (Thermo Scientific Pierce). The qRT-PCR analysis was performed using SYBR Green PCR Master Mix (Thermo Scientific Pierce) in PikoReal 96 (Thermo Scientific Pierce), following the manufacturer's instructions. The expression levels of target genes were normalized with those of the TATA box binding protein (TBP) [32]. The relative RNA expression levels were analyzed using the $2^{-(ave. \Delta\Delta CT)}$ method. The melting curve of each gene was examined to verify the amplification of a single product. The primers used for qRT-PCR analysis are presented in Table S1.

2.8. Trypan Blue Assay

Cell proliferation was evaluated with the trypan blue assay [11]. The 3T3-L1 preadipocytes plated in 6-well plates (5×10^4 cells/well) were differentiated as described in Section 2.3. The cells were harvested after 0, 24, and 48 h of stimulation with MDI by using trypsin-EDTA. Following the centrifugation (500× g, 5 min, 4 °C), collected pellets were suspended in growth medium and stained with 0.4% trypan blue solution. The viable cell numbers were counted using a hemocytometer.

2.9. Fluorescence-Activated Cell Sorting (FACS) Analysis

Cell cycle progression during MCE was investigated using FACS [7]. The 3T3-L1 preadipocytes plated in 60 mm culture dishes (1.0×10^5 cells/dish) were induced to differentiate, as described in Section 2.4. After stimulation with MDI for 16 h, cells were trypsinized and centrifuged (500× g, 5 min, 4 °C). The pellets were rinsed twice with PBS and fixed overnight in 70% ethyl alcohol at −20 °C. Following the removal of residual ethyl alcohol, cells were washed thrice with PBS and incubated in PBS containing 10 μg/mL RNase A and 50 μg/mL propidium iodide (PI) for 30 min. FACS analysis was performed using a CytoFLEX flow cytometer (Beckman Coulter, Brea, CA, USA). In total, 10,000 cells in each sample were used to measure the fluorescence of PI. The data were collected and analyzed by using CytExpert software (Beckman Coulter).

2.10. Ultra Performance Liquid Chromatography-Electrospray Ionization-Q/Orbitrap (UPLC-ESI-Q/Orbitrap) Tandem Mass Spectrometry (TEM), and High-Performance Liquid Chromatography (HPLC) Analysis

The UPLC-ESI-Q/Orbitrap tandem mass spectrometry analysis was conducted as previously described to identify the phenolic compounds of IAE [25]. Briefly, the UPLC analysis was performed using the Ultimate 3000 UPLC system (Thermo Fisher Scientific) equipped with a Hypersil GOLD™ C18 column (2.1 mm × 100 mm, 1.9 μm; Thermo Fisher Scientific). The binary mobile phase system (A, 0.1% formic acid in water; B, 0.1% formic acid in acetonitrile) was employed with the linear gradient program at a flow rate of 0.2 mL/min. The injection volume was 1 μL. Following ionization in negative mode, five ions were analyzed by using a Q-Exactive Orbitrap mass spectrometer (Thermo Fisher Scientific). The data were analyzed using Xcalibur™ software (Thermo Fisher Scientific).

Based on the results of UPLC-ESI-Q/Orbitrap tandem mass spectrometry analysis, the phenolic compounds of IAE were quantified using HPLC analysis [24]. Briefly, HPLC analysis was performed with Waters 600 HPLC system (Waters Corporation, Milford, MA, USA) equipped with an Eclipse XDB-C18 column (4.6 mm × 150 mm, 5 μm; Agilent Technologies, Santa Clara, MA, USA) and a Waters 2487 Dual-wavelength detector (Waters Corporation). The concentration of each compound was determined from the external regression curve, which was constructed with five concentrations of standards.

2.11. Statistical Analysis

The data were presented as mean ± standard deviation of three values obtained from the independent experiment conducted in triplicate at least. The values of respective experiments were determined by the mean of three measurements. The data were analyzed by using IBM SPSS version 24.0 (SPSS Inc., Chicago, IL, USA). Differences among multiple groups were evaluated with a one-tailed one-way analysis of variance (one-way ANOVA), followed by Tukey's multiple comparison test ($p < 0.05$). The differences were considered significant at $p < 0.05$.

3. Results

3.1. IAE Inhibits the Lipid Accumulation without Inducing Cytotoxic Effects

The dose-escalating cytotoxicity assessment was performed using the MTT assay. Compared with that in the control groups, IAE did not show significant adverse effect on the cell viability of undifferentiated preadipocytes or differentiated adipocytes up to concentrations of 500 μg/mL (Figure 1A). The effect of IAE on lipid accumulation in the differentiated adipocytes was examined. The Oil Red O staining showed that treatment with IAE dose-dependently inhibited the MDI-induced intracellular lipid accumulation (Figure 1B,C). Correspondingly, the intracellular triglyceride levels were significantly decreased upon treatment with IAE (Figure 1D). These results indicated that IAE inhibits lipogenesis in the MDI-induced 3T3-L1 preadipocytes without exerting cytotoxic effects. Therefore, the cytotoxicity of IAE was not considered in the subsequent experiments.

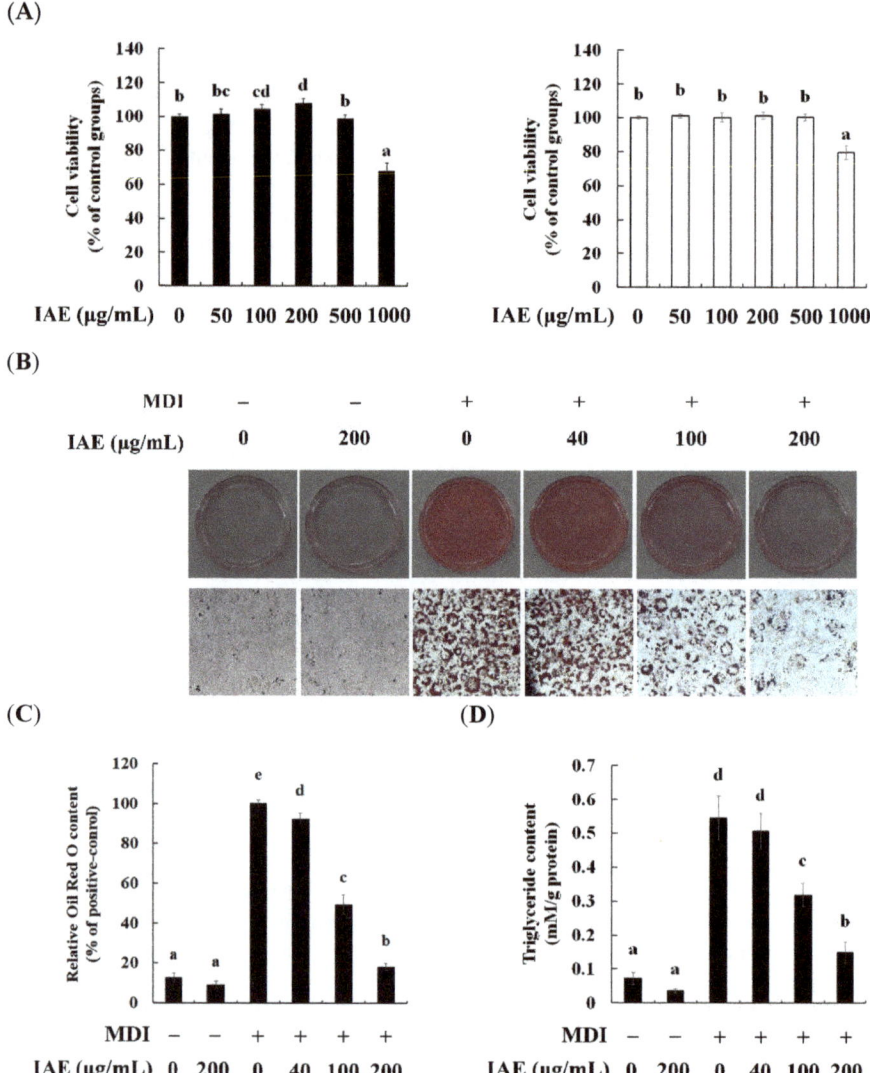

Figure 1. *Inula britannica* flower aqueous extract (IAE) inhibits lipid accumulation without exerting cytotoxic effects during the differentiation of 3T3-L1 preadipocytes. The cells were induced to differentiate by the MDI (differentiation medium) upon treatment with IAE in indicated concentrations. (**A**) The effect of IAE on cell viability was evaluated with the MTT assay (■, cell viability of preadipocytes; □, cell viability of differentiated preadipocytes). (**B**) Oil Red O staining of intracellular lipids on day 8. (**C**) Relative absorbance of Oil Red O eluted from intracellular lipids at 500 nm. (**D**) Measurement of intracellular triglyceride levels on day 8. The data are presented as mean ± standard deviation. Values labeled with different letters (a–e) are significantly different ($p < 0.05$). Differences among the multiple groups were determined based on one-tailed one-way analysis of variance, followed by Tukey's post hoc test.

3.2. IAE Exhibits Anti-Adipogenic Effect during Adipocyte Differentiation

To evaluate the effect of IAE on adipogenesis, the expression levels of lipogenesis- and adipogenesis-associated mediators were investigated in differentiated 3T3-L1 cells upon treatment with IAE. First, the effect of IAE on lipogenesis-related biomarkers was assessed. Consistent with the results of intracellular lipid contents, treatment with MDI markedly increased the protein expression levels of FAS, FABP4, perilipin, and SCD-1. However, the expression levels of those proteins were mitigated upon treatment with IAE (Figure 2A,B). Consistently, treatment with IAE downregulated the mRNA expression levels of FAS, FABP4, perilipin, and SCD-1 upon MDI stimulation (Figure S1A). Following this, the effect of IAE on the expression of adipogenesis-specific biomarkers was examined. As expected, IAE treatment significantly suppressed the expression levels of PPAR-γ, C/EBP-α, sterol regulatory element-binding protein (SREBP)-1c, and adiponectin following MDI treatment at both the protein (Figure 2C,D) and transcriptional levels (Figure S1B). These findings demonstrated that IAE inhibits the de novo lipogenesis by regulating the adipogenesis, which results in the inhibition of the accumulation of intracellular lipids.

To further examine the anti-adipogenic properties of IAE, the effect of IAE on the activation of the Akt/GSK-3β axis was investigated in the 3T3-L1 cells on day 8. Upon stimulation with insulin, the Akt/GSK-3β signaling pathways promote the terminal differentiation of adipocytes through the phosphorylation of C/EBP-α and modulation of glucose uptake [33]. Consistent with the preceding results, the MDI-induced phosphorylation of Akt and GSK-3β was significantly attenuated upon treatment with IAE (Figure 2E,F). These results indicated that IAE inhibits adipogenesis and subsequent intracellular lipid accumulation in differentiated 3T3-L1 cells through regulating the Akt/GSK-3β signaling pathways.

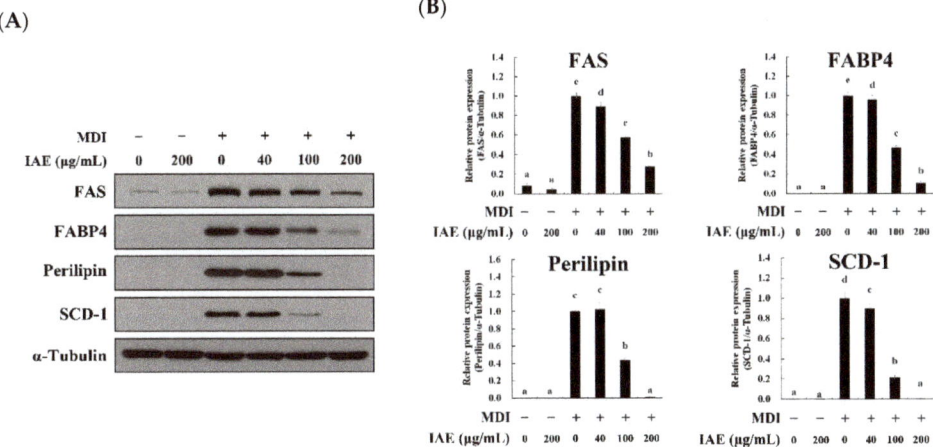

Figure 2. Cont.

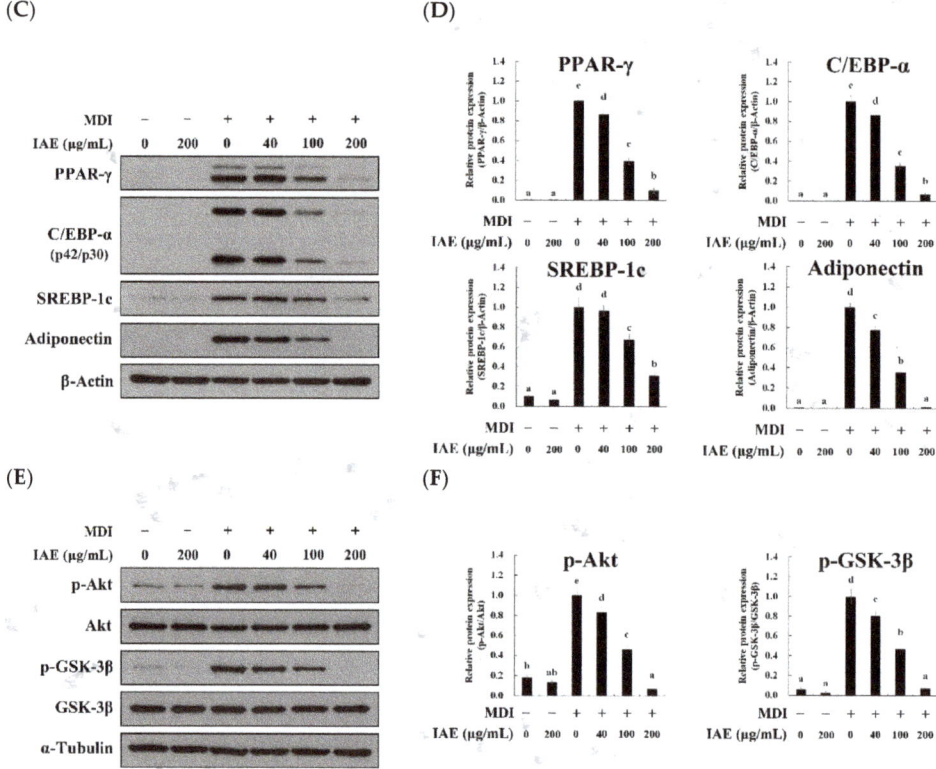

Figure 2. *Inula britannica* flower aqueous extract (IAE) exerts anti-adipogenic effects in MDI-induced differentiation of 3T3-L1 preadipocytes involving regulation of Akt/GSK-3β signaling pathways. The cells were differentiated for eight days with the indicated concentrations of IAE. The phosphorylation of Akt (Ser 473) and GSK-3β (Ser21/9) was examined to evaluate the activation of the Akt/GSK-3β signaling pathways. The protein expression levels of adipogenesis-associated biomarkers were determined by using western blotting. (**A**) Protein expression levels of lipogenesis-associated biomarkers. (**B**) Relative protein expression levels of lipogenesis-associated biomarkers. (**C**) Protein expression levels of adipogenesis-specific biomarkers. (**D**) Relative protein expression levels of adipogenesis-specific biomarkers. (**E**) Effect of IAE on the activation of Akt/GSK-3β signaling pathways. (**F**) Relative protein expression levels of phosphorylated Akt and GSK-3β. The data are presented as mean ± standard deviation. Values labeled with different letters (a–e) are significantly different ($p < 0.05$). Differences among the multiple groups were determined based on one-tailed one-way analysis of variance, followed by Tukey's post hoc test.

3.3. IAE Modulates the Early Phase of Adipogenesis

To elucidate the mechanism underlying the anti-adipogenic effect of IAE, the 3T3-L1 cells were treated with IAE at different time points during differentiation (Figure 3A). Compared with the control groups (treatment no. 1), treatment with IAE reduced the intracellular lipid accumulation irrespective of the treatment periods (Figure 3B,C). Additionally, the strongest inhibition of lipid accumulation was observed upon treatment with IAE during the first two days. The lipid accumulation in the cells treated with IAE for the first two days (treatment no. 3) was comparable to that in the cells treated with IAE for eight days (treatment no. 2). Consistent with the result of Oil Red O staining, the protein expression levels of FAS, PPAR-γ, C/EBP-α, and p-Akt were significantly downregulated upon treatment with IAE in MDI-stimulated 3T3-L1 preadipocytes (Figure 3D), which indicated that IAE modulates the early phase of adipogenesis. Based on these findings, we hypothesized that the anti-adipogenic effect of IAE was closely associated with the regulation of MCE, which is critical for the initiation of adipogenesis.

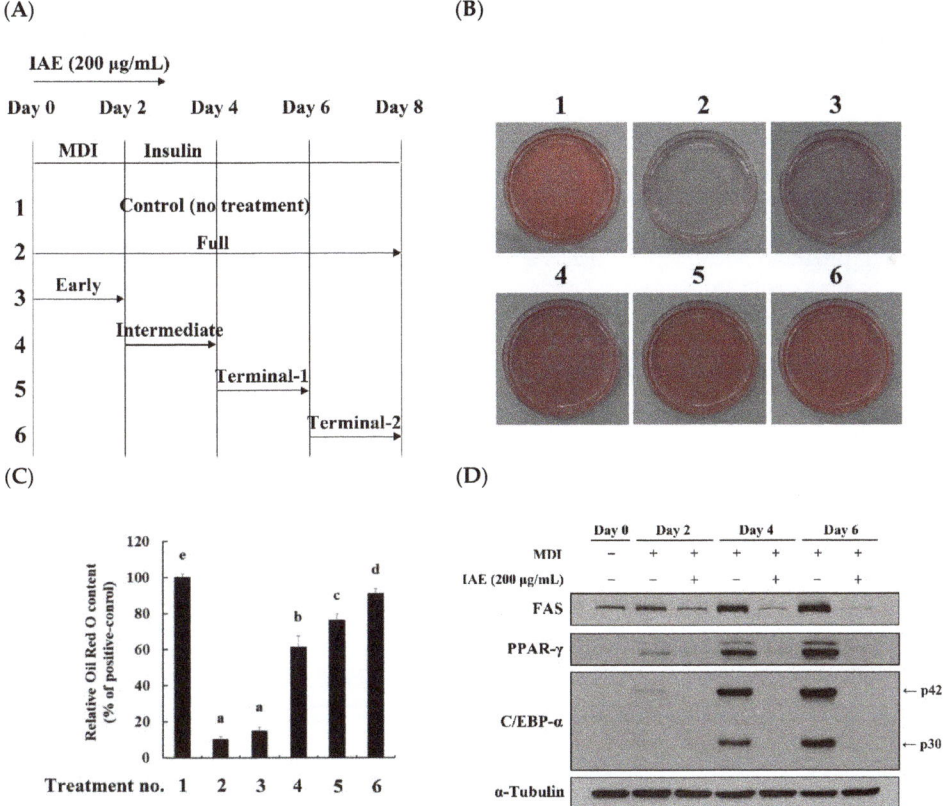

Figure 3. *Inula britannica* flower aqueous extract (IAE) affects the early phases of adipogenesis. During the eight days of 3T3-L1 differentiation, IAE (200 µg/mL) was treated at different time points as indicated. (**A**) Schematic depiction of different treatment intervals of IAE during 3T3-L1 differentiation. (**B**) Intracellular lipids were stained with Oil Red O on day 8. (**C**) Relative absorbance of Oil Red O dye eluted from intracellular lipids at 500 nm. (**D**) Expression levels of adipogenesis-associated proteins on day 0, 2, 4, and 6 of differentiation. The data are presented as mean ± standard deviation. Values labeled with different letters (a–d) are significantly different ($p < 0.05$). Differences among the multiple groups were determined based on one-tailed one-way analysis of variance, followed by Tukey's post hoc test.

3.4. IAE Inhibits the MCE by Arresting the Cell Cycle Progression

During the early phase of adipogenesis, MDI induction led the growth-arrested 3T3-L1 preadipocytes to undergo MCE, which involves synchronous re-entry into the cell cycle and cell proliferation [7]. Therefore, the effect of IAE on MDI-induced cell proliferation and cell cycle progression was investigated during early phases of 3T3-L1 preadipocyte differentiation. The result of the trypan blue assay revealed that treatment of IAE significantly inhibited the MDI-induced cell proliferation showing a 24.35% and 32.60% inhibition rate at 24 h and 48 h, respectively (Figure S2). Compared with the negative control group, the MDI-induced group exhibited 1.8- and 2.2-times higher cell numbers after 24 and 48 h, respectively, while the IAE (200 µg/mL)-treated group exhibited 1.4- and 1.5-times higher cell numbers at 24 and 48 h, respectively.

The role of cell cycle arrest in the inhibitory effect of IAE on cell proliferation was examined using FACS analysis and western blotting. The cell cycle of fully confluent 3T3-L1 preadipocytes was primarily remained at the G0/G1 phase. However, MDI stimulation promoted the entry of 3T3-L1 preadipocytes into the S phase. The analysis of cellular DNA content revealed that the proportions of cells at the G0/G1 and S phases in the negative control group were 78.05% and 6.98%, respectively, while those in the positive group were 51.56%, and 22.87%, respectively. This indicated that MDI induced a cell cycle transition from the G0/G1 phase to the S phase. However, IAE dose-dependently inhibited shift of cell cycle from the G0/G1 phase to the S phase (Figure 4A,B), as evidenced by a significant increase in the cell population remaining at the G0/G1 phase (ranging from 58.25 to 77.94%). In particular, the proportion of cells at S phase in the IAE (200 µg/mL)-treated group was 5.38%, which was comparable with that in the negative control groups. Next, the expression levels of cell cycle progression-associated proteins were evaluated. Consistent with the results of the FACS analysis, treatment with IAE suppressed the expression levels of cell cycle progression-related proteins in MDI-stimulated 3T3-L1 cells (Figure 4C,D). In particular, IAE dose-dependently suppressed the expression levels of S phase-mediating proteins (cyclin D1, cyclin A1, and CDK2) and significantly mitigated the degradation of p27 (CDK inhibitor 1B). Additionally, downregulated expression levels of G2/M-mediating proteins (cyclin B1 and p-cdc2) upon treatment of IAE corroborate the evidence that IAE inhibits cell cycle progression by arresting the cell cycle at the G0/G1 phase.

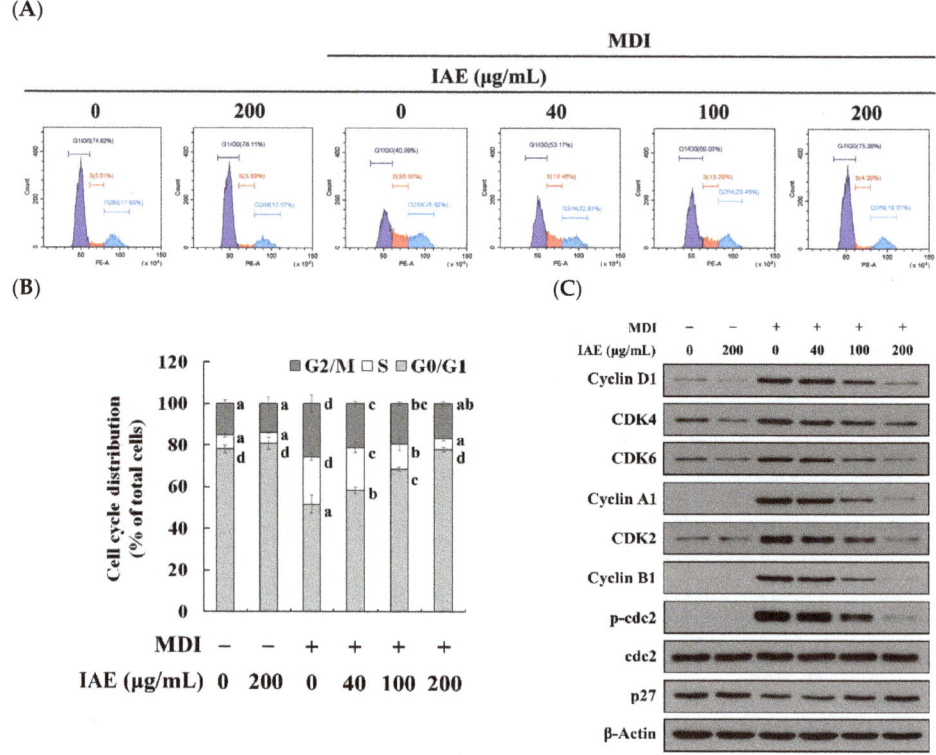

Figure 4. *Cont.*

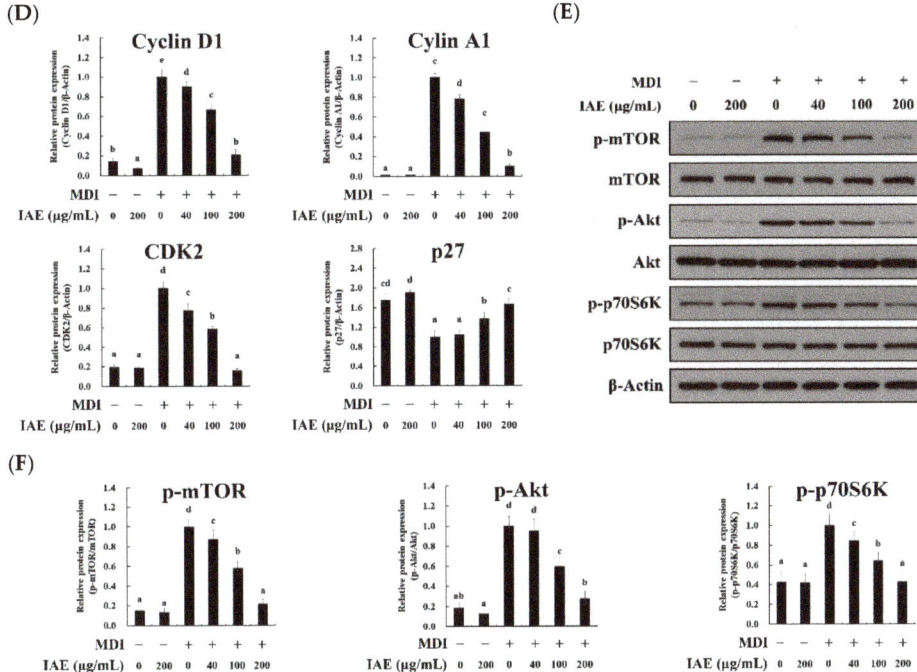

Figure 4. *Inula britannica* flower aqueous extract (IAE) inhibits the MCE involving Akt signaling pathways during early phase of adipogenesis. Growth-arrested 3T3-L1 preadipocytes were induced to differentiate by stimulating with MDI in the presence of indicated concentrations of IAE. The phosphorylation of cdc2 (Tyr15) and mTOR (Ser2448), Akt (Ser473), and p70S6K (Ser371) was examined to evaluate the activation of the G2/M phase and mTOR/Akt/p70S6K axis, respectively. (**A**) After 16 h of MDI treatment, cell cycle progression was investigated using FACS. (**B**) The cell distribution in the G0/G1, S, and G2/M phases was calculated as a percentage of total cell numbers based on the results of FACS analysis. (**C**) Western blotting was used to examine the expression of cell cycle progression-associated proteins after 18 h of MDI treatment. (**D**) Relative expression levels of representative proteins contributing to the transition of the cell cycle. (**E**) Effect of IAE on the activation of the mTOR/Akt/p70S6K axis after 18 h of MDI stimulation. (**F**) Relative expression levels of phosphorylated mTOR, Akt, and p70S6K. The data are presented as mean ± standard deviation. Values labeled with different letters (a–d) are significantly different ($p < 0.05$). Differences among the multiple groups were determined based on one-tailed one-way analysis of variance, followed by Tukey's post hoc test.

To further examine the cellular mechanisms involved in cell cycle progression, the effect of IAE on MDI-induced activation of mTOR/Akt/p70S6K axis was investigated. The mTOR/Akt/p70S6K axis plays a pivotal role in cell proliferation and metabolism by regulating the cell cycle progression and lipogenesis [34]. Consistent with previous findings, MDI stimulation markedly up-regulated the phosphorylation of mTOR/Akt/p70S6K (Figure 4E,F). However, IAE dose-dependently alleviated the MDI-induced phosphorylation of mTOR/Akt/p70S6K, which indicated that IAE inhibits MCE by causing the cell cycle arrest at the G0/G1 phase involving the mTOR/Akt/p70S6K signaling pathways. Based on these results, we hypothesized that the anti-mitotic effect of IAE is mediated through regulation of transcription factors involved in MCE during the early phases of adipogenesis.

3.5. IAE Regulates the Transcription Factors of the Early Phase of Adipogenesis

To determine whether the anti-mitotic effect was associated with alteration in the levels of adipogenic transcription factors, the effect of IAE on the activation of STAT3 and the expression of C/EBP-β was investigated in the MDI-stimulated 3T3-L1 preadipocytes during the early phase of differentiation. The activation of STAT3 and C/EBP-β mediates cell proliferation and activation of adipogenic transcription factors, thereby promoting MCE and adipogenesis [17,18,35]. Consistent with these findings, stimulation with MDI induced the phosphorylation of STAT3 and IAE attenuated the MDI-induced phosphorylation of STAT3 (Figure 5A). Additionally, IAE dose-dependently mitigated the MDI-induced phosphorylation of STAT3 (Figure 5B,C), which concurred with arrested cell cycle progression (Figure 4A–C) and downregulated expression of adipogenic transcription factors (Figure 2C and Figure S1B) following MDI stimulation in the presence of IAE. Similarly, IAE attenuated the MDI-induced expression of C/EBP-β isoforms, C/EBP-β/LAP, and C/EBP-β/LIP (Figure 5D–F). Both C/EBP-β isoforms were rapidly expressed following MDI stimulation and treatment with IAE mitigated the MDI-induced expression of C/EBP-β isoforms (Figure 5D). In addition, IAE showed dose-dependent inhibitory effects on the MDI-induced C/EBP-β expression (Figure 5E,F). These findings indicated that the inhibitory effect of IAE on adipogenesis of 3T3-L1 preadipocytes is associated with regulation of STAT3 and C/EBP-β.

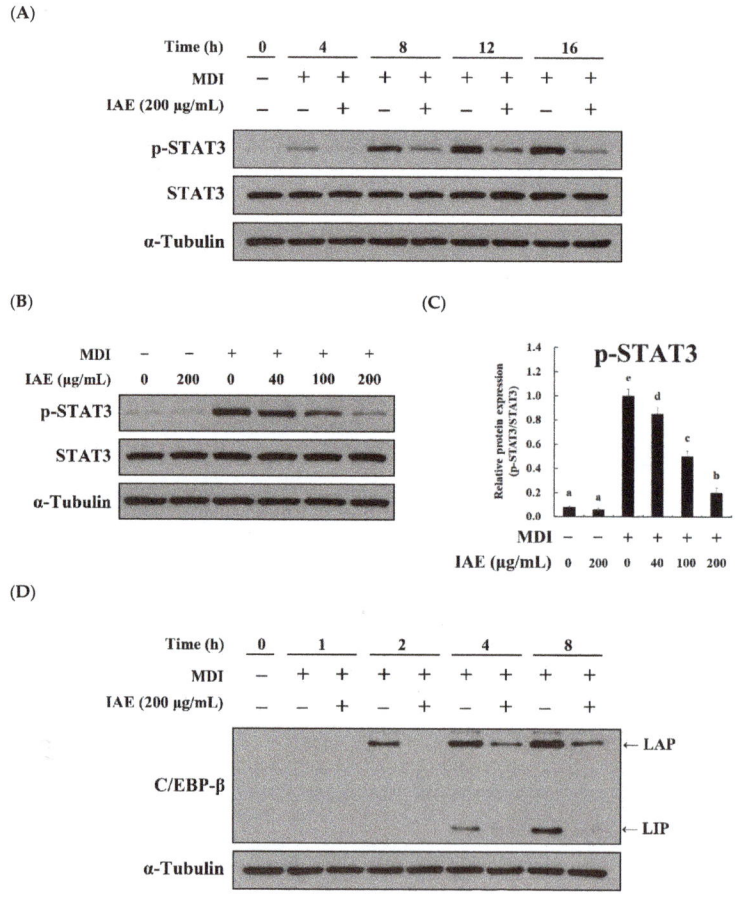

Figure 5. *Cont.*

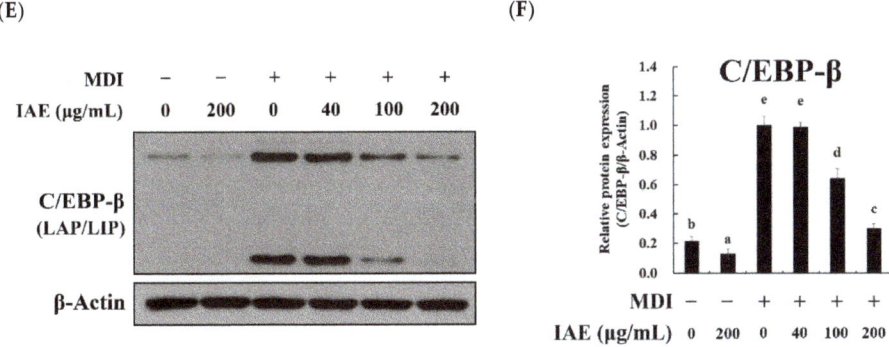

Figure 5. *Inula britannica* flower aqueous extract (IAE) inhibits the activation of STAT3 and C/EBP-β during the early phase of adipogenesis. Fully confluent 3T3-L1 preadipocytes were differentiated by MDI stimulation upon treatment with indicated concentrations of IAE. The phosphorylation of STAT3 (Tyr705) was examined to evaluate STAT3 activation. The expression levels of proteins were assessed with western blotting. (**A**) The time-course of MDI-induced STAT3 phosphorylation in the presence or absence of IAE. (**B**) The dose-dependent inhibitory effect of IAE on STAT3 activation was determined after 18 h of MDI stimulation. (**C**) Relative protein expressions of phosphorylated STAT3. (**D**) The time-course of MDI-induced C/EBP-β expression in the presence or absence of IAE. (**E**) The dose-dependent inhibitory effect of IAE on C/EBP-β was assessed after 4 h of MDI stimulation. (**F**) Relative protein expression levels of C/EBP-β. The data are presented as mean ± standard deviation. Values labeled with different letters (a–e) are significantly different ($p < 0.05$). Differences among the multiple groups were determined based on one-tailed one-way analysis of variance, followed by Tukey's post hoc test.

3.6. IAE Inhibits the Adipogenesis by Regulating the ERK 1/2 and Akt Signaling Pathways

The proliferation and differentiation of cells are modulated by cascades of transcription factors involving various cellular signaling pathways [9]. Insulin-like growth factor (IGF)-1, which is upregulated upon stimulation with MDI, activates the MEK-1/ERK 1/2 and Akt signaling pathways and consequently promotes activation of the adipogenic transcription factors [13,15,16]. Thus, the effect of IAE on MDI-induced activation of ERK 1/2 and Akt was investigated during the early phase of adipogenesis. Compared to MDI-treated groups, MDI-induced activation of MEK-1, ERK 1/2, and Akt was attenuated upon treatment with IAE during early phases of differentiation (Figure 6A). Additionally, IAE exhibited a dose-dependent inhibitory effects on the phosphorylation of MEK-1, ERK 1/2, and Akt (Figure 6B,C). Next, the ERK 1/2 and Akt signaling pathways in adipogenesis of 3T3-L1 preadipocytes confirmed by using U0126 and LY294002 inhibitors, respectively. The U0126 inhibits the MDI-induced ERK 1/2 activation by inactivating MEK-1 and MEK-2, which are the kinase of ERK 1/2, and consequently suppresses the activation of PPAR-γ and C/EBP-α [15]. Similarly, inactivation of Akt upon treatment LY294002 results in the inhibition of adipogenesis as well as lipogenesis [16]. Consistent with previous findings, the inhibition of ERK 1/2 and Akt upon pre-treatment with U0126 and LY294002 (Figure S3A) resulted in suppression of MCE by arresting the cell cycle progression (Figure S3B and Figure 6D) and mitigating the STAT3 activation (Figure 6E). Following this, U0126 and LY294002 inhibited the accumulation of intracellular lipids (Figure S3C) and expression of adipogenic biomarkers, FAS, PPAR-γ, and C/EBP-α (Figure 6F). These results suggest that the anti-adipogenic effect of IAE is associated with regulation of the MEK-1/ERK 1/2 and Akt signaling pathways.

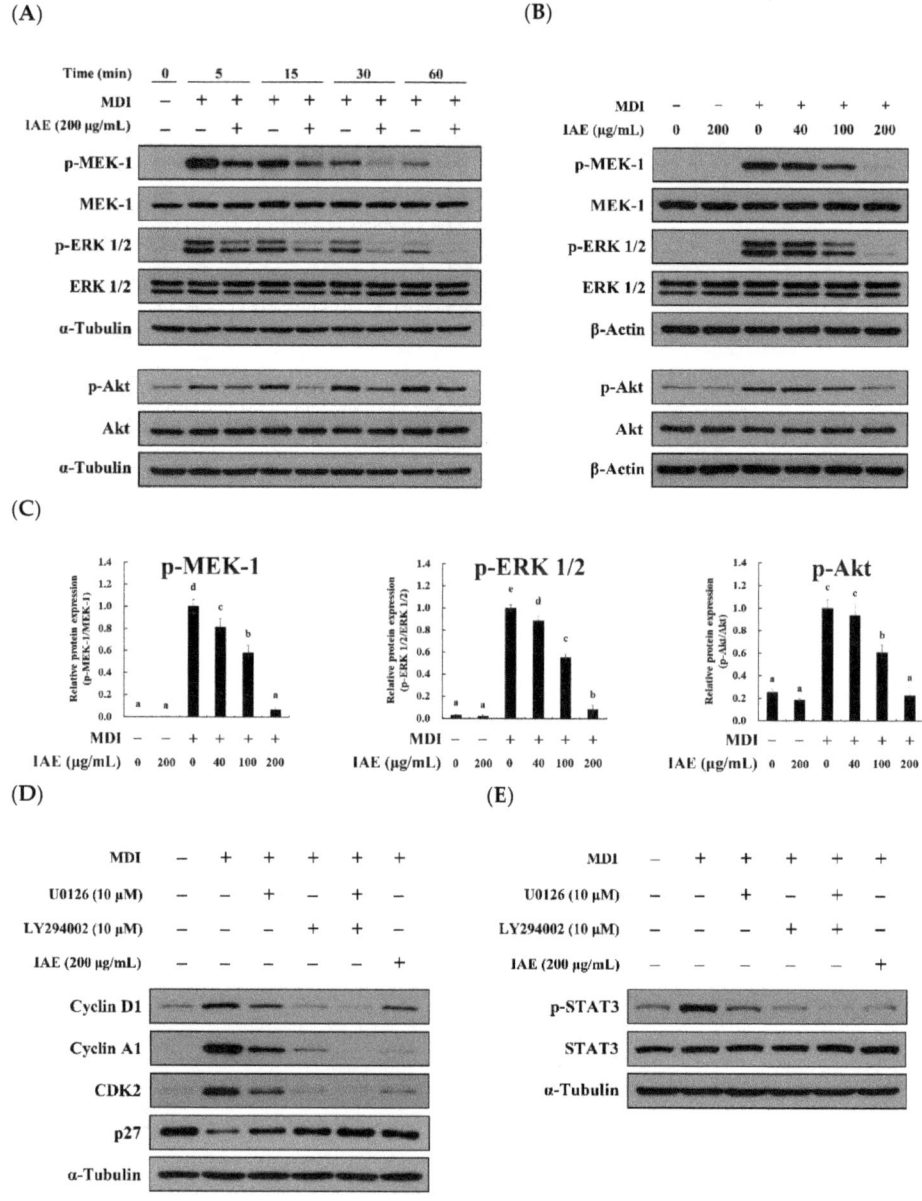

Figure 6. Cont.

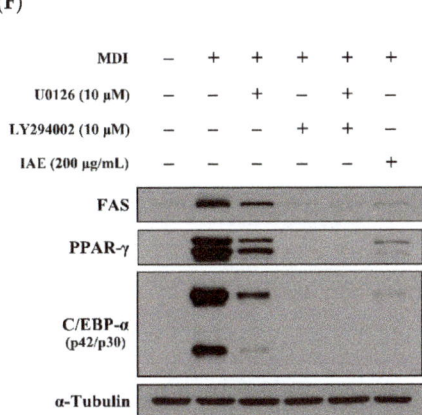

Figure 6. *Inula britannica* flower aqueous extract (IAE) inhibits the adipogenesis of 3T3-L1 preadipocytes through regulation of the ERK 1/2 and Akt signaling pathways. The 3T3-L1 preadipocytes were induced to differentiate by MDI in the presence of indicated concentrations of IAE or specific inhibitors (U0126 and LY294002). Cells were treated with specific inhibitors for 1 h prior to MDI stimulation. The phosphorylation of MEK-1 (Ser217/221), ERK 1/2 (Thr202/Tyr204), and Akt (Ser473) was examined to evaluate activation of these proteins. Western blotting was performed to examine the expression levels of proteins. (**A**) Inhibitory effect of IAE on activation of MEK-1/ERK and Akt during early phase of adipogenesis. (**B**) The dose-dependent inhibitory effect of IAE on MDI-induced MEK/Akt activation was investigated following 30 min of MDI induction. (**C**) Relative protein expression levels of MEK-1, ERK 1/2, and Akt. (**D,E**) After 18 h of MDI treatment, the effect of ERK 1/2 and Akt signaling pathways on the expression of proteins mediating the cell cycle progression was assessed. (**F**) Effect of ERK 1/2 and Akt signaling pathways on adipogenesis-associated biomarkers was assessed on day 8. The data are presented as mean ± standard deviation. Values labeled with different letters (a–e) are significantly different ($p < 0.05$). Differences among the multiple groups were determined based on one-tailed one-way analysis of variance, followed by Tukey's post hoc test.

3.7. Determination of Phenolic Compounds of IAE

The phenolic compounds of IAE were examined using UPLC-ESI-Q/Orbitrap tandem mass spectrometry analysis and quantified using HPLC analysis (Table 1). IAE comprised gallic acid (m/z [M-H] = 169.08749), protocatechuic acid (m/z [M-H] = 153.00632), chlorogenic acid (m/z [M-H] = 353.34218), kaempferol-3-O-glucoside (m/z [M-H] = 447.35581), and 6-methoxyluteolin (m/z [M-H] = 315.25656), which was consistent with the results of previous studies on the major phenolic compounds of *I. britannica* flower [24–28]. Additionally, these phenolic compounds were reported to exhibit anti-obesogenic properties through the regulation of adipogenesis and lipogenesis [22]. The phenolic compounds were quantified using a HPLC system. The most abundant phenolic compound was kaempferol-3-O-glucoside (54.842 ± 0.191 µg/mg), followed by chlorogenic acid (16.540 ± 0.094 µg/mg), 6-methoxyluteolin (6.669 ± 0.286 µg/mg), and protocatechuic acid (3.998 ± 0.027 µg/mg). However, the levels of gallic acid were lower than the limit of quantification. These results suggest that IAE suppresses lipid accumulation by inhibiting the development of adipogenesis, which may be mediated by identified anti-obesogenic phenolic compounds in the extract.

Table 1. Ultra-performance liquid chromatography-electrospray ionization-Q/Orbitrap tandem mass spectrometry analysis of *Inula britannica* flower aqueous extract.

Compounds	Retention Time (min)	m/z [M-H]	MS^2 Fragment	Molecular Formula	Contents (µg/mg)	References
Gallic acid	0.08	169.08749	125.09668	$C_7H_6O_5$	<LOQ ^{1}	
Protocatechuic acid	0.34	153.00632	109.06452	$C_7H_6O_4$	3.998 ± 0.027	[25,26]
Chlorogenic acid	3.65	353.34218	168.98956	$C_{16}H_{18}O_9$	16.540 ± 0.094	[25,27]
Kaempferol-3-*O*-glucoside	4.13	447.35581	168.98952	$C_{21}H_{20}O_{11}$	54.842 ± 0.191	[25]
6-Methoxyluteolin	14.50	315.25656	96.96816	$C_{16}H_{12}O_7$	6.669 ± 0.286	[25]

The experiment was independently performed in triplicate. The concentration of phenolic compounds is presented as mean ± standard deviation. ^{1} LOQ, limit of quantification.

4. Discussion

Obesity is reported to be associated with increased risk of onset of various degenerative diseases including metabolic syndrome morbidities. The aberrant growth of adipose tissue, which is a characteristic feature of obesity, is dependent on the hypertrophy and/or hyperplasia of adipocytes [7]. Adipocyte hypertrophy is an enlargement in size of pre-existed mature adipocytes, resulting from an accumulation of intracellular lipids in individual adipocytes. In contrast, adipocyte hyperplasia is an increased number of adipocytes due to the development of new adipocytes, which results from adipogenesis [36]. Adipocyte hyperplasia is a crucial process in determining the adipocyte numbers, which is primarily established in childhood and adolescence. The adipocyte number is sustained in adults even after weight loss, which indicates weight loss mainly results from the decreased volume of established adipocytes [22]. Following this, upregulated adipogenesis leads to the growth of adipose tissue by promoting the hyperplasia and hypertrophy of adipocytes and consequently results in the development of obesity. Therefore, the regulation of adipogenesis is a potential therapeutic strategy for obesity. Plant materials, which are a source of phenolic compounds with anti-obesogenic efficacy, are of increasing interest for prophylactic and therapeutic options in obesity and obesity-related disorders [37–39]. This study revealed the anti-obesity potential of *I. britannica* by demonstrating the anti-adipogenic effect of IAE and its underlying cellular mechanisms in the 3T3-L1 preadipocytes. Additionally, phenolic constituents of IAE were identified.

The differentiation of adipocytes accompanies upregulated de novo lipogenesis, which is modulated by various transcription factors such as C/EBPs and PPARs and results in the accumulation of intracellular lipids [40]. In particular, C/EBP-α and PPAR-γ are both anti-mitotic and essential for the development of adipogenesis, in addition to the maintenance of a differentiated state. These transcription factors terminate the MCE and reciprocally promote triacylglycerol synthesis, which is dependent on the transcriptional modulation of lipogenesis-associated genes such as *Srebp1c* (SREBP-1c), *Fasn* (FAS), *Fabp4* (FABP4), *Plin1* (perilipin), and *Scd1* (SCD-1), thereby establishing an adipocyte phenotype [12,22]. Numerous studies have demonstrated that these transcription factors play critical roles in adipogenesis and the development of obesity. For example, a previous study reported that the white adipose tissues of C/EBP-α knockout mice exhibited deficient metabolism and lipid storage [41]. Similarly, mice with adipocyte-specific deletion of PPAR-γ were resistant to high-fat diet (HFD)-induced obesity as the development of adipose tissue was impaired [42]. Therefore, the inhibition of these transcription factors is a potential therapeutic strategy for obesity with respect to the regulation of adipogenesis. Consistently, the *Edgeworthia gardineri* flower, *Aster spathulifolius*, and *Viburnum opulus* fruit extracts have been reported to inhibit development of adipogenesis by regulating the expression of C/EBP-α and PPAR-γ, which results in decreased accumulation of intracellular lipids [37,40,43]. Our data demonstrated that IAE inhibited intracellular lipid accumulation through suppressing the expression levels of lipogenesis- and adipogenesis-associated biomarkers including C/EBP-α and PPAR-γ. Additionally, the IAE-mediated inhibition of lipid accumulation was associated with the regulation of early phases of adipogenesis.

This indicated that IAE inhibits intracellular lipid accumulation by suppressing adipogenesis rather than direct regulation of lipogenesis.

During the early phases of adipogenesis, quiescent preadipocytes are induced to undergo MCE upon hormonal stimulation. Hence, growth-arrested preadipocytes synchronously re-enter the cell cycle and consequently undergo one or two rounds of mitosis, which increases the numbers of adipocytes and results in adipocyte hyperplasia [9,22]. Despite several controversies regarding the role of MCE in adipogenesis, numerous studies have reported that MCE is a prerequisite for the terminal phases of adipogenesis by demonstrating the correlation between MCE and adipogenesis, which is dependent on the activation of adipogenic transcriptional cascades [13,18,44,45]. C/EBP-β and STAT3, which are early adipogenic transcription factors, are involved in development of MCE and adipogenesis [17,46]. Activated C/EBP-β develops MCE by mediating DNA replication and promotes adipogenesis by activating the transcription of C/EBP-α and PPAR-γ. Consistently, 3T3-L1 preadipocytes following knockdown of C/EBP-β genes, neither undergo MCE nor develop into adipocytes [46,47]. In addition to activating C/EBP-β and PPAR-γ, STAT3 is involved in cell proliferation by promoting cell cycle progression [7,17]. The growth-arrested preadipocytes remained predominantly at the G0/G1 phase due to upregulated cell cycle suppressor proteins such as hypo-phosphorylated retinoblastoma (Rb), a tumor suppressor protein, and $p27^{KIP1}$, a CDK inhibitor protein. However, hormonal stimulation induces the degradation of CDK inhibitor proteins and consequently promotes cell cycle progression by sequential activation and assembly of cyclin D1/CDK4/CDK6, cyclin E/CDK2, cyclin A1/CDK2, and cyclin B1/CDK1 (cdc2) complexes. In particular, cyclin E/CDK2 and cyclin A1/CDK2 complexes play crucial roles in cell cycle progression by mediating the G1/S phase transition and S phase progression. Furthermore, C/EBP-β and STAT3 are activated by acquiring DNA-binding capacity during the S phase [7,12,22,46]. A previous study has demonstrated that cell cycle arrest leads to the disruption of transactivation domains of C/EBP-β, which results in the inhibition of adipogenesis [18]. Several studies have demonstrated that the upregulated expression of $p27^{KIP1}$ contributes to the inhibition of MCE and adipocyte differentiation, whereas the degradation of $p27^{KIP1}$ promotes adipogenesis and increases fat mass, indicating that $p27^{KIP1}$ potentially inhibits hyperplasia [48,49]. Therefore, inhibition or delaying the cell cycle progression by regulating the cell cycle modulators during MCE as well as inactivating the early transcription factors could be efficacious strategies to inhibit adipogenesis and mitigate obesity. Our data showed that IAE inhibited cell proliferation by arresting the cell cycle at the G0/G1 phase, which was corroborated by inactivated cell cycle modulators and upregulated expression levels of $p27^{KIP1}$. Additionally, IAE inhibited the expression of C/EBP-β and the activation of STAT3. Consistent with preceding results, previous studies have reported that plant extracts and their phytochemicals inhibit adipogenesis and lipid accumulation through suppression of MCE, which was dependent on the regulation of cell cycle progression and/or suppression of transcription factors [50–52]. For instance, *Gleditsia sinensis* fruit extract suppressed MCE and adipogenesis through the inhibition of $p27^{KIP1}$ degradation and the activation of STAT3 [7].

The ERK 1/2 and Akt cellular signaling pathways are involved in MCE and adipogenesis, depending on the modulation of proliferation, differentiation, and lipid metabolism of adipocytes [11,33,34,53]. The activation of the MEK-1/ERK 1/2 signaling pathways promotes cell cycle progression by activating the cell cycle modulators such as the cyclin D1 and Rb [15,53]. Similarly, the activation of the mTOR/Akt/p70S6K axis mediates cell proliferation by modulating cyclin D1 and $p27^{KIP1}$ [34]. Additionally, the phosphorylation cascades of MEK-1/ERK 1/2 and Akt/GSK-3β sequentially lead to the phosphorylation and acquisition of DNA-binding activity of C/EBP-β, which promotes adipogenesis [18,22,33]. Thus, the ERK 1/2 and Akt signaling pathways are potential molecular therapeutic targets for obesity. Correspondingly, mice with the deletion of ERK genes are resistant to HFD-induced obesity, which was consistent with the suppressed expression of C/EBP-α and PPAR-γ in 3T3-L1 preadipocytes upon blockage of MEK/ERK cascades [15,49]. Our data indicated that IAE inhibits adipogenesis including MCE by regulating the activation of the ERK 1/2 and Akt signaling pathways. Consistent with these results, *Clitoria ternatea* flower and coffee extracts inhibited MDI-induced phosphorylation of ERK 1/2 and Akt, which resulted in the inhibition of adipogenesis development [41,50].

Phenolic compounds including phenolic acids and flavonoids have been demonstrated to exhibit anti-obesogenic properties such as the suppression of adipogenesis and the degradation of intracellular lipids [22,38,39]. The phytochemical analysis of IAE revealed the presence of protocatechuic acid, chlorogenic acid, kaempferol-3-O-glucoside, and 6-methoxyluteolin. Dietary flavonoids such as kaempferol, quercetin, and curcumins inhibited the adipogenesis of 3T3-L1 preadipocytes by suppressing MCE and regulating adipogenic transcriptional cascades [22,49]. For instance, kaempferol induced cell cycle arrest at the S phase by inactivating the mTOR/p70S6K/Akt axis, thereby inhibiting the adipogenesis accompanied by the downregulated expression of C/EBP-α and PPAR-γ [34]. Similarly, phenolic acids such as chlorogenic acid, ellagic acid, and p-coumaric acid suppressed intracellular lipid accumulation by inhibiting the expression of lipogenic enzymes, which results from the downregulated expression of C/EBP-α and PPAR-γ [18,39]. Moreover, previous studies have demonstrated that chlorogenic acid and luteolin alleviate obesity in HFD-induced mice by improving lipid metabolism, in addition to exercise endurance [54,55]. Additionally, flavonoids and phenolic acids regulate the activity of PPAR-γ by interacting with receptors as an agonist, which is attributable to their amino acid residue-dependent binding affinity to PPAR-γ, thereby inhibiting adipogenesis [39]. Our results indicate that anti-obesogenic phenolic compounds are potentially involved in mediating the anti-adipogenic effect of IAE.

5. Conclusions

This study revealed the anti-obesity potential of IAE by demonstrating the anti-adipogenic effects of IAE and elucidating the underlying mechanisms during the differentiation of 3T3-L1 preadipocytes. The inhibitory effect of IAE on MCE during the early phases of adipogenesis primarily contributed to the suppressed expression of adipogenesis-associated biomarkers, which resulted in the inhibition of adipogenesis and lipogenesis. Additionally, IAE exerted an anti-adipogenic effect through the regulation of the ERK 1/2 and Akt cellular signaling pathways. Furthermore, IAE comprised anti-obesogenic phenolic compounds. Although further in vivo studies are needed to confirm the anti-obesity properties of IAE, the findings of this study indicate that IAE can potentially prevent obesity by regulating the hyperplasia and hypertrophy of adipocytes. Thus, IAE might be considered as a potential therapeutic agent for obesity. Overall, IAE could be potentially used for the development of prophylactic and therapeutic products for obesity.

Supplementary Materials: The following materials are available online at http://www.mdpi.com/2072-6643/12/10/3037/s1, Table S1: Primer sequences employed in quantitative real-time PCR, Figure S1: *Inula britannica* flower aqueous extract (IAE) inhibits adipogenesis of 3T3-L1 preadipocytes via modulating the transcriptional expression, Figure S2: *Inula britannica* flower aqueous extract (IAE) inhibits proliferation of the 3T3-L1 preadipocytes during the MDI-induced MCE development, Figure S3: *Inula britannica* flower aqueous extract (IAE) inhibits the MDI-induced adipogenesis of 3T3-L1 preadipocytes by regulating the ERK 1/2 and Akt signaling pathways.

Author Contributions: Conceptualization, H.-S.Y. and H.-D.P.; Investigation, H.-S.Y., W.-J.K., and W.-Y.B.; Validation, H.-S.Y. and N.-K.L.; Supervision, N.-K.L. and H.-D.P.; Writing—original draft preparation, H.-S.Y.; Writing—review and editing, N.-K.L and H.-D.P. All authors have read and agreed to the published version of the manuscript.

Funding: This research received no external funding.

Conflicts of Interest: The authors declare no conflict of interest.

References

1. Konige, M.; Wang, H.; Szalryd, C. Role of adipose specific lipid droplet proteins in maintaining whole body energy homeostasis. *Biochim. Biophys. Acta Mol. Basis Dis.* **2014**, *1842*, 393–401. [CrossRef] [PubMed]
2. Graham, M.R.; Baker, J.S.; Davies, B. Causes and consequences of obesity: Epigenetics or hypokinesis? *Diabetes Meab. Syndr. Obes. Targets Ther.* **2015**, *8*, 455–460.

3. Apovian, C.M. Obesity: Definition, comorbidities, causes, and burden. *Am. J. Manag. Care* **2016**, *22*, s176–s185. [PubMed]
4. Jang, Y.J.; Koo, H.J.; Sohn, E.H.; Kang, S.C.; Rhee, D.K.; Pyo, S. Theobromine inhibits differentiation of 3T3-L1 cells during the early stage of adipogenesis via AMPK and MAPK signaling pathways. *Food Funct.* **2015**, *6*, 2365. [CrossRef]
5. Hales, C.; Carroll, M.; Fryar, C.; Ogden, C. Prevalence of Obesity and Severe Obesity among Adults: United States, 2017–2018. Available online: https://www.cdc.gov/nchs/products/databriefs/db360.htm (accessed on 27 September 2020).
6. Finkelstein, E.A.; Khavjou, O.A.; Thompson, H.; Trogdon, J.G.; Pan, L.; Sherry, B.; Dietz, W. Obesity and severe obesity forcasts through 2030. *Am. J. Prev. Med.* **2012**, *42*, 563–570. [CrossRef]
7. Lee, J.H.; Go, Y.; Lee, B.; Wang, Y.H.; Park, K.I.; Cho, W.K.; Ma, J.Y. The fruits of *Gleditsia sinensis* Lam. inhibits adipogenesis through modulation of mitotic clonal expansion and STAT3 activation in 3T3-L1 cells. *J. Ethnopharmacol.* **2018**, *222*, 61–70. [CrossRef]
8. Green, H.; Kehinde, O. Sublines of mouse 3T3 cells that accumulate lipid. *Cell* **1974**, *1*, 113–116. [CrossRef]
9. Gao, Y.; Koppen, A.; Rakhshandehroo, M.; Tasdelen, I.; van de Graaf, S.F.; van Loosdregt, J.; van Beekum, O.; Hamers, N.; van Leenen, D.; Berkers, C.R.; et al. Early adipogenesis is regulated through USP7-mediated deubiquitination of the histone acetyltransferase TIP60. *Nat. Commun.* **2013**, *4*, 1–10. [CrossRef]
10. Cristancho, A.G.; Lazar, M.A. Forming functional fat: A growing understanding of adipocyte differentiation. *Nat. Rev. Mol. Cell Biol.* **2011**, *12*, 722–734. [CrossRef]
11. Chae, S.Y.; Seo, S.G.; Yang, H.; Yu, J.G.; Suk, S.J.; Jung, E.S.; Ji, H.; Kwon, J.Y.; Lee, H.J.; Lee, K.W. Anti-adipogenic effect of erucin in early stage of adipogenesis by regulating Ras activity in 3T3-L1 preadipocytes. *J. Funct. Foods* **2015**, *19*, 700–709. [CrossRef]
12. Moseti, D.; Regassa, A.; Kim, W.K. Molecular regulation of adipogenesis and potential anti-adipogenic bioactive molecules. *Int. J. Mol. Sci.* **2016**, *17*, 124. [CrossRef]
13. Tang, Q.Q.; Otto, T.C.; Lane, M.D. Mitotic clonal expansion: A synchronous process required for adipogenesis. *Proc. Natl. Acad. Sci. USA* **2003**, *100*, 44–49. [CrossRef]
14. Chen, Q.; Hao, W.; Xiao, C.; Wang, R.; Xu, X.; Lu, H.; Chen, W.; Deng, C.X. SIRT6 is essential for adipocyte differentiation by regulating the mitotic clonal expansion. *Cell Rep.* **2017**, *18*, 3155–3166. [CrossRef]
15. Prusty, D.; Park, B.H.; Davis, K.E.; Farmer, S.R. Activation of MEK/ERK signaling promotes the adipogenesis by enhancing peroxisome proliferator-activated receptor γ (PPARγ) and C/EBPα gene expression during the differentiation of 3T3-L1 preadipocytes. *J. Biol. Chem.* **2002**, *277*, 46226–46232. [CrossRef] [PubMed]
16. Xu, J.; Liao, K. Protein kinase B/Akt 1 plays a pivotal role in insulin-like growth factor-1 receptor signaling induced 3T3-L1 adipocyte differentiation. *J. Biol. Chem.* **2004**, *279*, 35914–35922. [CrossRef] [PubMed]
17. Kang, H.J.; Seo, H.A.; Go, Y.; Oh, C.J.; Jeoung, N.H.; Park, K.G.; Lee, I.K. Dimethylfumarate suppresses adipogenic differentiation in 3T3-L1 preadipocytes through inhibition of STAT3 activity. *PLoS ONE* **2013**, *8*, e61411. [CrossRef] [PubMed]
18. Zhang, J.W.; Tang, Q.Q.; Vinson, C.; Lane, M.D. Dominant-negative C/EBP disrupts mitotic clonal expansion and differentiation of 3T3-L1 preadipocytes. *Proc. Natl. Acad. Sci. USA* **2004**, *101*, 43–47. [CrossRef]
19. Bae, W.Y.; Kim, H.Y.; Park, E.H.; Kim, K.T.; Paik, H.D. Improved in vitro antioxidant properties and hepatoprotective effects of a fermented *Inula britannica* extract on ethanol-damaged HepG2 cells. *Mol. Biol. Rep.* **2019**, *46*, 6053–6063. [CrossRef]
20. Zhang, H.; Tsao, R. Dietary polyphenols, oxidative stress and antioxidant and anti-inflammatory effects. *Curr. Opin. Food Sci.* **2016**, *8*, 33–42. [CrossRef]
21. Granato, D.; Mocan, A.; Câmara, J.S. Is a higher ingestion of phenolic compounds the best dietary strategy? A scientific opinion on the deleterious effects of polyphenols in vivo. *Trends Food Sci. Technol.* **2020**, *98*, 162–166. [CrossRef]
22. Chang, E.; Kim, C.Y. Natural products and obesity: A focus on the regulation of mitotic clonal expansion during adipogenesis. *Molecules* **2019**, *24*, 1157. [CrossRef] [PubMed]
23. Kim, H.Y.; Bae, W.Y.; Yu, H.S.; Chang, K.H.; Hong, Y.H.; Lee, N.K.; Paik, H.D. *Inula britannica* fermented with probiotic *Weissella cibaria* D30 exhibited anti-inflammatory effect and increased viability in RAW 264.7 cells. *Food Sci. Biotechnol.* **2020**, *29*, 569–578. [CrossRef] [PubMed]

24. Bae, W.Y.; Kim, H.Y.; Kim, K.T.; Paik, H.D. Inhibitory effects of *Inula britannica* extract fermented by *Lactobacillus plantarum* KCCM 11613P on coagulase activity and growth of *Staphylococcus aureus* including methicillin-resistant strains. *J. Food Biochem.* **2019**, *43*, e12785. [CrossRef]
25. Bae, W.Y.; Kim, H.Y.; Choi, K.S.; Chang, K.H.; Hong, Y.H.; Eun, J.; Lee, N.K.; Paik, H.D. Investigation of *Brassicajuncea, Forsythia suspensa*, and *Inula britannica*: Phytochemical properties, antiviral effects, and safety. *BMC Complement. Altern. Med.* **2019**, *19*, 253. [CrossRef]
26. Khan, A.L.; Hussain, J.; Hamayun, M.; Gilani, S.A.; Ahmad, S.; Rehman, G.; Kim, Y.H.; Kang, S.M.; Lee, I.J. Secondary metabolites from *Inula britannica* L. and their biological activities. *Molecules* **2010**, *15*, 1562–1577. [CrossRef] [PubMed]
27. Cai, Y.; Luo, Q.; Sun, M.; Corke, H. Antioxidant activity and phenolic compounds of 112 traditional Chinese medicinal plants associated with anticancer. *Life Sci.* **2004**, *74*, 2157–2184. [CrossRef]
28. Bai, N.; Zhou, Z.; Znu, N.; Zhang, L.; Quan, Z.; He, K.; Zheng, Q.Y.; Ho, C.T. Antioxidative flavonoids from the flower of *Inula britannica*. *J. Food Lipids* **2005**, *12*, 141–149. [CrossRef]
29. Hong, T.; Zhao, J.; Dong, M.; Meng, Y.; Mu, J.; Yang, Z. Composition and bioactivity of polysaccharides from *Inula britannica* flower. *Int. J. Biol. Macromol.* **2012**, *51*, 550–554. [CrossRef]
30. Kim, H.S.; Yu, H.S.; Lee, J.H.; Lee, G.H.; Choi, S.J.; Chang, P.S.; Paik, H.D. Application of stabilizer improves stability of nanosuspended branched-chain amino acids and anti-inflammatory effect in LPS-induced RAW 264.7 cells. *Food Sci. Biotechnol.* **2018**, *27*, 451–459. [CrossRef]
31. Yu, H.S.; Lee, N.K.; Choi, A.J.; Choe, J.S.; Bae, C.H.; Paik, H.D. Anti-inflammatory potential of probiotic strain *Weissella cibaria* JW15 isolated from kimchi through regulation of NF-κB and MAPKs pathways in LPS-induced RAW 264.7 cells. *J. Microbiol. Biotechnol.* **2019**, *29*, 1022–1032. [CrossRef]
32. Cabiati, M.; Raucci, S.; Caselli, C.; Guzzardi, M.A.; D'Amico, A.; Prescimone, T.; Giannessi, D.; del Ry, S. Tissue-specific selection of stable reference genes for real-time PCR normalization in an obese rat model. *J. Mol. Endocrinol.* **2012**, *48*, 251–260. [CrossRef] [PubMed]
33. Ross, S.E.; Erickson, R.L.; Hemati, N.; MacDougald, O.R. Glycogen synthase kinase 3 is an insulin-regulated C/EBPα kinase. *Mol. Cell. Biol.* **1999**, *19*, 8433–8441. [CrossRef]
34. Lee, Y.J.; Choi, H.S.; Seo, M.J.; Jeon, H.J.; Kim, K.J.; Lee, B.Y. Kaempferol suppresses lipid accumulation by inhibiting early adipogenesis in 3T3-L1 cells and zebrafish. *Food Funct.* **2015**, *6*, 2824. [CrossRef] [PubMed]
35. Kim, C.Y.; Kang, B.; Hong, J.; Choi, H.S. Parthenolide inhibits lipid accumulation via activation of Nrf2/Keap1 signaling during adipocyte differentiation. *Food Sci. Biotechnol.* **2020**, *29*, 431–440. [CrossRef] [PubMed]
36. Spalding, K.L.; Arner, E.; Westermark, P.O.; Bernard, S.; Buchholz, B.A.; Bergmann, O.; Blomqvist, L.; Hoffstedt, J.; Naslund, E.; Britton, T.; et al. Dynamics of fat cell turnover in humans. *Nature* **2008**, *453*, 783–787. [CrossRef]
37. Zakłos-Szyda, M.; Pietrzyk, N.; Szustak, M.; Podsedek, A. *Viburnum opulus* L. juice phenolics inhibits Mouse 3T3-L1 cells adipogenesis and pancreatic lipase activity. *Nutrients* **2020**, *12*, 2003. [CrossRef]
38. Rayalam, S.; Della-Fera, A.D.; Baile, C.A. Phytochemicals and regulation of the adipocyte life cycle. *J. Nutr. Biochem.* **2008**, *19*, 717–726. [CrossRef]
39. Feng, S.; Reuss, L.; Wang, Y. Potential of natural products in the inhibition of adipogenesis through regulation of PPARγ expression and/or its transcriptional activity. *Molecules* **2016**, *21*, 1278. [CrossRef]
40. Kim, S.J.; Choung, S.Y. Inhibitory effects of *Aster spathulifolius* extract on adipogenesis and lipid accumulation in 3T3-L1 preadipocytes. *J. Pharm. Pharmacol.* **2016**, *68*, 107–118. [CrossRef]
41. Darlington, G.J.; Wang, N.; Hanson, R.W. C/EBP α: A critical regulator of genes governing integrative metabolic processes. *Curr. Opin. Gent. Dev.* **1995**, *5*, 565–570. [CrossRef]
42. Jones, J.R.; Barrick, C.; Kim, K.A.; Lindner, J.; Blondeau, B.; Fujimoto, Y.; Shiota, M.; Kesterson, R.A.; Kahn, B.B.; Magnuson, M.A. Deletion of PPAR in adipose tissues of mice protects against high fat diet-induced obesity and insulin resistance. *Proc. Natl. Acad. Sci. USA* **2005**, *102*, 6207–6212. [CrossRef] [PubMed]
43. Gao, D.; Zhang, Y.; Yang, F.; Li, F.; Zhang, Q.; Xia, Z. The flower of *Edgeworthia gardneri* (wall.) Meisn. suppresses adipogenesis through modulation of the AMPK pathway in 3T3-L1 adipocytes. *J. Ethnopharmacol.* **2016**, *191*, 379–386. [CrossRef] [PubMed]
44. Merkestein, M.; Laber, S.; McMurray, F.; Andrew, D.; Sachse, G.; Sanderson, J.; Li, M.; Usher, S.; Sellaya, D.; Ashcroft, F.M.; et al. FTO influences adipogenesis by regulating mitotic clonal expansion. *Nat. Commun.* **2015**, *6*, 6792. [CrossRef] [PubMed]

45. Qiu, Z.; Wei, Y.; Chen, N.; Jiang, M.; Wu, J.; Liao, K. DNA synthesis and mitotic clonal expansion is not a required step for 3T3-L1 preadipocyte differentiation into adipocytes. *J. Biol. Chem.* **2001**, *276*, 11988–11995. [CrossRef]
46. Tang, Q.Q.; Ott, T.C.; Lane, M.D. CCAT/enhancer-binding protein β is required for mitotic clonal expansion during adipogenesis. *Proc. Natl. Acad. Sci. USA* **2003**, *100*, 850–855. [CrossRef]
47. Guo, L.; Li, X.; Huang, J.X.; Huang, H.Y.; Zhang, Y.Y.; He, Q.; Liu, Y.; Ma, C.G.; Tang, Q.Q. Transcriptional activation of histone H4 by C/EBPβ during the mitotic clonal expansion of 3T3-L1 adipocyte differentiation. *Cell Death Differ.* **2012**, *19*, 1917–1927. [CrossRef]
48. Sakai, T.; Sakaue, H.; Nakamura, T.; Okada, M.; Matsuki, Y.; Watanabe, E.; Hiramatsu, R.; Nakayama, K.; Nakayama, K.I.; Kasuga, M. Skp2 controls adipocyte proliferation during the development of obesity. *J. Biol. Chem.* **2007**, *282*, 2038–2046. [CrossRef]
49. Ferguson, B.S.; Nam, H.; Morrison, R.F. Curcumin inhibits 3T3-L1 preadipocyte proliferation by mechanisms involving post-transcriptional p27 regulation. *Biochem. Biophys. Rep.* **2016**, *5*, 16–21. [CrossRef]
50. Maki, C.; Funakoshi-Tago, M.; Aoyagi, R.; Ueda, F.; Kumura, M.; Kobata, K.; Tago, K.; Tamura, H. Coffee extract inhibits adipogenesis in 3T3-L1 preadipocyes by interrupting insulin signaling through the downregulation of IRS1. *PLoS ONE* **2017**, *12*, e0173264. [CrossRef]
51. Chayaratanasin, P.; Caobi, A.; Suparpprom, C.; Saense, S.; Pasukamonset, P.; Suanpairintr, N.; Barbieri, M.A.; Adisakwattana, S. *Clitoria ternatea* flower petal extract inhibits adipogenesis and lipid accumulation in 3T3-L1 preadipocytes by downregulating adipogenic gene expression. *Molecules* **2019**, *24*, 1894. [CrossRef]
52. Abood, S.; Veisaga, M.; López, L.; Barbieri, M. Dehydroleucodine inhibits mitotic clonal expansion during adipogenesis through cell cycle arrest. *Phytother. Res.* **2018**, *32*, 1583–1592. [CrossRef] [PubMed]
53. Bost, F.; Aouadi, M.; Caron, L.; Even, P.; Belmonte, N.; Prot, M.; Dani, C.; Hofman, P.; Pagès, G.; Pouysségur, J.; et al. The extracellular signal-regulated kinase isoform ERK1 is specifically required for in vitro and in vivo adipogenesis. *Diabetes* **2005**, *54*, 402–411. [CrossRef] [PubMed]
54. Cho, A.S.; Jeon, S.M.; Kim, M.J.; Yeo, J.; Seo, K.I.; Choi, M.S.; Lee, M.K. Chlorogenic acid exhibits anti-obesity property and improves lipid metabolism in high-fat diet-induced-obese mice. *Food Chem. Toxicol.* **2010**, *48*, 937–943. [CrossRef] [PubMed]
55. Park, S.H.; Lee, D.H.; Kim, M.J.; Ahn, J.; Jang, Y.J.; Ha, T.Y.; Jung, C.H. *Inula japonica* Thunb. flower ethanol extract improves obesity and exercise endurance in mice fed a high-fat diet. *Nutrients* **2019**, *11*, 17. [CrossRef] [PubMed]

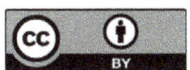

© 2020 by the authors. Licensee MDPI, Basel, Switzerland. This article is an open access article distributed under the terms and conditions of the Creative Commons Attribution (CC BY) license (http://creativecommons.org/licenses/by/4.0/).

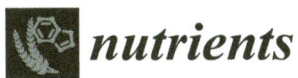

Review

Nutraceutical Properties of Polyphenols against Liver Diseases

Jorge Simón [1,2,*,†], **María Casado-Andrés** [3,†], **Naroa Goikoetxea-Usandizaga** [1,2], **Marina Serrano-Maciá** [1,2] **and María Luz Martínez-Chantar** [1,2]

1. Liver Disease Laboratory, Center for Cooperative Research in Biosciences (CIC bioGUNE), Basque Research and Technology Alliance (BRTA), Bizkaia Technology Park, Building 801A, 48160 Derio, Bizkaia, Spain; ngoikoetxea@cicbiogune.es (N.G.-U.); mserrano@cicbiogune.es (M.S.-M.); mlmartinez@cicbiogune.es (M.L.M.-C.)
2. Centro de Investigación Biomédica en Red de Enfermedades Hepáticas y Digestivas (CIBERehd), 48160 Derio, Bizkaia, Spain
3. Cell Biology and Histology Department, University of the Basque Country (UPV/EHU), Barrio Sarriena, S/N, 48940 Leioa, Spain; mdcasado002@gmail.com
* Correspondence: jsimon@cicbiogune.es; Tel.: +34-944-061304
† These authors contributed equally to this work.

Received: 14 October 2020; Accepted: 12 November 2020; Published: 15 November 2020

Abstract: Current food tendencies, suboptimal dietary habits and a sedentary lifestyle are spreading metabolic disorders worldwide. Consequently, the prevalence of liver pathologies is increasing, as it is the main metabolic organ in the body. Chronic liver diseases, with non-alcoholic fatty liver disease (NAFLD) as the main cause, have an alarming prevalence of around 25% worldwide. Otherwise, the consumption of certain drugs leads to an acute liver failure (ALF), with drug-induced liver injury (DILI) as its main cause, or alcoholic liver disease (ALD). Although programs carried out by authorities are focused on improving dietary habits and lifestyle, the long-term compliance of the patient makes them difficult to follow. Thus, the supplementation with certain substances may represent a more easy-to-follow approach for patients. In this context, the consumption of polyphenol-rich food represents an attractive alternative as these compounds have been characterized to be effective in ameliorating liver pathologies. Despite of their structural diversity, certain similar characteristics allow to classify polyphenols in 5 groups: stilbenes, flavonoids, phenolic acids, lignans and curcuminoids. Herein, we have identified the most relevant compounds in each group and characterized their main sources. By this, authorities should encourage the consumption of polyphenol-rich products, as most of them are available in quotidian life, which might reduce the socioeconomical burden of liver diseases.

Keywords: polyphenols; liver; stilbenes; flavonoids; phenolic acids; lignans; curcuminoids; NAFLD; HCC; DILI; ALF; ALD

1. Introduction

Current food tendencies and suboptimal dietary habits, together with an unhealthy lifestyle, are leading to the development of metabolic pathologies and their spreading worldwide [1,2]. In this context, the prevalence of liver pathologies is increasing among population, as this organ is responsible for the metabolism of exogenous substances in the organism [3]. Chronic liver pathologies, one of the leading mortality causes in USA and Europe, have on nutritional imbalances and sedentary habits their main causative agent nowadays. Non-alcoholic fatty liver disease (NAFLD) has emerged as the most frequent form of chronic liver disease worldwide, with an estimated prevalence of around 25% of general population [4,5]. Indeed, such elevated prevalence is expected to even increase within next years due to the rising of comorbidities from metabolic syndrome (MetS), making NAFLD a global health problem [6,7]. The term NAFLD is used to define a group of hepatic disorders that go from a simple lipid accumulation in the hepatocyte (steatosis) to its progression into more severe stages as non-alcoholic steatohepatitis (NASH), characterized by lipid-derived inflammation, hepatocellular ballooning and fibrosis. In case of a chronic fibrosis development, hepatocyte cell death and extracellular matrix (ECM) deposition, NASH may turn into cirrhosis. Moreover, the risk of developing NAFLD highly rises up the risk of developing hepatocellular carcinoma (HCC), the most frequent form of liver cancer [6,8–10].

Until date, the two-hit or multiple-hit hypothesis is the most extended explanation for the progression of NAFLD, in which a first hit induced steatosis and the aberrant lipid homeostasis leads to derived complications that contribute to its aggravation [11]. Related to the first hit, two imbalances have been reported to promote hepatic lipid accumulation, between: (i) fatty acid uptake and very-low-density lipoprotein (VLDL) export and (ii) de novo lipogenesis and fatty acid oxidation (FAO). Indeed, the metabolic triggering of the pathology has led to propose a new term MAFLD, metabolic-associated fatty liver disease, to define this group of pathologies [12]. Then, the appearance of second hits such as peroxidation, oxidative and reticulum stress development and mitochondrial dysfunction triggers an inflammatory response that may result in fibrosis development. In this process, the hepatocyte suffers from an antioxidant machinery depletion that finally leads to its death and, in the meantime, macrophage activation by pro-inflammatory cytokines such as tumor-necrosis factor (TNF) or several interleukine (IL) isoforms. Thus, hepatic stellate cells (HSC) are activate and proliferate by several signaling pathways such as transforming growth factor-beta (TGF-β)/SMAD, promoting collagen synthesis and ECM deposition, in which the matrix metalloproteinases (MMP)/tissue inhibitor of metalloproteinases (TIMP) is essential [13]. Regarding HCC development, the heterogeneity of the disease implies different molecular signaling pathways activated at the same time to deregulate hepatocyte growth, proliferation, differentiation and apoptosis. Several pro-proliferative pathways and signaling occur such as protein kinase B (AKT), nuclear factor-kappa B (NF-κB), mammalian target of rapamycin (mTOR) or c-MYC [14].

Furthermore, unhealthy lifestyle does not necessarily mean an inadequate food intake, but also into the excessive consumption of certain prescription and non-prescription medications or toxic compounds. As a consequence, liver can suffer from an acute liver failure (ALF) with drug-induced liver injury (DILI) as its main cause [15–17]. DILI is estimated to affect 14 of 100,000 inhabitants worldwide and it presents a real challenge to gastroenterologists when diagnosing the pathology [18]. The liver is the organ responsible of the metabolism of exogenous compounds. Under overdose conditions, compounds such as acetaminophen or carbon tetrachloride are converted by cytochrome P450 2E1 (CYP2E1) into toxic compounds by the hepatocyte [19]. These toxic compounds deplete the anti-oxidant machinery of the cell, mainly composed by reduced glutathione (GSH), catalase (CAT) and superoxide dismutase (SOD). The direct impact they have over mitochondrial integrity causes a damage that finally results on the necrosis of the hepatocyte [20,21]. During DILI, the release of mitochondrial pro-apoptotic proteins such as BAX or BCL-2 and the TNF- or NF-κB-mediated pro-inflammatory signaling are key hallmarks [22].

Additionally, the chronic and heavy consumption of alcohol leads to the development of steatosis in 90% of patients who drink over 60 g of alcohol per day and cirrhosis in 30% cases [23], making alcoholic liver disease (ALD) to follow a similar pattern of progression as NAFLD. Similarly to DILI, CYP2E1-mediated metabolism of ethanol leads to the production of acetaldehyde that leads to mitochondrial dysfunction [24] that impairs lipid homeostasis in the hepatocyte causing steatosis. The increased oxidative stress and depletion of anti-oxidant activity of the hepatocyte, together with aberrant lipid metabolism by peroxidation, induce a hepatocellular damage that promotes the progression of the disease from alcoholic steatosis to hepatitis and finally cirrhosis [24]. The molecular basis of ALD progression from steatosis to cirrhosis follow similar molecular mechanisms to NAFLD, including an inflammatory environment and HSC proliferation and activation [24].

Considering the elevated prevalence of aforementioned liver pathologies and their expected increase, together with the lack of awareness of general population, authorities are focusing on reducing their prevalence and improving their prognosis [25]. Clinical and scientific studies point out lifestyle modifications as the mainstay and cornerstone in treating these pathologies, comprising adequate meal plans and physical activity [26,27]. Although behavioral interventions attempt to guarantee the adherence of the patients, in most of cases it is hard to achieve so they do not follow the designed plans.

Therefore, the supplementation with certain products may offer a more easy-to-adhere approach in order to prevent or improve liver pathologies. In this context, current evidence highlights the beneficial properties associated to polyphenols, a group of natural metabolites contained in plants that own a variety of beneficial effects for the liver and associated comorbidities. They play a role in the regulation of oxidative stress, the lipid metabolism, the development of insulin resistance, inflammation or body weight among others [28,29]. Moreover, they are capable of attenuate drug-induced toxicity by reducing apoptosis and enhancing the expression of antioxidant enzymes [30]. Thus, they offer an attractive nutraceutical approach not only for reducing the impact and prevalence of chronic liver diseases, but also for ameliorating the prognosis of acute liver alterations.

The aim of the present review is to highlight the benefits of polyphenols intake and identify the main polyphenol-rich sources. By this, we propose a change in dietary lifestyle pattern by presenting such polyphenol-rich foods, which can be easily introduced in the diet. Considering their nutraceutical value, they may represent a strategic approach in which future dietary guidelines and public health recommendations should be based on.

2. Polyphenols and Their Nutraceutical Value

Polyphenols are a large group of at least 10,000 different naturally occurring phytochemicals, with one or more aromatic rings and with one or more hydroxyl functional groups attached. They are secondary metabolites that represent a large and diverse group of substances abundantly present in vegetables, fruits, cereals, spices, teas, rizhomes, medical plants and flowers [29,31].

Although the diversity of their chemical structure makes their classification difficult, the number of phenol rings and the structural elements allows to distinguish between certain groups of polyphenols. So that, according to their structural similarities polyphenols can be grouped in stilbenes, flavonoids, phenolic acids, lignans and curcuminoids [31,32]. In the following work, the main polyphenolic compounds of each group, their beneficial properties for certain liver pathologies and their main food source will be deeply described.

2.1. Stilbenes

Stilbenes are phytochemicals, some of which are considered phytoalexins, mainly present in berries, grapes, peanuts and red wine. This group of polyphenols is composed by three main compounds: resveratrol and its derived compounds pterostilbene and piceatannol [32,33].

Resveratrol may be one of the most popular polyphenols in our society and it is found in coco, mulberries, peanuts, soy and grapes [34]. Preclinical studies have characterized its protective features at multiple levels, by modulating oxidative stress and hepatocellular damage in order to ameliorate NAFLD through the reduction of free radicals and pro-inflammatory cytokines and the increased response of anti-oxidant enzymes such as glutathione (GSH) and cytochrome P450 (CYP) 2E1 [35,36]. Moreover, resveratrol reduces hepatic lipid content by reducing sirtuin 1 (SIRT1)-mediated lipogenic activity through the modulation of acyl-coA carboxylase (ACC), peroxisome proliferation activity receptor γ (PPARγ) and sterol response element binding protein-1 (SREBP-1) [37].

As aforementioned, pterostilbene is a derivate from resveratrol which is mainly present in blueberries [38]. This compound is also reported to reduce steatosis and modify hepatic fatty acid profile stimulating carnitine-palmitoyltransferase-1 (CPT1)-mediated FAO, stimulating microsomal triglyceride transfer protein (MTP)-mediated very-low-density lipoprotein (VLDL) export and reducing lipid uptake by CD36 [39]. Likewise, it enhances liver glucokinase and glucose-6-phosphatase activity to ameliorate insulin resistance and hepatic glycogen homeostasis and, therefore, lowering total cholesterol and triglyceride levels in serum [40].

Another derivate from the hydroxylation of resveratrol is piceatannol, present in grapes, passion fruit and peanut calluses [33]. Although this compound has been less studied than resveratrol due to its lower concentration in food, it has been reported to have a higher activity [41]. Thus, piceatannol also improves hepatic glycemic control by activating adenosine monophosphate-activated protein kinase (AMPK) through phosphorylation while ameliorating serum lipid profile in mice inhibiting the lipogenic flux mediated by ACC and fatty acid synthase (FAS) expression [42] Piceatannol-mediated AMPK phosphorylation also induces autophagy, a process reported to be dysregulated in NAFLD [43].

Regarding the effects of stilbenes among human population, clinical trials have been carried out only by evaluating the properties of resveratrol in NAFLD, liver cancer and hepatitis patients. Remarkably, the dietary supplementation with resveratrol has been shown to be effective in improving the inflammatory marker profile in NAFLD patients [44].

2.2. Flavonoids

Flavonoids comprise the larger group of polyphenols and the most abundant compounds in human diet. They are characterized by a C6-C3-C6 backbone structure and appear in almost all foods of vegetable origin and, particularly, in apples, berries, citrus fruits, onions, red wine, grapes, tea or olive oil [31]. Flavonoids are classified into six additional subgroups: anthocyanins, flavanols, flavanones, flavonols, flavones and isoflanoids. In the following section a detailed description of each subgroup and their main compounds is provided.

First, the subgroup of anthocyanins is composed by water-soluble flavonoid species as delphinidin, pelargonidin, cyanidin and malvidin. Delphinidin appears in flowers and berries as blueberry, Saskatoon berry, raspberry, strawberry or chokecherry, being its richest natural source the Maqui berry [45]. They have been reported to have anti-inflammatory properties targeting nuclear factor kappa-B (NF-κB), activator protein-1 (AP-1) and cyclooxygenase-2 (COX-2) [46]. Moreover, delphindin prevents triglyceride accumulation in in vitro NASH models modulating AMPK and FAS [47] or to downregulate fibrogenic stimuli to prevent fibrosis development in preclinical models [48]. Therein, fibrogenic response is attenuated by a decreased oxidative stress development, increasing matrix metalloproteinase (MMP)-9 and metallothionein (MT) I/II expression [48]. Although pelargonidins have been less studied, their protective properties against lipopolysaccharide (LPS)-induced liver injury have been characterized by modulating the inflammatory pathway mediated by toll-like receptor (TLR) [49]. This polyphenolic compound is mainly present in orange- or red-color fruits as raspberries, blackberries, strawberries or plums [50]. On another hand, cyanidin have been reported to promote lipid oxidative flux by increasing CPT1 and PPARα expression to enhance FAO and by decreasing FAS and SREBP-1 expression to downregulate lipogenesis [51]. Cyanidin prevents fibrosis development inhibiting collagen type I synthesis and downregulating extracellular-regulated kinase 1/2 (ERK1/2) [52], while promotes cAMP-mediated protein kinase A (PKA) activation to induce glutathione (GSH) synthesis and protect the hepatocyte [53]. Additionally, hepatocellular damage derived from alcoholic toxicity is also prevented by activating AMPK, that induces autophagy [54]. Cyanidins are present in red berries, grapes, bilberry, blackberry, blueberry, cherry, cranberry, elderberry, hawthorn, loganberry, açaai berry and raspberry [55]. Similar to cyanidin, malvidin is present in red grapes, cranberries, blueberries and black rice. They have been reported to increase FAO in the same way as cyanidins [51], and, remarkably, to attenuate tumor growth in HCC by regulating BAX and caspase-3 for apoptosis; several cyclin isoforms and phosphatase and tensin homolog (PTEN) for proliferation and metastasis derived from MMP-2/9 activity [56].

Secondly, flavanols share a general chemical structure of two rings linked by three carbons forming an oxygenated heterocyclic ring [57]. Among them epicatechin, epigallocatechin and its gallate derivate (EGCG) and procyanidins are the most popular compounds. Epicatechin is mainly present in dark chocolate and cocoa [58] and it has been reported to regulate lipid profile in serum and liver through regulating SREBP, FAS, liver X receptor (LXR) and SIRT [59]; as well as to attenuate oxidative stress and inflammatory injury via abrogation of NF-κB signaling pathway [60]. EGCGs, mainly present in green tea [61], may be another one of the most popular polyphenols in society normally sold as green tea extract. Their biological effects on NAFLD have been characterized in terms of lipid metabolism via pAMPK, SREBP-1, FAS and ACC; the oxidative response mediated by CYP2E1 or malonaldehyde production; TNF and IL-mediated inflammation and the fibrosis development induced by TGF-β/SMAD pathway [62]. EGCG also decreases body weight and reduces liver injury mediated by oxidative stress and inflammatory response, reducing the formation of collagen and alpha-smooth muscle actin (αSMA) in the liver and the expression of tissue inhibitor of metalloproteinase-2 (TIMP-2) in preclinical studies [63]. Moreover, EGCG has a protective effect on hepatotoxicity by decreasing bile acid and lipid absorption [60] and lowering cytochrome P450 (CYP)-mediated activation and toxicity of acetaminophen in DILI [64]. Related to HCC, EGCG has been also characterized to promote apoptosis in cancer cells in a multifactor way targeting genes involved in initiation (like NF-κB or BCL-2), proliferation (like cMyc, ERK1/2 or DDR mechanisms) and invasion (like MMPs or COX-2). [65]. The antioxidant properties of the last compound, procyanidins, have been also reported in fibrosis animal models via inhibition of CYP2E1-mediated metabolism of toxic compounds and improving antioxidant capacity through GSH or superoxide dismutase (SOD) [66]. Additionally, procyanidins exert a protective effect against ALD ameliorating SREBP-1-mediated steatosis and inflammation via IL-6 or TNF [67], with a possible involvement in preventing mitochondrial dysfunction and apoptosis [68]. Procyanidins are present in chocolate, apples, red grapes and cranberries [69].

The subgroup of flavanones is smaller than the previous one, as only hesperidin and naringenin compose it. Both compounds are characterized by a double bond between C2 and C3 and the lack of the oxygenation in C3 [70]. On one hand, hesperidin is mainly found in citrus fruits (grapefruit, lemon, lime or orange) and peppermint [71,72]. Similarly to other flavonoids, this compound has been found to protect against fibrosis enhancing GSH and decreasing catalase (CAT) and SOD levels [73]. Likewise, hesperidin reduced development of hepatic oxidative stress, dyslipidemia and histological changes via decreasing lipid peroxidation and recovering hepatocyte antioxidant properties [74]. On the other hand, naringenin is mainly found in Mexican oregano [75]. This flavanone's beneficial effects have been studied over DILI by downregulating caspase-3, BAX and BCL [76]. Hepatoxocity-induced fibrosis is also inhibited by naringenin, that inhibits the development of oxidative stress, the activation of HSC mediated TGF-β and the synthesis of ECM [77].

Flavonols present a large group of polyphenols in which quercetin is one of the most important flavonoids and, in addition, kaempferol, myricetin, isorhamnetin and galangin also compose this group. Quercetin is found in a variety of food that includes apples, berries, brassica vegetables, capers, grapes, onions, shallots, tea, tomatoes, many seeds and nuts [78,79]. This flavonol has been characterized to ameliorate fibrosis development by targeting NF-κB-mediated signal transduction, downregulating TNF, IL-6, IL-1β and IL-8 cytokines production [78], together with an increase of the antioxidant mechanisms mediated by GSH and IL-10 and decreasing lipid peroxidation in ALD [79]. Kampferol, present in tea, broccoli, apples, strawberries and beans [80] prevents tumor development by enhancing PTEN expression and inactivate PI3K/Akt/mTOR signaling in order to inhibit migration, proliferation and invasion [81]. Otherwise, CYP2E1 inhibition by kaempferol protects the hepatocyte against ALD development [82], whereas fibrosis development is attenuated by the inhibition of SMAD2/3 via the direct interaction between kaempferol and ATP-binding pocker of activing receptor-like kinase 5 (ALK5) [83]. Myricetin is found in berries, honey, vegetables, teas and wines [84]. This flavonolic compound has a regressive effect on steatosis development in preclinical NASH models by promoting NRF2-mediated mitochondrial functionality, which increases antioxidative enzyme activities and PPAR-mediated fat decomposition [85]. Miricetin-mediated YAP downregulation also leads this polyphenol to exert anti-tumoral properties [86]. Isorhamnetin also alleviates steatosis decreasing FAS activity and fibrosis development via TGF-β-mediated HSC activation and proliferation [87], while decreasing the production of lipoperoxide compounds in serum and liver [88]. This compound is present in pears, onion, olive oil, grapes, tomato and the spice, Mexican Tarragon [80,89]. The last flavonol, galangin, is less abundant in nature as it is mainly present in galangal rizhome and propolis [90]. Similar to myricetin, galangin-mediated NRF2 activation attenuates oxidative damage, inflammation and apoptosis during hepatotoxicity [91], while inhibiting the proliferation of HCC cells through the combined activation of NRF2 and hemooxygenase-1 (HO-1) [92].

The fifth flavonoid subgroup are flavones, distinguished by their double bond between C2 and C3, the lack of substitution at the C3 and the oxidation in C4 [93]. In this subgroup apigenin, chrysin and luteolin are the most relevant compounds. Apigenin is present in vegetables as parsley, broccoli, celery and onions; in fruits as oranges, olives, cherries and tomatoes; in herbs as chamomile, thyme, oregano, basil; and plant-based beverages as tea [93]. Between the beneficial properties of apigenin, it should be noted its anti-inflammatory properties against ALD by regulating CYP2E1-mediated oxidative stress and PPARα-mediated lipogenic gene expression [94] and the prospective effect for the damage induced by ischemia-reperfusion by suppressing inflammation, oxidative stress and apoptosis mediated by BAX and BCL-2 [95]. Additionally, this compound has been also characterized to ameliorate serum and hepatic lipid profile via metabolic and transcriptional modulations in the liver in genes involves in FAO, tricarboxylic acid cycle and oxidative phosphorylation among other [96]. Chrysin is specially present in honey and propolis [97] and this flavone has been reported to ameliorate NAFLD by modulating TNF- and IL-6-derived inflammatory response and SREBP-1-mediated lipogenesis in rats [98] and to reduce fibrosis development in a dose-dependent way via regulating MMP/TIMP imbalance [99]. Otherwise, luteolin is found in vegetables and fruits such as celery, parsley, broccoli, onion, carrots, peppers, cabbages or apple skins [100]. The protective properties of luteolin have been studied in DILI, where it restores the synthesis of antioxidant compounds as GSH while decreasing the inflammation signaling via TNF, NF-κB and IL-6 signaling and decreasing endoplasmic reticulum stress as well [101]. It also protects from developing liver pathologies derived from the chronic consumption of toxic substances as mercury, promoting mitochondrial functionality via NRF-2/NF-κB/P53 signaling [102] or alcoholic liver disease (ALD), where it downregulates the expression of SREBP-1 and recovers the AMPK activity [103].

The last subclass of flavonoids are isoflavonoids, where genistein and daidzein are the most common compounds. Genistein is found in soybeans and soy-based food and formulas, nuts and legumes as peas or lentils [104]. Its protective properties have been characterized on NAFLD by modulating PPARα-mediated lipid metabolism [105], while it also ameliorates hepatic inflammation by reducing TLR4 expression [106] and fibrosis development by decreasing lipid peroxidation and increasing GSH levels [107]. Similarly to genistein, daidzein is also found in the same food sources and the supplementation of daidzein, although it is less effective [108], has been reported to alleviate NAFLD by upregulating FAO and downregulating TNF expression [109].

Regarding the clinical trials carried out to determine the effect of flavonoids in human population, the effect of hesperidin supplementation has been studied in NASH development finding an improvement in steatosis, hepatic enzymes and several parameters as glycaemia [110]. A clinical study about naringenin has proposed this compound as an attractive approach for treating hepatitis C [111], while quercetin has been characterized to attenuate the secretion of the virus [112]. Additional clinical studies expected within next years will evaluate the effect of camu, a food rich in procyanidins, in obesity-related disorders as NAFLD and the effect of EGCG in cancer development from cirrhosis.

2.3. Phenolic Acids

This group of polyphenols is constituted by phenolic compounds, having one carboxylic group and typically in bound form as amides, esters or glycosides. They are found in a variety of plant-based foods, seeds, skins or fruits and leaves of vegetables [113]. In the meantime, phenolic acids are divided into hydroxibenzoic acids, hydroxycinnamic acids and oleuropeunosides.

On one hand, hydroxibenzoic acids possess a common structure of C6-C1 derived from benzoic acid [113], being ellagic and gallic the most common compounds. Ellagic acid may be the most common compound in this subclass and it is present in nuts, walnuts, berries and fruits as pomegranates or berries [114]. This molecule has been reported to normalize the activity of antioxidative enzymes and to ameliorate histopathology by reducing inflammatory response via modulating oxidative stress [115], also reducing oxidative stress after ischemia-reperfusion liver injury [116] or impeding hepatotoxicity-derived fibrosis development in preclinical studies via downregulating caspase-3, BCL-2 and NF-κB expression while elevating NRF-2-mediated mitochondrial functionality [117]. Similarly to ellagic acid, gallic acid is found in berries as blueberries and strawberries, and fruits as mango [118]. This compound has been reported to exert protective properties in liver damage induced by drug abuse by reducing TNF-mediated inflammation and lipid peroxidation [119]. Moreover, gallic acid increases GSH and CAT antioxidative activities to protect the hepatocyte from ischemia-reperfusion [120] and decreases fibrosis development by restoring GSH and TGF-β levels while normalizing HSC activation and proliferation [121].

On the other hand, hydroxycinnamic acids derive from cinnamic acid and they are often present in food as simple esters with quinic acid or glucose [113], being ferulic and chlorogenic acids the most frequent compounds. Ferulic acid is found in commelinid plants as rice, wheat, oats or grains, and in vegetables, pineapple, beans, coffee, artichoke, peanut or nuts [122]. Similarly to hydroxybenzoic compounds, it upregulates NRF-2/HO-1 signaling to restore mitochondrial integrity and reduce the development of oxidative stress and inflammation in DILI [123], whereas it prevents fibrosis development by interfering in TGF-β/SMAD-mediated activation of HSCs [124]. Chlorogenic acid is particularly found in the coffee grain but it is also present in beans, potato tubers, fruits as apple and prunes [125]. This hydroxycinnamic compound also fibrosis development mediated by pro-inflammatory citokines such as TNF, IL-6 and IL-1β [126] and scavenges ROS production in alcohol consumption, reducing the steatosis, apoptosis and fibrosis development pathways mediated by TNF and TGF-β [127].

Oleuropein is mainly present in olive leaves, olives, virgin olive oil and olive mill waste [128]. Interestingly, this polyphenol has been shown to exert anti-inflammatory properties by scavenging ROS production under hepatotoxic conditions [129] and reduce lipid-derived inflammatory processes to prevent NASH progression such as TLR-mediated response [130].

Concerning the properties of phenolic acids in the human organism, clinical trials have been only developed by evaluating NAFLD development with a gallic acid-rich compound (Ajwa Date) and coffee supplementation, rich in chlorogenic acid. Although liver diseases were studied in the clinical trial evaluating Ajwa Date, outcomes have been focused on the prevention of atherosclerosis development. The results from the other clinical trial with coffee supplementation have not been published yet.

2.4. Lignans

Lignans are characterized by two phenylpropane units linked by a C6-C3 bond between the central atoms of the respective side chains. This group of polyphenols is present in a wide variety of plans in which latter, flaxseed and sesame seed represent the richest sources [131]. Moreover, lignans can be also found in fish, whole-grain cereals (as wheat or oats), meat, oilseed (as flax or soy) and beverages (as coffee, tea or wine) [131]. Although it can be distinguished among classical lignans, neolignans, flavonolignans and carbohydrate-conjugates, the main compounds present in nature are sesamin and diglucoside.

Sesamin is mainly present in sesame seeds and preclinical studies have reported metabolic properties in liver pathologies by preventing from ACC- [132] and SREBP-1-mediated fatty acid synthesis [133], while enhances FAO mediated by CPT1 or 3-hydroxyacyl-coA dehydrogenase [132]. Otherwise, diglucoside is found in flaxseed [134] and this compound has been also reported to downregulate hepatic lipid accumulation, while downregulating hepatic lipid peroxidation and decreasing cholesterol in serum [135].

Until date, no clinical trials for evaluating lignans have been carried out.

2.5. Curcuminoids

Regarding the group of curcuminoids, curcumin is the main compound as it gives the name to this group. This compound is the principal extract from the turmeric (Curcumula longa) herb [136] and preclinical approaches have characterized its anti-inflammatory and anti-oxidant properties derived from the intake of hepatotoxic compounds [137]. Curcumin alleviates hepatic dyslipidemia by inhibiting lipogenesis and promoting FAO, while enhancing cholesterol efflux and, in the meantime, reducing the lipid imbalance-derived oxidative stress [137]. By this, the expression of NRF-2 restores mitochondrial integrity in the hepatocyte, while GSH increase leads to an enhanced antioxidant capacity thus downregulating HSC activation [137].

There are currently three clinical trials under recruitment in order to evaluate the effects of different forms of curcumin, as dietary supplement or conjugated to phosphatidylcholine, in the development of NAFLD and insulin resistance. Another clinical trial has proven its effectivity in reducing steatosis, reducing body-mass index and improving serum profile in terms of cholesterol, triglycerides and transaminases [138].

3. Discussion

It is a fact that current unhealthy food tendencies, accompanied by a more sedentary lifestyle, have a direct impact over the health of global population [1]. Metabolic disorders are spreading worldwide and, among them, liver pathologies are on the most extended ones. Non-alcoholic fatty liver disease or NAFLD has an alarming prevalence of 25% worldwide and it is even expected to increase within next years due to such unhealthy lifestyle [5]. Otherwise, the excessive drug consumption that sometimes takes place can also lead to other liver pathologies, reaching an acute liver failure (ALF) in which drug-induced liver injury (DILI) is the main cause affecting [18] and chronic alcohol consumption leads to the development of alcoholic liver diseases (ALD) [23]. The management of liver pathologies presents a challenge to authorities and, although dietary and behavioral plans are currently being carried out, the long-term compliance of population sometimes presents the true challenge. Therefore, the supplementation or feeding with certain products can offer a more easy-to-adhere strategy in terms of preventing or ameliorating both chronic and acute liver diseases. Related to this, in the present work the role of different polyphenols has been described in detail as well as the most relevant clinical trials about them (Table 1). Overall, all polyphenols [26,31] described in the present review are reported to have beneficial properties towards either preventing or ameliorating NAFLD, DILI or ALD. Although some of them as resveratrol, EGCG, or curcumin are more popular in society, any of these compounds may offer healthy properties for the liver.

Thus, the consumption of polyphenol-rich food is a suitable option when planning a diet. As it can be observed in Table 2, most of them are present in foods that can be easily found in any supermarket so general population might not have problems when acquiring them. Therefore, it is an interesting point that authorities promote the consumption of these kind of foods when designing their programs for creating awareness, especially in such patients of liver diseases who are under treatment. Reducing their prize or promoting their inclusion in certain products or meals (e.g., strawberries in yogurts or coffee in some drinks) might be adequate options. Moreover, as it can be observed in Table 2, most part of the polyphenol-rich foods are not high-calorie so their inclusion should not have an impact over total daily calorie intake, another concern in the development of MetS and related metabolic disorders [139]. Furthermore, it must be always taken into account that not only polyphenols but also other micronutrients present beneficial properties, and the existence of variety in a diet is which makes it healthy.

Table 1. Clinical trials testing polyphenols against liver pathologies.

Polyphenol	Group/Subgroup	Pathology	Outcome
Resveratrol	Stilbenes	NAFLD, HCC, Hepatitis	Improved inflammatory profile in NAFLD [44].
Hesperidin	Flavonoids/Flavanones	NASH	Ameliorated steatosis, hepatic enzymes and glycaemia [110].
Naringenin	Flavonoids/Flavanones	Hepatitis C	Ameliorated phenotype [111].
Quercetin	Flavonoids/Flavonols	Hepatitis C	Attenuated secretion of the virus [112]
Procyanidins	Procyanidins/Flavanols	NAFLD	Not finished
EGCG	Flavonoids/Flavanols	Cirrhosis-derived HCC	Not finished
Gallic acid	Phenolic acids/Hydroxibenzoic acids	NAFLD	Atherosclerosis reduction.
Chlorogenic acid	Phenolic acids/Hydroxicinnamic acids	NAFLD	Not published
Curcumin	Curcuminoids	NAFLD	Reduction in steatosis and body-mass index and improved serum profile [138]

Table 2. List of most relevant polyphenols, their richest sources and pathologies with potential beneficial properties with each respective molecular target.

Polyphenol	Group/Subgroup	Source	Liver Pathology	Molecular Targets
Resveratrol	Stilbenes	Coco, mulberries, peanuts, soy and grapes [34]	Steatosis/NASH	Glutathione, CYP2E1 [35,36]
			Steatosis	SIRT1, ACC, PPARγ, SREBP-1 [37]
Pterostilbene	Stilbenes	Blueberries [38]	Steatosis	Glucokinase, Glucose-6-phosphatase [40]
			Steatosis	CPT1, MTP, CD36 [39]
Piceatannol	Stilbenes	Grapes, passion fruit and peanut calluses [33]	Steatosis	AMPK, ACC, FAS and autophagy [42]
			NASH/ALD	NF-κB, AP-1, COX-2 [46]
Delphinidin	Flavonoids/anthocyanins	Flowers, blueberry, Saskatoon berry, raspberry, strawberry, chokecherry, Maqui berry [45]	Steatosis	AMPK, FAS [47]
			Fibrosis	Oxidative stress, MMP-9 and MT [48]
Pelargonidin	Flavonoids/Anthocyanins	Raspberries, blackberries, strawberries or plums [50]	NASH/ALD	TLR [49]
			Steatosis	CPT1, PPARα, FAS, SREBP-1 [51]
Cyanidin	Flavonoids/Anthocyanins	Red berries, grapes, bilberry, blackberry, blueberry, cherry, cranberry, elderberry, hawthorn, loganberry, açaai berry and raspberry [55]	Fibrosis	Collagen I, ERK 1/2 [52]
			NASH/Fibrosis	PKA, GSH [53]
			ALD	AMPK [54]
Malvidin	Flavonoids/Anthocyanins	Red grapes, cranberries, blueberries and black rice [80]	Steatosis	CPT1, PPARα, FAS, SREBP-1 [51]
			HCC	BAX, Caspase-3, Cyclin, PTEN, MMP-2/9 [56]
Epicatechin	Flavonoids/Flavanols	Dark chocolate and cocoa [58]	Steatosis	SREBP-1, FAS, LXR, SIRT [59]
			DILI/ALD	Bile acid and lipid absorption [60]
			NASH	NF-κB [60]
Epigallocatechin/EGCG	Flavonoids/Flavanols	Green tea [61]	Steatosis/NASH	AMPK, SREBP-1, FAS, ACC; CYP2E1, malonaldehyde, TNF, IL; TGF/SMAD [62]
			Fibrosis	Collagen, αSMA, TIMP-2 [63]
			DILI	CYP [64]
			HCC	NF-κB, BCL2; cMYC, ERK1/2, DDR; MMP, COX-2 [65]
Procyanidins	Flavonoids/Flavanols	Chocolate, apples, red grapes and cranberries [69]	NASH/Fibrosis	CYP2E1, GSH, SOD [66]
			ALD	SREBP-1, IL-6, TNF [67]
			NASH/ALD/DILI	Mitochondrial dysfunction and apoptosis [68]
Hesperidin	Flavonoids/Flavanones	Citrus fruits and peppermint [71,72]	NASH/Fibrosis	GSH, CAT, SOD [73]
			Steatosis/NASH	Lipoperoxidation [74]
Naringenin	Flavonoids/Flavanones	Mexican oregano [75]	DILI	Caspase-3, BAX, BCL [76]
			Fibrosis	TGF-β, ECM deposition [77]
Quercetin	Flavonoids/Flavonols	Apples, berries, brassica vegetables, capers, grapes, onions, shallots, tea, tomatoes, seeds and nuts [78,79]	Fibrosis	NF-κB, TNF, IL-1β, IL-6, IL-8 [78]
			ALD	GSH, IL-10, lipid peroxidation [79]
			Fibrosis	ALK5, SMAD 2/3
Kaempferol	Flavonoids/Flavonols	Tea, broccoli, apples, strawberries and beans [80]	HCC	PTEN, PI3K/AKT/mTOR [81]
			ALD	CYP2E1 [82]

Table 2. Cont.

Polyphenol	Group/Subgroup	Source	Liver Pathology	Molecular Targets
Myricetin	Flavonoids/Flavonols	Berries, honey, vegetables, teas and wines [84]	Steatosis/NASH	NRF-2, mitochondrial functionality, PPAR [85]
			HCC	YAP [86]
Isorhamnetin	Flavonoids/Flavonols	Pears, onion, olive oil, grapes, tomato, Mexican Tarragon [80,89]	Steatosis/NASH/Fibrosis	FAS, TGF-β, HSC activation [87]
			NASH	Lipoperoxidation [88]
Galangin	Flavonoids/Flavonols	Rizhome and propolis [90]	NASH/DILI	NRF-2, apoptosis [91]
			HCC	NRF-2, HO-1 [92]
Apigenin	Flavonoids/Flavones	Parsley, broccoli, celery, onions, oranges, olives, cherries, tomatoes, chamomile, thyme, oregano, basil, tea [93]	ALD	CYP2E1, PPARα [94]
			Steatosis	FAO, Tricarboxylic acid cycle, oxidative phosphorylation [96]
Chrysin	Flavonoids/Flavones	Honey and propolis [97]	Steatosis/NASH	TNF, IL-6, SREBP-1 [98]
			Fibrosis	MMP, TIMP [99]
Luteolin	Flavonoids/Flavones	Celery, parsley, broccoli, onion, carrots, peppers, cabbages and apple [100]	DILI	GSH, TNF, NF-κB, IL-6, ER stress [101]
			Fibrosis/DILI	NRF-2, NF-κB, P53 [102]
			ALD	SREBP-1, AMPK [103]
			Steatosis	PPARα [105]
Genistein	Flavonoids/Isoflanoids	Soybeans, nuts and legumes [104]	NASH	TLR4 [106]
			Fibrosis	Lipoperoxidation, GSH [107]
Daidzein	Flavonoids/Isoflanoids	Soybeans, nuts and legumes [104]	Steatosis/NASH	FAO, TNF [109]
			NASH/DILI/ALD	Oxidative stress [115]
Ellagic acid	Phenolic acids/Hydroxibenzoic acids	Nuts, walnuts, berries, pomegranades or berries [114]	IR	Oxidative stress [116]
			Fibrosis	Caspase-3, BCL-2, NF-kB, NRF-2 aslan [117]
Gallic acid	Phenolic acids/Hydroxibenzoic acids	Blueberries, strawberries and mango [118]	Fibrosis	GSH, TGF-β [121]
			DILI/ALD	TNF, lipoperoxidation [119]
			IR	GSH and CAT [120]
Ferulic acid	Phenolic acids/Hydroxycinnamic acids	Rice, wheat, oats, grains, vegetables, pineapple, beans, coffee, artichoke, peanut, nuts [122]	DILI	NRF-2/HO-1 [123]
			Fibrosis	TGF-β/SMAD [124]
Cholorogenic acid	Phenolic acids/Hydroxycinnamic acids	Coffee, beans, potato, apple and prunes [125]	Fibrosis	TNF, IL-6 and IL-1β [126]
			ALD	ROS, TNF, TGF-β [127]
Oleuropein	Phenolic acids/Oleuropeunosides	Olive leaves, olives, virgin olive oil and olive mill waste [128]	DILI/ALD	ROS [129]
			NASH	TLR [130]
Sesamin	Lignans	Flaxseed and sesame seeds [131]	Steatosis	ACC, CPT1, 3-hydroxyacyl-coA dehydrogenase [132]
			Steatosis	SREBP-1 [133]
Diglucoside	Lignans	Flaxseed [134]	Steatosis/NASH	Lipoperoxidation [135]
Curcumin	Curcuminoids	Curcuma longa [136]	Steatosis	FAO [137]
			Fibrosis/DILI/ALD	NRF-2, GSH, HSC activation [137]

4. Conclusions

The supplementation with polyphenols has an effect in treating liver pathologies: non-alcoholic fatty liver disease, drug-induced liver injury, hepatocellular carcinoma and alcoholic liver disease. The inclusion of polyphenol-rich foods is an attractive approach when developing a nutritional program. Authorities should encourage their consumption. Polyphenols and other micronutrients are essential for an equilibrated diet, where variety is an essential feature.

Author Contributions: Conceptualization, J.S., M.C.-A. and M.L.M.-C.; methodology, J.S. and M.C.-A.; investigation, J.S. and M.C.-A.; writing—original draft preparation, M.C.-A., N.G.-U. and M.S.-M.; writing—review and editing, J.S., M.C.-A. and M.S.-M.; supervision, J.S. and M.L.M.-C.; project administration, J.S. and M.L.M.-C. All authors have read and agreed to the published version of the manuscript.

Funding: This research received no external funding.

Acknowledgments: We thank University of Basque Country (UPV/EHU), Basque Government and Asociación Española Contra el Cáncer (AECC) for the Pre-doctoral grants to M.C.-A., N.G.-U. and M.S.-M., respectively. Ciberehd_ISCIII_MINECO is funded by the Instituto de Salud Carlos III. We thank MINECO for the Severo Ochoa Excellence Accreditation to CIC bioGUNE (SEV-2016-0644).

Conflicts of Interest: M.L.M.-C. advises for Mitotherapeutix LLC.

References

1. Yasutake, K.; Kohjima, M.; Kotoh, K.; Nakashima, M.; Nakamuta, M.; Enjoji, M. Dietary habits and behaviors associated with nonalcoholic fatty liver disease. *World J. Gastroenterol.* **2014**, *20*, 1756–1767. [CrossRef]
2. Micha, R.; Shulkin, M.L.; Peñalvo, J.L.; Khatibzadeh, S.; Singh, G.M.; Rao, M.; Fahimi, S.; Powles, J.; Mozaffarian, D. Etiologic effects and optimal intakes of foods and nutrients for risk of cardiovascular diseases and diabetes: Systematic reviews and meta-analyses from the Nutrition and Chronic Diseases Expert Group (NutriCoDE). *PLoS ONE* **2017**, *12*, e0175149. [CrossRef]
3. Tarasenko, T.N.; McGuire, P.J. The liver is a metabolic and immunologic organ: A reconsideration of metabolic decompensation due to infection in inborn errors of metabolism (IEM). *Mol. Genet. Metab.* **2017**, *121*, 283–288. [CrossRef]
4. Vernon, G.; Baranova, A.; Younossi, Z.M. Systematic review: The epidemiology and natural history of non-alcoholic fatty liver disease and non-alcoholic steatohepatitis in adults. *Aliment. Pharmacol. Ther.* **2011**, *34*, 274–285. [CrossRef]
5. Younossi, Z.M.; Koenig, A.B.; Abdelatif, D.; Fazel, Y.; Henry, L.; Wymer, M. Global epidemiology of nonalcoholic fatty liver disease—Meta-analytic assessment of prevalence, incidence, and outcomes. *Hepatology* **2016**, *64*, 73–84. [CrossRef]
6. Loomba, R.; Sanyal, A.J. The global NAFLD epidemic. *Nat. Rev. Gastroenterol. Hepatol.* **2013**, *10*, 686–690. [CrossRef]
7. Mishra, A.; Younossi, Z.M. Epidemiology and Natural History of Non-alcoholic Fatty Liver Disease. *J. Clin. Exp. Hepatol.* **2012**, *2*, 135–144. [CrossRef]
8. Adams, L.A.; Lymp, J.F.; St. Sauver, J.; Sanderson, S.O.; Lindor, K.D.; Feldstein, A.; Angulo, P. The natural history of nonalcoholic fatty liver disease: A population-based cohort study. *Gastroenterology* **2005**, *129*, 113–121. [CrossRef]
9. Day, C.P. From fat to inflammation. *Gastroenterology* **2006**, *130*, 207–210. [CrossRef]
10. Noureddin, M.; Rinella, M.E. Nonalcoholic Fatty Liver Disease, Diabetes, Obesity, and Hepatocellular Carcinoma. *Clin. Liver Dis.* **2015**, *19*, 361–379. [CrossRef]
11. Neuschwander-Tetri, B.A. Hepatic lipotoxicity and the pathogenesis of nonalcoholic steatohepatitis: The central role of nontriglyceride fatty acid metabolites. *Hepatology* **2010**, *52*, 774–788. [CrossRef]
12. Eslam, M.; Sanyal, A.J.; George, J. MAFLD: A Consensus-Driven Proposed Nomenclature for Metabolic Associated Fatty Liver Disease. *Gastroenterology* **2020**, *158*, 1999–2014. [CrossRef]
13. Friedman, S.L. Mechanisms of hepatic fibrogenesis. *Gastroenterology* **2008**, *134*, 1655–1669. [CrossRef]
14. Kim, E.; Lisby, A.; Ma, C.; Lo, N.; Ehmer, U.; Hayer, K.E.; Furth, E.E.; Viatour, P. Promotion of growth factor signaling as a critical function of β-catenin during HCC progression. *Nat. Commun.* **2019**, *10*. [CrossRef]
15. David, S.; Hamilton, J.P. Drug-induced Liver Injury. *US Gastroenterol. Hepatol.* **2010**, *6*, 73–80.

16. He, Y.; Jin, L.; Wang, J.; Yan, Z.; Chen, T.; Zhao, Y. Mechanisms of fibrosis in acute liver failure. *Liver Int.* **2015**, *35*, 1877–1885. [CrossRef]
17. Giordano, C.; Rivas, J.; Zervos, X. An Update on Treatment of Drug-Induced Liver Injury. *J. Clin. Transl. Hepatol.* **2014**, *2*, 74–79.
18. Bell, L.N.; Chalasani, N. Epidemiology of idiosyncratic drug-induced liver injury. *Semin. Liver Dis.* **2009**, *29*, 337–347. [CrossRef]
19. Ye, H.; Nelson, L.J.; Gómez Del Moral, M.; Martínez-Naves, E.; Cubero, F.J. Dissecting the molecular pathophysiology of drug-induced liver injury. *World J. Gastroenterol.* **2018**, *24*, 1373–1385. [CrossRef]
20. Bajt, M.L.; Ramachandran, A.; Yan, H.-M.; Lebofsky, M.; Farhood, A.; Lemasters, J.J.; Jaeschke, H. Apoptosis-Inducing Factor Modulates Mitochondrial Oxidant Stress in Acetaminophen Hepatotoxicity. *Toxicol. Sci.* **2011**, *122*, 598–605. [CrossRef]
21. Jaeschke, H.; Duan, L.; Akakpo, J.Y.; Farhood, A.; Ramachandran, A. The role of apoptosis in acetaminophen hepatotoxicity. *Food Chem. Toxicol.* **2018**, *118*, 709–718. [CrossRef] [PubMed]
22. Cao, L.; Quan, X.-B.; Zeng, W.-J.; Yang, X.-O.; Wang, M.-J. Mechanism of Hepatocyte Apoptosis. *J. Cell Death* **2016**, *9*, 19–29. [CrossRef] [PubMed]
23. Basra, S.; Anand, B.S. Definition, epidemiology and magnitude of alcoholic hepatitis. *World J. Hepatol.* **2011**, *3*, 108–113. [CrossRef] [PubMed]
24. Osna, N.A.; Donohue, T.M., Jr.; Kharbanda, K.K. Alcoholic Liver Disease: Pathogenesis and Current Management. *Alcohol Res.* **2017**, *38*, 147–161.
25. Asrani, S.K.; Devarbhavi, H.; Eaton, J.; Kamath, P.S. Burden of liver diseases in the world. *J. Hepatol.* **2019**, *70*, 151–171. [CrossRef]
26. Finicelli, M.; Squillaro, T.; Di Cristo, F.; Di Salle, A.; Melone, M.A.B.; Galderisi, U.; Peluso, G. Metabolic syndrome, Mediterranean diet, and polyphenols: Evidence and perspectives. *J. Cell. Physiol.* **2019**, *234*, 5807–5826. [CrossRef]
27. Petrides, J.; Collins, P.; Kowalski, A.; Sepede, J.; Vermeulen, M. Lifestyle Changes for Disease Prevention. *Prim. Care* **2019**, *46*, 1–12. [CrossRef]
28. Al-Dashti, Y.A.; Holt, R.R.; Stebbins, C.L.; Keen, C.L.; Hackman, R.M. Dietary Flavanols: A Review of Select Effects on Vascular Function, Blood Pressure, and Exercise Performance. *J. Am. Coll. Nutr.* **2018**, *37*, 553–567. [CrossRef]
29. Li, A.-N.; Li, S.; Zhang, Y.-J.; Xu, X.-R.; Chen, Y.-M.; Li, H.-B. Resources and biological activities of natural polyphenols. *Nutrients* **2014**, *6*, 6020–6047. [CrossRef]
30. Nguyen, N.U.; Stamper, B.D. Polyphenols reported to shift APAP-induced changes in MAPK signaling and toxicity outcomes. *Chem. Biol. Interact.* **2017**, *277*, 129–136. [CrossRef]
31. Manach, C.; Scalbert, A.; Morand, C.; Rémésy, C.; Jiménez, L. Polyphenols: Food sources and bioavailability. *Am. J. Clin. Nutr.* **2004**, *79*, 727–747. [CrossRef] [PubMed]
32. Li, S.; Tan, H.Y.; Wang, N.; Cheung, F.; Hong, M.; Feng, Y. The Potential and Action Mechanism of Polyphenols in the Treatment of Liver Diseases. *Oxid. Med. Cell. Longev.* **2018**, *2018*. [CrossRef] [PubMed]
33. Lee, H.J.; Kang, M.-G.; Cha, H.Y.; Kim, Y.M.; Lim, Y.; Yang, S.J. Effects of Piceatannol and Resveratrol on Sirtuins and Hepatic Inflammation in High-Fat Diet-Fed Mice. *J. Med. Food* **2019**, *22*, 833–840. [CrossRef] [PubMed]
34. Burns, J.; Yokota, T.; Ashihara, H.; Lean, M.E.J.; Crozier, A. Plant foods and herbal sources of resveratrol. *J. Agric. Food Chem.* **2002**, *50*, 3337–3340. [CrossRef]
35. Bishayee, A.; Darvesh, A.S.; Politis, T.; McGory, R. Resveratrol and liver disease: From bench to bedside and community. *Liver Int.* **2010**, *30*, 1103–1114. [CrossRef]
36. Peiyuan, H.; Zhiping, H.; Chengjun, S.; Chunqing, W.; Bingqing, L.; Imam, M.U. Resveratrol Ameliorates Experimental Alcoholic Liver Disease by Modulating Oxidative Stress. *Evidence-Based Complement. Altern. Med.* **2017**, *2017*. [CrossRef]
37. Andrade, J.M.O.; Paraíso, A.F.; de Oliveira, M.V.M.; Martins, A.M.E.; Neto, J.F.; Guimarães, A.L.S.; de Paula, A.M.; Qureshi, M.; Santos, S.H.S. Resveratrol attenuates hepatic steatosis in high-fat fed mice by decreasing lipogenesis and inflammation. *Nutrition* **2014**, *30*, 915–919. [CrossRef]
38. Paul, S.; DeCastro, A.J.; Lee, H.J.; Smolarek, A.K.; So, J.Y.; Simi, B.; Wang, C.X.; Zhou, R.; Rimando, A.M.; Suh, N. Dietary intake of pterostilbene, a constituent of blueberries, inhibits the beta-catenin/p65 downstream signaling pathway and colon carcinogenesis in rats. *Carcinogenesis* **2010**, *31*, 1272–1278. [CrossRef]

39. Aguirre, L.; Palacios-ortega, S.; Fernández-Quintela, A.; Hijona, E.; Bujanda, L.; Portillo, M.P. Pterostilbene reduces liver steatosis and modifies hepatic fatty acid profile in obese rats. *Nutrients* **2019**, *11*, 961. [CrossRef]
40. Gomez-Zorita, S.; Milton-Laskibar, I.; Aguirre, L.; Fernandez-Quintela, A.; Xiao, J.; Portillo, M.P. Effects of Pterostilbene on Diabetes, Liver Steatosis and Serum Lipids. *Curr. Med. Chem.* **2019**. [CrossRef]
41. Matsui, Y.; Sugiyama, K.; Kamei, M.; Takahashi, T.; Suzuki, T.; Katagata, Y.; Ito, T. Extract of passion fruit (Passiflora edulis) seed containing high amounts of piceatannol inhibits melanogenesis and promotes collagen synthesis. *J. Agric. Food Chem.* **2010**, *58*, 11112–11118. [CrossRef] [PubMed]
42. Tung, Y.-C.; Lin, Y.-H.; Chen, H.-J.; Chou, S.-C.; Cheng, A.-C.; Kalyanam, N.; Ho, C.-T.; Pan, M.-H. Piceatannol Exerts Anti-Obesity Effects in C57BL/6 Mice through Modulating Adipogenic Proteins and Gut Microbiota. *Molecules* **2016**, *21*, 1419. [CrossRef] [PubMed]
43. Zubiete-Franco, I.; Garcia-Rodriguez, J.L.; Martinez-Una, M.; Martinez-Lopez, N.; Woodhoo, A.; Juan, V.G.-D.; Beraza, N.; Lage-Medina, S.; Andrade, F.; Fernandez, M.L.; et al. Methionine and S-adenosylmethionine levels are critical regulators of PP2A activity modulating lipophagy during steatosis. *J. Hepatol.* **2016**, *64*, 409–418. [CrossRef] [PubMed]
44. Faghihzadeh, F.; Adibi, P.; Rafiei, R.; Hekmatdoost, A. Resveratrol supplementation improves inflammatory biomarkers in patients with nonalcoholic fatty liver disease. *Nutr. Res.* **2014**, *34*, 837–843. [CrossRef] [PubMed]
45. Hosseinian, F.S.; Beta, T. Saskatoon and wild blueberries have higher anthocyanin contents than other Manitoba berries. *J. Agric. Food Chem.* **2007**, *55*, 10832–10838. [CrossRef]
46. Watson, R.R.; Schönlau, F. Nutraceutical and antioxidant effects of a delphinidin-rich maqui berry extract Delphinol®: A review. *Minerva Cardioangiol.* **2015**, *63*, 1–12.
47. Parra-Vargas, M.; Sandoval-Rodriguez, A.; Rodriguez-Echevarria, R.; Dominguez-Rosales, J.A.; Santos-Garcia, A.; Armendariz-Borunda, J. Delphinidin ameliorates hepatic triglyceride accumulation in human HepG2 cells, but not in diet-induced obese mice. *Nutrients* **2018**, *10*, 1060. [CrossRef]
48. Domitrovic, R.; Jakovac, H. Antifibrotic activity of anthocyanidin delphinidin in carbon tetrachloride-induced hepatotoxicity in mice. *Toxicology* **2010**, *272*, 1–10. [CrossRef]
49. Lee, W.; Lee, Y.; Kim, J.; Bae, J.-S. Protective Effects of Pelargonidin on Lipopolysaccharide-induced Hepatic Failure. *Nat. Prod. Commun.* **2018**, *13*, 1934578X1801300114. [CrossRef]
50. Andersen, Ø; Jordheim, M. Basic Anthocyanin Chemistry and Dietary Source. In *Anthocyanins in Health and Disease*; CRC Press: Boca Raton, FL, USA, 2013; pp. 13–90. ISBN 9781439894712.
51. Park, S.; Kang, S.; Jeong, D.-Y.Y.; Jeong, S.-Y.Y.; Park, J.J.; Yun, H.S. Cyanidin and malvidin in aqueous extracts of black carrots fermented with Aspergillus oryzae prevent the impairment of energy, lipid and glucose metabolism in estrogen-deficient rats by AMPK activation. *Genes Nutr.* **2015**, *10*, 455. [CrossRef]
52. Bendia, E.; Benedetti, A.; Baroni, G.S.; Candelaresi, C.; Macarri, G.; Trozzi, L.; Di Sario, A. Effect of cyanidin 3-O-beta-glucopyranoside on hepatic stellate cell proliferation and collagen synthesis induced by oxidative stress. *Dig. Liver Dis.* **2005**, *37*, 342–348. [CrossRef] [PubMed]
53. Zhu, W.; Jia, Q.; Wang, Y.; Zhang, Y.; Xia, M. The anthocyanin cyanidin-3-O-beta-glucoside, a flavonoid, increases hepatic glutathione synthesis and protects hepatocytes against reactive oxygen species during hyperglycemia: Involvement of a cAMP-PKA-dependent signaling pathway. *Free Radic. Biol. Med.* **2012**, *52*, 314–327. [CrossRef] [PubMed]
54. Wan, T.; Wang, S.; Ye, M.; Ling, W.; Yang, L. Cyanidin-3-O-β-glucoside protects against liver fibrosis induced by alcohol via regulating energy homeostasis and AMPK/autophagy signaling pathway. *J. Funct. Foods* **2017**, *37*, 16–24. [CrossRef]
55. Tulio, A.Z.J.; Reese, R.N.; Wyzgoski, F.J.; Rinaldi, P.L.; Fu, R.; Scheerens, J.C.; Miller, A.R. Cyanidin 3-rutinoside and cyanidin 3-xylosylrutinoside as primary phenolic antioxidants in black raspberry. *J. Agric. Food Chem.* **2008**, *56*, 1880–1888. [CrossRef] [PubMed]
56. Wang, Y.; Lin, J.; Tian, J.; Si, X.; Jiao, X.; Zhang, W.; Gong, E.; Li, B. Blueberry Malvidin-3-galactoside Suppresses Hepatocellular Carcinoma by Regulating Apoptosis, Proliferation, and Metastasis Pathways In Vivo and In Vitro. *J. Agric. Food Chem.* **2019**, *67*, 625–636. [CrossRef]
57. Jaramillo Flores, M.E. Cocoa Flavanols: Natural Agents with Attenuating Effects on Metabolic Syndrome Risk Factors. *Nutrients* **2019**, *11*, 751. [CrossRef] [PubMed]

58. Dower, J.I.; Geleijnse, J.M.; Kroon, P.A.; Philo, M.; Mensink, M.; Kromhout, D.; Hollman, P.C.H. Does epicatechin contribute to the acute vascular function effects of dark chocolate? A randomized, crossover study. *Mol. Nutr. Food Res.* **2016**, *60*, 2379–2386. [CrossRef] [PubMed]
59. Cheng, H.; Xu, N.; Zhao, W.; Su, J.; Liang, M.; Xie, Z.; Wu, X.; Li, Q. (-)-Epicatechin regulates blood lipids and attenuates hepatic steatosis in rats fed high-fat diet. *Mol. Nutr. Food Res.* **2017**, *61*, 1700303. [CrossRef]
60. Huang, Z.; Jing, X.; Sheng, Y.; Zhang, J.; Hao, Z.; Wang, Z.; Ji, L. (-)-Epicatechin attenuates hepatic sinusoidal obstruction syndrome by inhibiting liver oxidative and inflammatory injury. *Redox Biol.* **2019**, *22*, 101117. [CrossRef]
61. Naumovski, N.; Blades, B.L.; Roach, P.D. Food Inhibits the Oral Bioavailability of the Major Green Tea Antioxidant Epigallocatechin Gallate in Humans. *Antioxidants* **2015**, *4*, 373–393. [CrossRef]
62. Chen, C.; Liu, Q.; Liu, L.; Hu, Y.Y.; Feng, Q. Potential Biological Effects of (-)-Epigallocatechin-3-gallate on the Treatment of Nonalcoholic Fatty Liver Disease. *Mol. Nutr. Food Res.* **2018**, *62*, 1–11. [CrossRef] [PubMed]
63. Tipoe, G.L.; Leung, T.M.; Liong, E.C.; Lau, T.Y.H.; Fung, M.L.; Nanji, A.A. Epigallocatechin-3-gallate (EGCG) reduces liver inflammation, oxidative stress and fibrosis in carbon tetrachloride (CCl4)-induced liver injury in mice. *Toxicology* **2010**, *273*, 45–52. [CrossRef] [PubMed]
64. Yao, H.T.; Li, C.C.; Chang, C.H. Epigallocatechin-3-gallate reduces hepatic oxidative stress and lowers cyp-mediated bioactivation and toxicity of acetaminophen in rats. *Nutrients* **2019**, *11*, 1862. [CrossRef] [PubMed]
65. Bimonte, S.; Albino, V.; Piccirillo, M.; Nasto, A.; Molino, C.; Palaia, R.; Cascella, M. Epigallocatechin-3-gallate in the prevention and treatment of hepatocellular carcinoma: Experimental findings and translational perspectives. *Drug Des. Devel. Ther.* **2019**, *13*, 611–621. [CrossRef]
66. Dai, N.; Zou, Y.; Zhu, L.; Wang, H.F.; Dai, M.G. Antioxidant properties of proanthocyanidins attenuate carbon tetrachloride (CCl4)-induced steatosis and liver injury in rats via CYP2E1 regulation. *J. Med. Food* **2014**, *17*, 663–669. [CrossRef]
67. Wang, Z.; Su, B.; Fan, S.; Fei, H.; Zhao, W. Protective effect of oligomeric proanthocyanidins against alcohol-induced liver steatosis and injury in mice. *Biochem. Biophys. Res. Commun.* **2015**, *458*, 757–762. [CrossRef]
68. Miltonprabu, S.; Nazimabashir; Manoharan, V. Hepatoprotective effect of grape seed proanthocyanidins on Cadmium-induced hepatic injury in rats: Possible involvement of mitochondrial dysfunction, inflammation and apoptosis. *Toxicol. Rep.* **2016**, *3*, 63–77. [CrossRef]
69. Hammerstone, J.F.; Lazarus, S.A.; Schmitz, H.H. Procyanidin content and variation in some commonly consumed foods. *J. Nutr.* **2000**, *130*, 2086S–2092S. [CrossRef]
70. Habtemariam, S. The Nrf2/HO-1 Axis as Targets for Flavanones: Neuroprotection by Pinocembrin, Naringenin, and Eriodictyol. *Oxid. Med. Cell. Longev.* **2019**, *2019*, 4724920. [CrossRef]
71. Guedon, D.J.; Pasquier, B.P. Analysis and Distribution of Flavonoid Glycosides and Rosmarinic Acid in 40 Mentha x piperita Clones. *J. Agric. Food Chem.* **1994**, *42*, 679–684. [CrossRef]
72. Ooghe, W.C.; Detavernier, C.M. Detection of the Addition of Citrus reticulata and Hybrids to Citrus sinensis by Flavonoids. *J. Agric. Food Chem.* **1997**, *45*, 1633–1637. [CrossRef]
73. Çetin, A.; Çiftçi, O.; Otlu, A. Protective effect of hesperidin on oxidative and histological liver damage following carbon tetrachloride administration in Wistar rats. *Arch. Med. Sci.* **2016**, *12*, 486–493. [CrossRef] [PubMed]
74. Pari, L.; Karthikeyan, A.; Karthika, P.; Rathinam, A. Protective effects of hesperidin on oxidative stress, dyslipidaemia and histological changes in iron-induced hepatic and renal toxicity in rats. *Toxicol. Rep.* **2015**, *2*, 46–55. [CrossRef] [PubMed]
75. Lin, L.-Z.; Mukhopadhyay, S.; Robbins, R.J.; Harnly, J.M. Identification and quantification of flavonoids of Mexican oregano (*Lippia graveolens*) by LC-DAD-ESI/MS analysis. *J. Food Compos. Anal. Off. Publ. United Nations Univ. Int. Netw. Food Data Syst.* **2007**, *20*, 361–369. [CrossRef] [PubMed]
76. Ahmed, O.M.; Fahim, H.I.; Ahmed, H.Y.; Al-Muzafar, H.M.; Ahmed, R.R.; Amin, K.A.; El-Nahass, E.S.; Abdelazeem, W.H. The preventive effects and the mechanisms of action of navel orange peel hydroethanolic extract, naringin, and naringenin in N-Acetyl-p-aminophenol-induced liver injury in wistar rats. *Oxid. Med. Cell. Longev.* **2019**, *2019*. [CrossRef]
77. Hernández-Aquino, E.; Muriel, P. Beneficial effects of naringenin in liver diseases: Molecular mechanisms. *World J. Gastroenterol.* **2018**, *24*, 1679–1707. [CrossRef]

78. Li, Y.; Yao, J.; Han, C.; Yang, J.; Chaudhry, M.T.; Wang, S.; Liu, H.; Yin, Y. Quercetin, Inflammation and Immunity. *Nutrients* **2016**, *8*, 167. [CrossRef]
79. Chen, X. Protective effects of quercetin on liver injury induced by ethanol. *Pharmacogn. Mag.* **2010**, *6*, 135–141. [CrossRef]
80. Somerset, S.M.; Johannot, L. Dietary flavonoid sources in Australian adults. *Nutr. Cancer* **2008**, *60*, 442–449. [CrossRef]
81. Zhu, G.; Liu, X.; Li, H.; Yan, Y.; Hong, X.; Lin, Z. Kaempferol inhibits proliferation, migration, and invasion of liver cancer HepG2 cells by down-regulation of microRNA-21. *Int. J. Immunopathol. Pharmacol.* **2018**, *32*. [CrossRef]
82. Wang, M.; Sun, J.; Jiang, Z.; Xie, W.; Zhang, X. Hepatoprotective effect of kaempferol against alcoholic liver injury in mice. *Am. J. Chin. Med.* **2015**, *43*, 241–254. [CrossRef] [PubMed]
83. Xu, T.; Huang, S.; Huang, Q.; Ming, Z.; Wang, M.; Li, R.; Zhao, Y. Kaempferol attenuates liver fibrosis by inhibiting activin receptor–like kinase 5. *J. Cell. Mol. Med.* **2019**, *23*, 6403–6410. [CrossRef] [PubMed]
84. Semwal, D.K.; Semwal, R.B.; Combrinck, S.; Viljoen, A. Myricetin: A Dietary Molecule with Diverse Biological Activities. *Nutrients* **2016**, *8*, 90. [CrossRef] [PubMed]
85. Xia, S.F.; Le, G.W.; Wang, P.; Qiu, Y.Y.; Jiang, Y.Y.; Tang, X. Regressive effect of myricetin on hepatic steatosis in mice fed a high-fat diet. *Nutrients* **2016**, *8*, 799. [CrossRef] [PubMed]
86. Li, M.; Chen, J.; Yu, X.; Xu, S.; Li, D.; Zheng, Q.; Yin, Y. Myricetin Suppresses the Propagation of Hepatocellular Carcinoma via Down-Regulating Expression of YAP. *Cells* **2019**, *8*, 358. [CrossRef] [PubMed]
87. Ganbold, M.; Owada, Y.; Ozawa, Y.; Shimamoto, Y.; Ferdousi, F.; Tominaga, K.; Zheng, Y.W.; Ohkohchi, N.; Isoda, H. Isorhamnetin Alleviates Steatosis and Fibrosis in Mice with Nonalcoholic Steatohepatitis. *Sci. Rep.* **2019**, *9*, 1–11. [CrossRef]
88. Igarashi, K.; Ohmuma, M. Effects of isorhamnetin, rhamnetin, and quercetin on the concentrations of cholesterol and lipoperoxide in the serum and liver and on the blood and liver antioxidative enzyme activities of rats. *Biosci. Biotechnol. Biochem.* **1995**, *59*, 595–601. [CrossRef]
89. Yang, J.H.; Kim, S.C.; Kim, K.M.; Jang, C.H.; Cho, S.S.; Kim, S.J.; Ku, S.K.; Cho, I.J.; Ki, S.H. Isorhamnetin attenuates liver fibrosis by inhibiting TGF-beta/Smad signaling and relieving oxidative stress. *Eur. J. Pharmacol.* **2016**, *783*, 92–102. [CrossRef]
90. Huang, H.; Chen, A.Y.; Ye, X.; Guan, R.; Rankin, G.O.; Chen, Y.C. Galangin, a Flavonoid from Lesser Galangal, Induced Apoptosis via p53-Dependent Pathway in Ovarian Cancer Cells. *Molecules* **2020**, *25*, 1579. [CrossRef]
91. Aladaileh, S.H.; Abukhalil, M.H.; Saghir, S.A.M.; Hanieh, H.; Alfwuaires, M.A.; Almaiman, A.A.; Bin-Jumah, M.; Mahmoud, A.M. Galangin activates Nrf2 signaling and attenuates oxidative damage, inflammation, and apoptosis in a rat model of cyclophosphamide-induced hepatotoxicity. *Biomolecules* **2019**, *9*, 346. [CrossRef]
92. Su, L.; Chen, X.; Wu, J.; Lin, B.; Zhang, H.; Lan, L.; Luo, H. Galangin inhibits proliferation of hepatocellular carcinoma cells by inducing endoplasmic reticulum stress. *Food Chem. Toxicol.* **2013**, *62*, 810–816. [CrossRef] [PubMed]
93. Hostetler, G.L.; Ralston, R.A.; Schwartz, S.J. Flavones: Food Sources, Bioavailability, Metabolism, and Bioactivity. *Adv. Nutr.* **2017**, *8*, 423–435. [CrossRef] [PubMed]
94. Wang, F.; Liu, J.-C.; Zhou, R.-J.; Zhao, X.; Liu, M.; Ye, H.; Xie, M.-L. Apigenin protects against alcohol-induced liver injury in mice by regulating hepatic CYP2E1-mediated oxidative stress and PPARalpha-mediated lipogenic gene expression. *Chem. Biol. Interact.* **2017**, *275*, 171–177. [CrossRef] [PubMed]
95. Tsaroucha, A.K.; Tsiaousidou, A.; Ouzounidis, N.; Tsalkidou, E.; Lambropoulou, M.; Giakoustidis, D.; Chatzaki, E.; Simopoulos, C. Intraperitoneal administration of apigenin in liver ischemia/reperfusion injury protective effects. *Saudi J. Gastroenterol.* **2016**, *22*, 415–422. [PubMed]
96. Jung, U.J.; Cho, Y.-Y.; Choi, M.-S. Apigenin Ameliorates Dyslipidemia, Hepatic Steatosis and Insulin Resistance by Modulating Metabolic and Transcriptional Profiles in the Liver of High-Fat Diet-Induced Obese Mice. *Nutrients* **2016**, *8*, 305. [CrossRef]
97. Balam, F.H.; Ahmadi, Z.S.; Ghorbani, A. Inhibitory effect of chrysin on estrogen biosynthesis by suppression of enzyme aromatase (CYP19): A systematic review. *Heliyon* **2020**, *6*, e03587. [CrossRef]
98. Pai, S.A.; Munshi, R.P.; Panchal, F.H.; Gaur, I.-S.; Juvekar, A.R. Chrysin ameliorates nonalcoholic fatty liver disease in rats. *Naunyn. Schmiedebergs. Arch. Pharmacol.* **2019**, *392*, 1617–1628. [CrossRef]

99. Balta, C.; Ciceu, A.; Herman, H.; Rosu, M.; Boldura, O.M.; Hermenean, A. Dose-dependent antifibrotic effect of chrysin on regression of liver fibrosis: The role in extracellular matrix remodeling. *Dose-Response* **2018**, *16*, 1–8. [CrossRef]
100. Lin, Y.; Shi, R.; Wang, X.; Shen, H.-M. Luteolin, a flavonoid with potential for cancer prevention and therapy. *Curr. Cancer Drug Targets* **2008**, *8*, 634–646. [CrossRef]
101. Tai, M.; Zhang, J.; Song, S.; Miao, R.; Liu, S.; Pang, Q.; Wu, Q.; Liu, C. Protective effects of luteolin against acetaminophen-induced acute liver failure in mouse. *Int. Immunopharmacol.* **2015**, *27*, 164–170. [CrossRef]
102. Zhang, H.; Tan, X.; Yang, D.; Lu, J.; Liu, B.; Baiyun, R.; Zhang, Z. Dietary luteolin attenuates chronic liver injury induced by mercuric chloride via the Nrf2/NF-κB/P53 signaling pathway in rats. *Oncotarget* **2017**, *8*, 40982–40993. [CrossRef] [PubMed]
103. Liu, G.; Zhang, Y.; Liu, C.; Xu, D.; Zhang, R.; Cheng, Y.; Pan, Y.; Huang, C.; Chen, Y. Luteolin alleviates alcoholic liver disease induced by chronic and binge ethanol feeding in mice. *J. Nutr.* **2014**, *144*, 1009–1015. [CrossRef] [PubMed]
104. Ritchie, M.R.; Cummings, J.H.; Morton, M.S.; Steel, C.M.; Bolton-Smith, C.; Riches, A.C. A newly constructed and validated isoflavone database for the assessment of total genistein and daidzein intake. *Br. J. Nutr.* **2006**, *95*, 204–213. [CrossRef] [PubMed]
105. Xin, X.; Chen, C.; Hu, Y.-Y.; Feng, Q. Protective effect of genistein on nonalcoholic fatty liver disease (NAFLD). *Biomed. Pharmacother.* **2019**, *117*, 109047. [CrossRef]
106. Yin, Y.; Liu, H.; Zheng, Z.; Lu, R.; Jiang, Z. Genistein can ameliorate hepatic inflammatory reaction in nonalcoholic steatohepatitis rats. *Biomed. Pharmacother.* **2019**, *111*, 1290–1296. [CrossRef]
107. Kuzu, N.; Metin, K.; Dagli, A.F.; Akdemir, F.; Orhan, C.; Yalniz, M.; Ozercan, I.H.; Sahin, K.; Bahcecioglu, I.H. Protective role of genistein in acute liver damage induced by carbon tetrachloride. *Mediators Inflamm.* **2007**, *2007*. [CrossRef]
108. Takahashi, Y.; Odbayar, T.O.; Ide, T. A comparative analysis of genistein and daidzein in affecting lipid metabolism in rat liver. *J. Clin. Biochem. Nutr.* **2009**, *44*, 223–230. [CrossRef]
109. Kim, M.-H.; Park, J.-S.; Jung, J.-W.; Byun, K.-W.; Kang, K.-S.; Lee, Y.-S. Daidzein supplementation prevents non-alcoholic fatty liver disease through alternation of hepatic gene expression profiles and adipocyte metabolism. *Int. J. Obes. (Lond.)* **2011**, *35*, 1019–1030. [CrossRef]
110. Cheraghpour, M.; Imani, H.; Ommi, S.; Alavian, S.M.; Karimi-Shahrbabak, E.; Hedayati, M.; Yari, Z.; Hekmatdoost, A. Hesperidin improves hepatic steatosis, hepatic enzymes, and metabolic and inflammatory parameters in patients with nonalcoholic fatty liver disease: A randomized, placebo-controlled, double-blind clinical trial. *Phytother. Res.* **2019**, *33*, 2118–2125. [CrossRef]
111. Nahmias, Y.; Goldwasser, J.; Casali, M.; van Poll, D.; Wakita, T.; Chung, R.T.; Yarmush, M.L. Apolipoprotein B-dependent hepatitis C virus secretion is inhibited by the grapefruit flavonoid naringenin. *Hepatology* **2008**, *47*, 1437–1445. [CrossRef]
112. Gonzalez, O.; Fontanes, V.; Raychaudhuri, S.; Loo, R.; Loo, J.; Arumugaswami, V.; Sun, R.; Dasgupta, A.; French, S.W. The heat shock protein inhibitor Quercetin attenuates hepatitis C virus production. *Hepatology* **2009**, *50*, 1756–1764. [CrossRef] [PubMed]
113. Kumar, N.; Goel, N. Phenolic acids: Natural versatile molecules with promising therapeutic applications. *Biotechnol. Rep. (Amsterdam, Netherlands)* **2019**, *24*, e00370. [CrossRef] [PubMed]
114. Kang, I.; Buckner, T.; Shay, N.F.; Gu, L.; Chung, S. Improvements in Metabolic Health with Consumption of Ellagic Acid and Subsequent Conversion into Urolithins: Evidence and Mechanisms. *Adv. Nutr.* **2016**, *7*, 961–972. [CrossRef] [PubMed]
115. Chen, P.; Chen, F.; Zhou, B. Antioxidative, anti-inflammatory and anti-apoptotic effects of ellagic acid in liver and brain of rats treated by D-galactose. *Sci. Rep.* **2018**, *8*, 2–11. [CrossRef]
116. Kapan, M.; Gumus, M.; Onder, A.; Firat, U.; Basarali, M.K.; Boyuk, A.; Aliosmanoglu, I.; Buyukbas, S. The effects of ellagic acid on the liver and remote organs' oxidative stress and structure after hepatic ischemia reperfusion injury caused by pringle maneuver in rats. *Bratisl. Lek. Listy* **2012**, *113*, 274–281. [CrossRef]
117. Aslan, A.; Gok, O.; Erman, O.; Kuloglu, T. Ellagic acid impedes carbontetrachloride-induced liver damage in rats through suppression of NF-kB, Bcl-2 and regulating Nrf-2 and caspase pathway. *Biomed. Pharmacother.* **2018**, *105*, 662–669. [CrossRef]

118. Setayesh, T.; Nersesyan, A.; Mišík, M.; Noorizadeh, R.; Haslinger, E.; Javaheri, T.; Lang, E.; Grusch, M.; Huber, W.; Haslberger, A.; et al. Gallic acid, a common dietary phenolic protects against high fat diet induced DNA damage. *Eur. J. Nutr.* **2019**, *58*, 2315–2326. [CrossRef]
119. Rasool, M.K.; Sabina, E.P.; Ramya, S.R.; Preety, P.; Patel, S.; Mandal, N.; Mishra, P.P.; Samuel, J. Hepatoprotective and antioxidant effects of gallic acid in paracetamol-induced liver damage in mice. *J. Pharm. Pharmacol.* **2010**, *62*, 638–643. [CrossRef]
120. Bayramoglu, G.; Kurt, H.; Bayramoglu, A.; Gunes, H.V.; Degirmenci, İ.; Colak, S. Preventive role of gallic acid on hepatic ischemia and reperfusion injury in rats. *Cytotechnology* **2015**, *67*, 845–849. [CrossRef]
121. El-Lakkany, N.M.; El-Maadawy, W.H.; Seif el-Din, S.H.; Saleh, S.; Safar, M.M.; Ezzat, S.M.; Mohamed, S.H.; Botros, S.S.; Demerdash, Z.; Hammam, O.A. Antifibrotic effects of gallic acid on hepatic stellate cells: In vitro and in vivo mechanistic study. *J. Tradit. Complement. Med.* **2019**, *9*, 45–53. [CrossRef]
122. Kumar, N.; Pruthi, V. Potential applications of ferulic acid from natural sources. *Biotechnol. Rep. (Amsterdam, Netherlands)* **2014**, *4*, 86–93. [CrossRef] [PubMed]
123. Mahmoud, A.M.; Hussein, O.E.; Hozayen, W.G.; Bin-Jumah, M.; Abd El-Twab, S.M. Ferulic acid prevents oxidative stress, inflammation, and liver injury via upregulation of Nrf2/HO-1 signaling in methotrexate-induced rats. *Environ. Sci. Pollut. Res.* **2020**, *27*, 7910–7921. [CrossRef] [PubMed]
124. Mu, M.; Zuo, S.; Wu, R.M.; Deng, K.S.; Lu, S.; Zhu, J.J.; Zou, G.L.; Yang, J.; Cheng, M.L.; Zhao, X.K. Ferulic acid attenuates liver fibrosis and hepatic stellate cell activation via inhibition of TGF-β/Smad signaling pathway. *Drug Des. Dev. Ther.* **2018**, *12*, 4107–4115. [CrossRef] [PubMed]
125. Nabavi, S.F.; Tejada, S.; Setzer, W.N.; Gortzi, O.; Sureda, A.; Braidy, N.; Daglia, M.; Manayi, A.; Nabavi, S.M. Chlorogenic Acid and Mental Diseases: From Chemistry to Medicine. *Curr. Neuropharmacol.* **2017**, *15*, 471–479. [CrossRef] [PubMed]
126. Shi, H.; Dong, L.; Jiang, J.; Zhao, J.; Zhao, G.; Dang, X.; Lu, X.; Jia, M. Chlorogenic acid reduces liver inflammation and fibrosis through inhibition of toll-like receptor 4 signaling pathway. *Toxicology* **2013**, *303*, 107–114. [CrossRef] [PubMed]
127. Kim, H.; Pan, J.H.; Kim, S.H.; Lee, J.H.; Park, J.-W. Chlorogenic acid ameliorates alcohol-induced liver injuries through scavenging reactive oxygen species. *Biochimie* **2018**, *150*, 131–138. [CrossRef]
128. Barbaro, B.; Toietta, G.; Maggio, R.; Arciello, M.; Tarocchi, M.; Galli, A.; Balsano, C. Effects of the olive-derived polyphenol oleuropein on human health. *Int. J. Mol. Sci.* **2014**, *15*, 18508–18524. [CrossRef]
129. Jemai, H.; Mahmoudi, A.; Feryeni, A.; Fki, I.; Bouallagui, Z.; Choura, S.; Chamkha, M.; Sayadi, S. Hepatoprotective Effect of Oleuropein-Rich Extract from Olive Leaves against Cadmium-Induced Toxicity in Mice. *BioMed Res. Int.* **2020**, *2020*, 4398924. [CrossRef]
130. Park, S.; Choi, Y.; Um, S.-J.; Yoon, S.K.; Park, T. Oleuropein attenuates hepatic steatosis induced by high-fat diet in mice. *J. Hepatol.* **2011**, *54*, 984–993. [CrossRef]
131. Durazzo, A.; Lucarini, M.; Camilli, E.; Marconi, S.; Gabrielli, P.; Lisciani, S.; Gambelli, L.; Aguzzi, A.; Novellino, E.; Santini, A.; et al. Dietary Lignans: Definition, Description and Research Trends in Databases Development. *Molecules* **2018**, *23*, 3251. [CrossRef]
132. Sirato-Yasumoto, S.; Katsuta, M.; Okuyama, Y.; Takahashi, Y.; Ide, T. Effect of Sesame Seeds Rich in Sesamin and Sesamolin on Fatty Acid Oxidation in Rat Liver. *J. Agric. Food Chem.* **2001**, *49*, 2647–2651. [CrossRef] [PubMed]
133. Ide, T.; Ashakumary, L.; Takahashi, Y.; Kushiro, M.; Fukuda, N.; Sugano, M. Sesamin, a sesame lignan, decreases fatty acid synthesis in rat liver accompanying the down-regulation of sterol regulatory element binding protein-1. *Biochim. Biophys. Acta* **2001**, *1534*, 1–13. [CrossRef]
134. Frank, J.; Eliasson, C.; Leroy-Nivard, D.; Budek, A.; Lundh, T.; Vessby, B.; Aman, P.; Kamal-Eldin, A. Dietary secoisolariciresinol diglucoside and its oligomers with 3-hydroxy-3-methyl glutaric acid decrease vitamin E levels in rats. *Br. J. Nutr.* **2004**, *92*, 169–176. [CrossRef] [PubMed]
135. Felmlee, M.A.; Woo, G.; Simko, E.; Krol, E.S.; Muir, A.D.; Alcorn, J. Effects of the flaxseed lignans secoisolariciresinol diglucoside and its aglycone on serum and hepatic lipids in hyperlipidaemic rats. *Br. J. Nutr.* **2009**, *102*, 361–369. [CrossRef] [PubMed]
136. Maiti, P.; Dunbar, G.L. Use of Curcumin, a Natural Polyphenol for Targeting Molecular Pathways in Treating Age-Related Neurodegenerative Diseases. *Int. J. Mol. Sci.* **2018**, *19*, 1637. [CrossRef] [PubMed]

137. Farzaei, M.H.; Zobeiri, M.; Parvizi, F.; El-Senduny, F.F.; Marmouzi, I.; Coy-Barrera, E.; Naseri, R.; Nabavi, S.M.; Rahimi, R.; Abdollahi, M. Curcumin in Liver Diseases: A Systematic Review of the Cellular Mechanisms of Oxidative Stress and Clinical Perspective. *Nutrients* **2018**, *10*, 855. [CrossRef]
138. Rahmani, S.; Asgary, S.; Askari, G.; Keshvari, M.; Hatamipour, M.; Feizi, A.; Sahebkar, A. Treatment of Non-alcoholic Fatty Liver Disease with Curcumin: A Randomized Placebo-controlled Trial. *Phytother. Res.* **2016**, *30*, 1540–1548. [CrossRef]
139. Saklayen, M.G. The Global Epidemic of the Metabolic Syndrome. *Curr. Hypertens. Rep.* **2018**, *20*, 12. [CrossRef]

Publisher's Note: MDPI stays neutral with regard to jurisdictional claims in published maps and institutional affiliations.

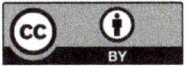

© 2020 by the authors. Licensee MDPI, Basel, Switzerland. This article is an open access article distributed under the terms and conditions of the Creative Commons Attribution (CC BY) license (http://creativecommons.org/licenses/by/4.0/).

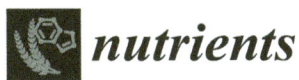 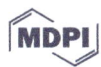

Article

A Ten-Day Grape Seed Procyanidin Treatment Prevents Certain Ageing Processes in Female Rats over the Long Term

Carme Grau-Bové, Marta Sierra-Cruz, Alba Miguéns-Gómez, Esther Rodríguez-Gallego, Raúl Beltrán-Debón, Mayte Blay, Ximena Terra, Montserrat Pinent * and Anna Ardévol

MoBioFood Research Group, Department of Biochemistry and Biotechnology, Universitat Rovira i Virgili, 43007 Tarragona, Spain; carme.grau@urv.cat (C.G.-B.); marta.sierra@urv.cat (M.S.-C.); alba.miguens@urv.cat (A.M.-G.); esther.rodriguez@urv.cat (E.R.-G.); raul.beltran@urv.cat (R.B.-D.); mteresa.blay@urv.cat (M.B.); ximena.terra@urv.cat (X.T.); anna.ardevol@urv.cat (A.A.)
* Correspondence: montserrat.pinent@urv.cat; Tel.: +34-977-559-566

Received: 27 October 2020; Accepted: 23 November 2020; Published: 27 November 2020

Abstract: Adaptive homeostasis declines with age and this leads to, among other things, the appearance of chronic age-related pathologies such as cancer, neurodegeneration, osteoporosis, sarcopenia, cardiovascular disease and diabetes. Grape seed-derived procyanidins (GSPE) have been shown to be effective against several of these pathologies, mainly in young animal models. Here we test their effectiveness in aged animals: 21-month-old female rats were treated with 500 mg GSPE/kg of body weight for ten days. Afterwards they were kept on a chow diet for eleven weeks. Food intake, body weight, metabolic plasma parameters and tumor incidence were measured. The GSPE administered to aged rats had an effect on food intake during the treatment and after eleven weeks continued to have an effect on visceral adiposity. It prevented pancreas dysfunction induced by ageing and maintained a higher glucagon/insulin ratio together with a lower decrease in ketonemia. It was very effective in preventing age-related tumor development. All in all, this study supports the positive effect of GSPE on preventing some age-related pathologies.

Keywords: ageing; procyanidins; food intake; adiposity; glucagon/insulin; tumor

1. Introduction

Adaptive homeostasis is a highly conserved process whereby cells, tissues and whole organisms transiently activate various signaling pathways in response to short-term mild internal or external perturbations, thereby resulting in transient changes in gene expression and stress resistance. There is a great deal of evidence that suggests that adaptive homeostasis declines with age. In fact, ageing is associated with a twofold detrimental impact on adaptive homeostasis [1]. Firstly, aged organisms lose their ability to rapidly modulate the adaptive homeostatic response and secondly, the compensatory basal increase in stress-responsive enzymes further compresses the maximal range of responses thus diminishing cellular ability to efficiently mitigate damage. All of this loss of adaptation leads to, among other things, chronic age-related pathologies such as cancer, neurodegeneration, osteoporosis, sarcopenia, cardiovascular disease and diabetes [2].

Metabolic derangement is one of the "seven pillars" considered among the basic mechanisms associated with age-related pathologies [3]. As glucose metabolism plays a key role in the energy management of the whole organism, its dysregulation with ageing affects several metabolic aspects [4]. Age changes in hepatic glucose output and peripheral insulin sensitivity seems to be more closely related to changes in body composition than to the ageing process itself [5]. Indeed, the intra-abdominal or visceral fat pad shows the highest association risk for diabetes mellitus, hypertension, atherosclerosis, dyslipidemia, cancers and mortality compared with peripheral obesity [6]. There is also controversy regarding the role of age in the ability of β-cells to function [5] and also its effect on β-cells although a few authors point to a higher hepatic sensitivity to plasma glucagon in older subjects [7].

Polyphenols are a broad spectrum of structures widely found in fruits and vegetables and derived products and also in beverages such as chocolate, green tea, coffee and wine [8]. They have been shown to protect against most age-related pathologies (cancer [9]; hypertension [10–12]; sarcopenia [13,14]; neurodegeneration [15–20], osteoporosis [21,22] and cataract formation [23]). One group of these polyphenols is grape seed-derived procyanidins (GSPE), which include several flavanols, procyanidins and some phenolic acids [24]. They have been widely studied as antiobesogenic and antidiabetic agents [8,25,26], as being protective against atherogenic indexes [27] and renal failure [28] and as anti-cancer agents [29]. However, their effectiveness on ageing processes in the metabolism has not been proved.

We have previously shown that some GSPE doses act as satiating agents in young healthy rats [30], limiting their body weight increase and adiposity [25] among other properties effective against metabolic syndrome [31,32]. Indeed, we have shown that their effects on body weight and adiposity [33] continue over the long term once the GSPE administration has finished [34]. Considering these beneficial effects of GSPE and the evidence that dietary restriction has been proven to extend lifespan [35], we hypothesize that the doses of GSPE with satiating properties may be beneficial in counteracting the ageing-induced loss of buffering in the body. We therefore aim to demonstrate this hypothesis after a 10-day GSPE oral treatment in aged rats and to observe its long term anti-ageing outcome, focusing our study on body weight and metabolism.

2. Materials and Methods

2.1. Proanthocyanidin Extract

The grape seed extract rich in proanthocyanidins (GSPE) came from Les Dérivés Résiniques et Terpéniques (Dax, France). According to the manufacturer, the GSPE used in this study (lot 207100) had a total proanthocyanidin content of 76.9% consisting of a mixture of monomers of flavan-3-ols (23.1%), dimers (21.7%), trimers (21.6%), tetramers (22.2%) and pentamers (11.4%).

2.2. Animal Model

In this study, 34 female Wistar rats were used, 10 of which were two months old (weighing 210–220 g) and 24 of which were 21 months old (weighing 300–350 g). The rats were obtained from Envigo (Barcelona, Spain). They were housed individually at a room temperature of 23 °C with a standard 12 h light-dark cycle, ventilation and ad libitum access to a standard chow diet (2014 Teklad Global 14% protein rodent maintenance diet, Envigo, Barcelona, Spain) and tap water.

2.3. Experimental Design

The experiment was divided into two parts (Figure 1). The first consisted of 10 days of treatment with GPSE by oral gavage and an evaluation of its immediate effects on food intake and body weight. The second consisted of an assessment of the long term effects of this 10-day GSPE treatment on the metabolism. All procedures were approved by the Experimental Animal Ethics Committee of the Generalitat de Catalunya, Spain (Department of Territory and Sustainability, General Directorate for Environmental and Natural Policy, project authorization code: 10183).

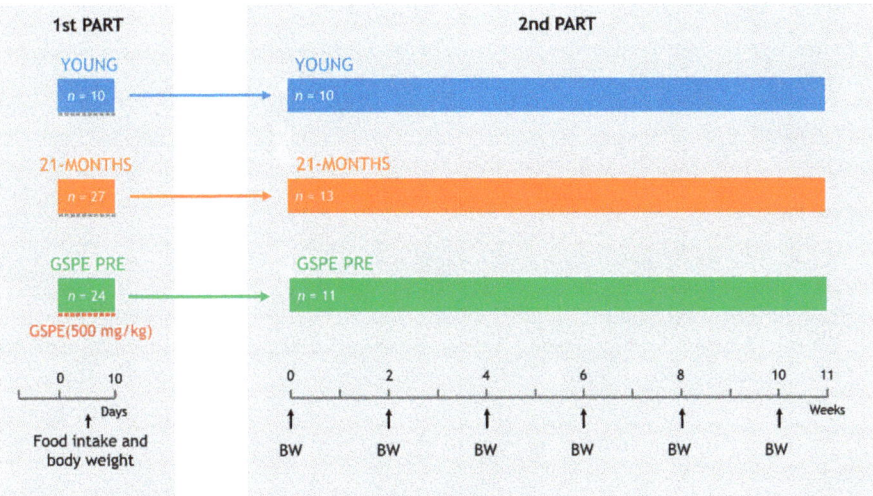

Figure 1. Schematic diagram of the experimental design. The experiment was divided into two parts. In the first part, the group named GSPE PRE animals were gavaged daily with a dose of 500 mg/kg of grape seed-derived procyanidins (GSPE) for 10 days while YOUNG and 21-MONTHS animals were gavaged with a vehicle. Food intake was recorded daily and body weight (BW) was measured after the 10 days of treatment. In the second part, all rats were maintained equally for 75 days and body weight was recorded every two weeks.

For the first part of the study, after a week of adaptation to the environment and another week of adaptation to oral gavage, the rats were weighed and divided into three experimental groups as follows:

(1) YOUNG, which consisted of 10 two-month-old rats.
(2) 21-MONTHS, which consisted of 27 twenty-one-month-old rats.
(3) GSPE PRE, which consisted of 24 twenty-one-month-old rats.

For 10 days, all of the animals were fasted from 15:00 h. The GSPE was dissolved in tap water and orally gavaged to the GSPE PRE animals at a dose of 500 mg GSPE/kg of body weight at 18:00 h, one hour before the dark onset. Animals in the YOUNG and 21-MONTHS groups received an equivalent volume of tap water at the same time points. The chow diet was administered at the dark onset (19:00 h). The chow intake was measured after 20 h, the next day at 15:00 h, when the animals were fasted again. At the beginning and end of the 10-day treatment, the rats were weighed.

After the treatment, 13 animals from the 21-MONTHS group and 11 animals from the GSPE PRE group together with all of the YOUNG animals ($n = 10$) entered the second part of the study, which consisted of maintaining them for 75 more days with a chow diet and body weight records every two weeks.

2.4. Blood and Tissue Collection

At the end of the study, the animals were fasted for 12 h and euthanized by decapitation. The blood was collected using heparin (Deltalab, Barcelona, Spain) as anticoagulant. Plasma was obtained by centrifugation (1500 g, 15 min, 4 °C) and stored at −80 °C until analysis. The different white adipose tissue depots (retroperitoneal (rWAT), mesenteric (mWAT) and periovaric (oWAT)) and the brown adipose tissue (BAT), liver, kidneys, spleen, stomach, caecum and femur were rapidly removed, weighed, snap-frozen in liquid nitrogen and stored at −80 °C. When identified, tumorous tissues were excised and weighed.

2.5. Biochemical Variables

Commercial colorimetric enzymatic kits were used to measure levels of glucose, triacylglycerol, cholesterol, urea, creatinine (QCA, Tarragona, Spain), non-esterified fatty acids (NEFAs) (Wako, Neuss, Germany) and β-hydroxybutyrate (Ben Biochemical Enterprise, Milano, Italy) in the plasma samples in accordance with the manufacturers' instructions. Commercial ELISA kits were used to quantify plasma levels of insulin (Millipore, Madrid, Spain) and glucagon (Mercodia, Uppsala, Sweden).

2.6. Statistical Analysis

At the end of the study, statistical analysis was performed with all collected data using one-way ANOVA with Dunnet's post-hoc test taking the 21-MONTHS group as control. A chi-squared test was used to assess the association between tumor incidence and the variables of interest (age, treatment) in XLSTAT 2020.1 (Addinsoft, Spain) statistical software. The statistical significance for both tests was set at $p < 0.05$.

3. Results

3.1. GSPE Reduces Food Intake and Body Weight in the Short-Term in Aged Rats

Our first goal was to find out whether a dose of GSPE with satiating properties in young animals [25] was also effective in aged rats. The daily food intake was equivalent between the YOUNG and 21-MONTHS groups (Figure 2a). In agreement, the accumulated food intake for the 10 days was not different between the two groups (Figure 2b). The GSPE treatment over 10 days reduced the 20 h food intake almost daily in comparison with the 21-MONTHS rats (Figure 2a). In this case, there was a statistically significant effect on the accumulated food intake for the 10-day GSPE treatment group versus the 21-MONTHS group, as shown in Figure 2b. This reduction in the energy entering the organism over these days brought about a slightly lower body weight after the end of the treatment in the GSPE PRE rats compared with the 21-MONTHS rats (Figure 2c). As expected, the young rats showed a lower body weight than the 21-MONTHS rats (Figure 2c).

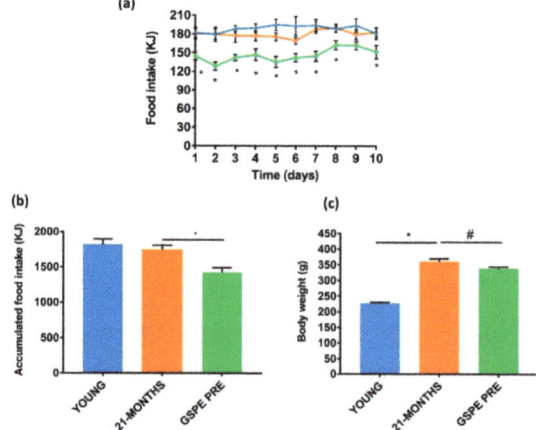

Figure 2. Effect of the 10-day treatment on food intake and body weight. (**a**) Daily food intake, where blue, orange and green represent YOUNG, 21-MONTHS and GSPE PRE groups, respectively. (**b**) Accumulated food intake over the 10 days of treatment. (**c**) Body weight at day 10. Values are means ± SEM. * p-value < 0.05, # p-value < 0.1 compared with 21-MONTHS rats.

3.2. The GSPE Effect on Body Weight and Adiposity Continued for Several Weeks after Administration

Once the GSPE treatment was finished, the rats were kept for eleven weeks to evaluate the long term effects of GSPE on the 21-MONTHS rats [33]. Figure 3a shows the percentage of body weight increase during this period. The highest percentage increase was found in the young rats because they were undergoing a growth period in their lives. The 21-MONTHS rats showed a significantly lower weight increase. Initially the GSPE-treated rats showed a body weight increase similar to that of the 21-MONTHS rats (Figure 3a). However, in the tenth and eleventh weeks they significantly increased their weight to reach a final body weight close to the 21-MONTHS group (Figure 3b).

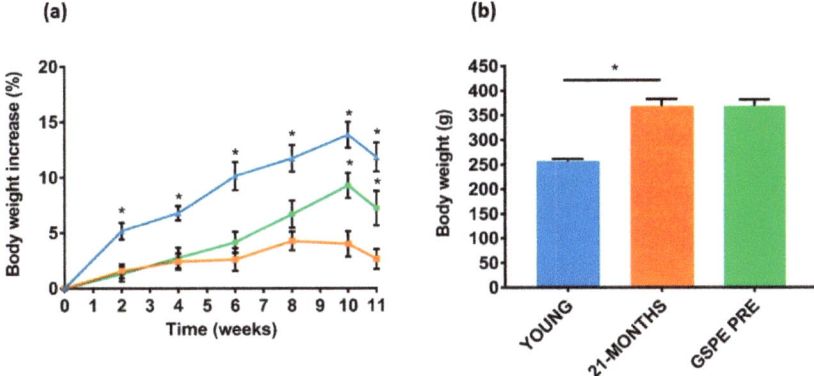

Figure 3. Body weight changes after GSPE pre-treatment. (**a**) Percentage of body weight increase from day 10 of the experiment. Body weight was measured once every two weeks throughout the whole experiment. Blue, orange and green represent YOUNG, 21-MONTHS and GSPE PRE groups, respectively. (**b**) Body weight at the end of the experiment. Values are means ± SEM. * $p < 0.05$ compared with 21-MONTHS rats.

Table 1 shows the weight of the tissues at the end of the experiment. As expected, due to their relative difference in size, all of the 21-MONTHS animals presented bigger organs than the young animals. When we compared the GSPE-treated rats with the untreated 21-MONTHS group, despite the similar body weight, the percentage of visceral adiposity was significantly lower in the GSPE PRE rats (Table 1). There were no differences in most of the other tissues except for the liver, which was also smaller in the GSPE-treated rats. The kidney showed a trend towards a lower size too.

Table 1. Morphometric characteristics at the end of the experiment (week 11).

Variable	YOUNG	21-MONTHS	GSPE PRE
n	10	13	11
Body weight (g)	256.6 ± 4.3 *	367.4 ± 15.0	366.8 ± 14.2
mWAT (g)	3.7 ± 0.2 *	13.1 ± 1.2	10.5 ± 1.3
oWAT (g)	6.8 ± 0.2 *	16.6 ± 1.5	15.5 ± 1.5
rWAT (g)	4.0 ± 0.3 *	11.1 ± 1.1	10.6 ± 1.1
Total visceral WAT (g)	14.6 ± 0.2 *	39.5 ± 3.4	34.8 ± 3.3
BAT (g)	0.4 ± 0.0 *	0.7 ± 0.1	0.7 ± 0.1
% visceral adiposity	5.4 ± 0.2 *	11.3 ± 0.6	9.5 ± 0.7 *
Liver (g)	6.2 ± 0.2 *	8.7 ± 0.4	7.7 ± 0.2 *
Spleen (g)	0.5 ± 0.0 *	0.8 ± 0.0	0.8 ± 0.0
Kidney (g)	0.8 ± 0.0 *	1.0 ± 0.0	0.9 ± 0.0 #

mWAT: mesenteric white adipose tissue; oWAT: periovaric white adipose tissue; rWAT: retroperitoneal white adipose tissue; BAT: brown adipose tissue; total visceral WAT: sum of all white adipose tissues. Values are means ± SEM. * $p < 0.05$ compared with 21-MONTHS rats. Trends: # $p < 0.1$ compared with 21-MONTHS rats.

3.3. Aged GSPE Pre-Treated Rats Showed a Higher Fasting Glucagon/Insulin Ratio Eleven Weeks after the Treatment

Looking at the biochemical parameters in the plasma of fasted YOUNG and 21-MONTHS rats, glucose, non-esterified fatty acids (NEFA), urea and creatinine levels were unaffected by ageing (Table 2). A GSPE pre-treatment (GSPE PRE) showed a trend towards increasing urea. Regarding endocrine pancreas hormones, plasma insulin and glucagon were greatly increased by the ageing process (Table 2) and the GSPE pre-treatment limited the increase in the insulinemia. To gain a better picture of the metabolic status of these animals, we worked on some ratios that provided us with more information. Figure 4a shows that the GSPE pre-treatment did not avoid the increase in insulin resistance brought about by the ageing processes as indicated by the index of insulin resistance HOMA-IR. Conversely, the GSPE pre-treated group (GSPE PRE) showed a normalized pancreatic response as indicated by the lower HOMA-β of this group versus the 21-MONTHS group (Figure 4b). When we compared the glucagon/insulin ratio in the plasma of fasted animals, we found no statistically different results due to the ageing process but we did find that the GSPE pre-treated group clearly showed a higher ratio (Figure 4c). To complete the picture, Figure 4d shows that the 21-MONTHS animals produced a limited amount of β-hydroxybutyrate derived from NEFA. Finally, there were no changes in renal functionality due to ageing or GSPE pre-treatment (GSPE PRE) as defined by the urea/creatinine ratio (Figure 4e).

Table 2. Plasma biochemical characteristics at the end of the experiment (week 11).

Variable	YOUNG	21-MONTHS	GSPE PRE
Plasma			
Glucose (mM)	7.3 ± 0.3	7.0 ± 0.3	8.1 ± 0.6
TAG (mM)	0.4 ± 0.1 #	0.6 ± 0.1	0.5 ± 0.1
NEFA (mM)	1.0 ± 0.1	1.0 ± 0.1	0.9 ± 0.1
Cholesterol (mM)	2.6 ± 0.1 *	4.5 ± 0.4	4.2 ± 0.4
β-Hydroxybutyrate (mM)	0.7 ± 0.1 *	0.3 ± 0.1	0.5 ± 0.1
Urea (mM)	4.2 ± 0.2	3.8 ± 0.2	4.3 ± 0.1 #
Creatinine (μM)	7.1 ± 0.3	7.7 ± 0.6	7.3 ± 0.7
Insulin (pM)	182.7 ± 1.0 *	322.2 ± 36.4	233.7 ± 13.4 *
Glucagon (pM)	7.2 ± 1.3 *	18.2 ± 2.5	18.8 ± 1.9

Values are means ± SEM. * $p < 0.05$ compared with 21-MONTHS rats. Trends: # $p < 0.1$ compared with 21-MONTHS rats. TAG: triglycerides; NEFA: non-esterified fatty acids.

3.4. GSPE Limits the Development of Tumors in 21-MONTHS Rats

One of the characteristics of ageing is an increase in the presence of tumors [36]. When the rats were dissected, all of the tumors found were counted, weighed and classified (Supplementary Table S1). Figure 5 shows that we found no tumors in the YOUNG rats but the incidence of spontaneous tumors in the 21-MONTHS rats was 46.2%. The GSPE pre-treatment limited their presence. The chi-squared test, comparing both aged groups, showed a significant reduction of the present of tumors with the GSPE pre-treatment of 9.1% (Fisher's exact test, $p < 0.078$).

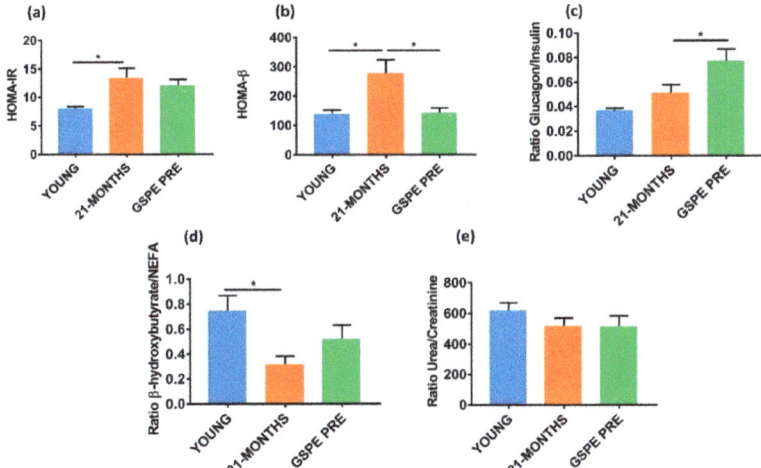

Figure 4. Biochemical characteristics of the groups analyzed at 13 weeks. (**a**) Insulin resistance HOMA-IR index. (**b**) Insulin resistance HOMA-β index. (**c**) Glucagon/insulin ratio. (**d**) β-hydroxybutyrate/non-esterified fatty acids (NEFA) ratio. (**e**) Urea/creatinine ratio. Values are means ± SEM. * $p < 0.05$ compared with 21-MONTHS rats.

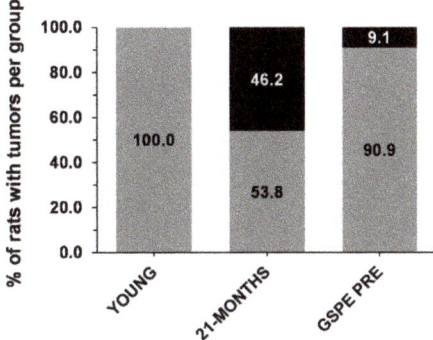

Figure 5. Percentage of tumors per group. Values are the percentage of rats without tumors (grey) and with tumors (black) per group studied.

4. Discussion

Ageing is a physiological process characterized by metabolic changes that lead to obesity, insulin resistance and dyslipidemia, which are risk factors for ageing-associated pathologies such as diabetes and cardiovascular disease [5,36]. GSPE has the ability to prevent several of these metabolic disruptions in young rats [33,34,37]. Here we have shown that GSPE maintains its ability in the 21-MONTHS animals. In addition, this GSPE treatment showed a trend to prevent the development of tumorigenic tissue growths, also closely associated with the ageing processes.

In previous studies, we defined a dose of 500 mg/kg GSPE as responsible for reducing food intake and body weight in young rats [25]. Here we have found a similar effect on food intake in aged animals over the 10 days that the treatment lasted. In this case, the food intake reduction of around 20% had only a slight effect on body weight immediately after the treatment because these animals had already reached adulthood and their body weight remained constant. In young rats, studies on a caloric restriction of 20% have shown reductions in body weight increase of around 40% in fifteen days [25,38]. In 21-month-old animals, the same caloric restriction takes several weeks to obtain a 30% decrease in body weight [35]. We found that in young rats the effects of GSPE were maintained for several weeks after the treatment had finished [33]. We have now shown that in aged rats, the GSPE effect limiting body weight increase was also maintained for eight more weeks after the end of the treatment. This was probably due to the ability of proanthocyanidins to limit adipose accrual several weeks after the end of the treatment [34]. Indeed, we also found that GSPE was able to maintain a lower percentage of visceral adiposity 11 weeks after the treatment. The effects of this GSPE dose as a preventive works in a similar way to caloric restriction interventions that reverse ageing-associated visceral fat increase and have an important impact on decreasing insulin resistance [39]. Our results eleven weeks after the end of the treatment with GSPE showed a preventive effect on the increase in the HOMA-β index as also found in some other models of caloric restriction [40]. However, it did not show any clear protective effect on the insulin resistance index (HOMA-IR). This lack of effect of GSPE on insulin resistance could be the explanation for the dyslipidemic profile found in the GSPE pre-treated group at the end of the study. There is a definite cause/effect associated with insulin resistance on muscle and adipose tissue [41] and dyslipidemia [42]. Dyslipidemia, together with a decreased ketosis, has also been observed in recent work with 24-month-old male Wistar rats [43,44] and is in line with what we saw in our 21-month-old female rats. There have been some controversial results regarding caloric restriction effects on ketone bodies. A lower ability with ageing to synthetize ketone bodies in the intestine has been reported [45] as has a lower consumption of ketone bodies in the kidney [46]. In both examples, these reductions were reverted by caloric intake restriction. We previously found a higher expression of HMGCS2 in the liver of young rats five weeks after the last GSPE dose [34] suggesting a greater ability in the GSPE-treated rats to produce ketone bodies. In the present study, we did not have a statistically different effect on plasma β-hydroxybutyrate but this could be due to the length of the study.

In a fasting situation when blood insulin is low, glucagon levels are high and therefore fat oxidation and ketosis are increased and hepatic lipogenesis is activated [47]. Glucagonemia was also increased in our 21-MONTHS rats as found by Fernández et al. [44], although there is no wide consensus on glucagonemia and ageing [7]. Here, GSPE brought about a situation different than the 20% caloric restriction of Fernández et al. [44]. This higher glucagonemia in GSPE pre-treated rats clearly produced a higher glucagon/insulin ratio despite the weeks without treatment. This could explain the trend found in the limited increase in visceral adiposity in these animals. A higher presence of glucagon versus insulin during a fasting situation favors higher fat oxidation [48], which together with a higher liver sensitivity to glucagon on ageing [7] would produce a higher hepatic gluconeogenesis. We did not find a statistical change on glycemia in these GSPE pre-treated rats sacrificed in a fasting situation, but we cannot discard that it happened at some point earlier than the several weeks post-treatment when we were measuring it.

One of the significant organ systems that declines with ageing is the kidney. Changes in renal structure (reduction in mass) and function (glomerular filtration rate (GFR)) accompany advancing age [49]. Here, we found no effect of age on kidney size nor did we find any on urea, creatinine or their ratio. However, we did observe a GSPE trend after several weeks towards a smaller kidney size and an increase in urea versus the 21-MONTHS group but without any significant change in the urea/creatinine ratio, suggesting the maintenance of the glomerular filtration rate. A similar dose of 500 mg/kg GSPE had beneficial effects on reducing induced acute renal injury and chronic kidney fibrosis in young mice [50] and diabetic-associated renal injury in young rats [28]. Our results therefore suggest no clear preventive effects on kidney functionality.

All in all, this GSPE pre-treatment produced a long term effect close to a caloric restriction state in the rats. Its preventive effect against tumorigenesis was also observed. Caloric restriction prevents tumorigenesis by decreasing the metabolic rate and oxidative damage [51]. Here, we found spontaneous tumors on 46.2% of the 25-month-old rats at the end of the study, a value that was lower than the reported number of age-associated tumors on female Wistar rats [52]. With the sample size used in this study, the GSPE treatment showed a trend towards a lowered incidence of tumors on GSPE PRE rats to 9.1%. A bigger sample size would be necessary to fully demonstrate this effect. Related to the possible reasons involving caloric restriction, the GSPE tumor suppressing effect may be explained by its modulation of antiproliferative and proapoptotic genes [53] such as the tumor suppressing factor p53 [54] and NF-κβ [55] observed in different cancerous cell lines, their anti-inflammatory properties [56] and antioxidant properties [57].

5. Conclusions

We can conclude that GSPE showed interesting properties on 21-MONTHS rats. It acted to limit food intake resulting in a decreased body weight after treatment. Eleven weeks after the treatment, GSPE maintained its effects on limiting visceral adipose tissue growth, prevented the increase in the HOMA-β index and maintained a higher glucagon/insulin ratio together with a reduced incidence of age-associated spontaneous tumors. A few of these effects might be related to their caloric restriction mimetic effect.

Supplementary Materials: The following are available online at http://www.mdpi.com/2072-6643/12/12/3647/s1, Table S1: Number, weight and classification of tumor per group.

Author Contributions: Conceptualization, A.A., M.P., X.T. and M.B.; Methodology and Investigation, C.G.-B., M.S.-C. and A.M.-G.; Data Curation, E.R.-G. and R.B.-D.; Writing—Original Draft Preparation, C.G.-B. and M.S.-C.; Writing—Review & Editing, E.R.-G., A.A. and M.P.; Visualization, R.B.-D., X.T. and M.B.; Supervision, M.B. and R.B.-D.; Project Administration, M.P. and E.R.-G.; Funding Acquisition, A.A. and X.T. All authors have read and agreed to the published version of the manuscript.

Funding: This research was funded by the Spanish Government grant number AGL2017-83477-R.

Acknowledgments: We would like to thank Niurka Llopiz for technical support. C. Grau-Bové and M. Sierra-Cruz received a doctoral research grant from the Marti Franques programme of the Universitat Rovira i Virgili. M. Pinent and X. Terra are Serra Húnter fellows.

Conflicts of Interest: The authors declare no conflict of interest.

References

1. Pomatto, L.C.D.; Davies, K.J.A. The role of declining adaptive homeostasis in ageing. *J. Physiol.* **2017**, *595*, 7275–7309. [CrossRef] [PubMed]
2. Campisi, J. Aging, Cellular Senescence, and Cancer. *Annu. Rev. Physiol.* **2013**, *75*, 685–705. [CrossRef]
3. Franceschi, C.; Garagnani, P.; Morsiani, C.; Conte, M.; Santoro, A.; Grignolio, A.; Monti, D.; Capri, M.; Salvioli, S. The continuum of aging and age-related diseases: Common mechanisms but different rates. *Front. Med.* **2018**, *5*. [CrossRef] [PubMed]
4. Elahi, D.; Muller, D.C. Carbohydrate metabolism in the elderly. *Eur. J. Clin. Nutr.* **2000**, *54* (Suppl. 3), S112–S120. [CrossRef] [PubMed]
5. Chia, C.W.; Egan, J.M.; Ferrucci, L. Age-Related Changes in Glucose Metabolism, Hyperglycemia, and Cardiovascular Risk. *Circ. Res.* **2018**, *123*, 886–904. [CrossRef]
6. Shuster, A.; Patlas, M.; Pinthus, J.H.; Mourtzakis, M. The clinical importance of visceral adiposity: A critical review of methods for visceral adipose tissue analysis. *Br. J. Radiol.* **2012**, *85*, 1–10. [CrossRef]
7. Simonson, D.C.; DeFronzo, R.A. Glucagon physiology and aging: Evidence for enhanced hepatic sensitivity. *Diabetologia* **1983**, *25*, 1–7. [CrossRef]
8. Bladé, C.; Aragones, G.; Arola-Arnal, A.; Muguerza, B.; Bravo, F.I.; Salvadó, M.J.; Arola, L.; Suárez, M. Proanthocyanidins in Health and Disease. *Biofactors* **2016**, *42*, 5–12.
9. Mirza-Aghazadeh-Attari, M.; Ekrami, E.M.; Aghdas, S.A.M.; Mihanfar, A.; Hallaj, S.; Yousefi, B.; Safa, A.; Majidinia, M. Targeting PI3K/Akt/mTOR signaling pathway by polyphenols: Implication for cancer therapy. *Life Sci.* **2020**, *255*, 117481. [CrossRef]
10. Tasatargil, A.; Tanriover, G.; Barutcigil, A.; Turkmen, E. Protective effect of resveratrol on methylglyoxal-induced endothelial dysfunction in aged rats. *Aging Clin. Exp. Res.* **2019**, *31*, 331–338. [CrossRef]

11. Dehghani, A.; Hafizibarjin, Z.; Najjari, R.; Kaseb, F.; Safari, F. Resveratrol and 1,25-dihydroxyvitamin D co-administration protects the heart against d-galactose-induced aging in rats: Evaluation of serum and cardiac levels of klotho. *Aging Clin. Exp. Res.* **2019**, *31*, 1195–1205. [CrossRef] [PubMed]
12. Masodsai, K.; Lin, Y.-Y.; Chaunchaiyakul, R.; Su, C.-T.; Lee, S.-D.; Yang, A.-L. Twelve-Week Protocatechuic Acid Administration Improves Insulin-Induced and Insulin-Like Growth Factor-1-Induced Vasorelaxation and Antioxidant Activities in Aging Spontaneously Hypertensive Rats. *Nutrients* **2019**, *11*, 699. [CrossRef] [PubMed]
13. Annunziata, G.; Jimenez-García, M.; Tejada, S.; Moranta, D.; Arnone, A.; Ciampaglia, R.; Tenore, G.C.; Sureda, A.; Novellino, E.; Capó, X. Grape Polyphenols Ameliorate Muscle Decline Reducing Oxidative Stress and Oxidative Damage in Aged Rats. *Nutrients* **2020**, *12*, 1280. [CrossRef]
14. Meador, B.M.; Mirza, K.A.; Tian, M.; Skelding, M.B.; Reaves, L.A.; Edens, N.K.; Tisdale, M.J.; Pereira, S.L. The Green Tea Polyphenol Epigallocatechin-3-Gallate (EGCg) Attenuates Skeletal Muscle Atrophy in a Rat Model of Sarcopenia. *J. Frailty Aging* **2015**, *4*, 209. [PubMed]
15. Sarubbo, F.; Ramis, M.R.; Aparicio, S.; Ruiz, L.; Esteban, S.; Miralles, A.; Moranta, D. Improving effect of chronic resveratrol treatment on central monoamine synthesis and cognition in aged rats. *Age* **2015**, *37*, 9777. [CrossRef] [PubMed]
16. Abhijit, S.; Subramanyam, M.V.V.; Devi, S.A. Grape Seed Proanthocyanidin and Swimming Exercise Protects Against Cognitive Decline: A Study on M1 Acetylcholine Receptors in Aging Male Rat Brain. *Neurochem. Res.* **2017**, *42*, 3573–3586. [CrossRef]
17. Abhijit, S.; Tripathi, S.J.; Bhagya, V.; Shankaranarayana Rao, B.S.; Subramanyam, M.V.; Asha Devi, S. Antioxidant action of grape seed polyphenols and aerobic exercise in improving neuronal number in the hippocampus is associated with decrease in lipid peroxidation and hydrogen peroxide in adult and middle-aged rats. *Exp. Gerontol.* **2018**, *101*, 101–112. [CrossRef]
18. Ksiezak-Reding, H.; Ho, L.; Santa-Maria, I.; Diaz-Ruiz, C.; Wang, J.; Pasinetti, G.M. Ultrastructural alterations of Alzheimer's disease paired helical filaments by grape seed-derived polyphenols. *Neurobiol. Aging* **2012**, *33*, 1427–1439. [CrossRef]
19. Santa-Maria, I.; Diaz-Ruiz, C.; Ksiezak-Reding, H.; Chen, A.; Ho, L.; Wang, J.; Pasinetti, G.M. GSPE interferes with tau aggregation in vivo: Implication for treating tauopathy. *Neurobiol. Aging* **2012**, *33*, 2072–2081. [CrossRef]
20. Asha Devi, S.; Sagar Chandrasekar, B.K.; Manjula, K.R.; Ishii, N. Grape seed proanthocyanidin lowers brain oxidative stress in adult and middle-aged rats. *Exp. Gerontol.* **2011**, *46*, 958–964. [CrossRef]
21. Graef, J.L.; Ouyang, P.; Wang, Y.; Rendina-Ruedy, E.; Lerner, M.R.; Marlow, D.; Lucas, E.A.; Smith, B.J. Dried plum polyphenolic extract combined with vitamin K and potassium restores trabecular and cortical bone in osteopenic model of postmenopausal bone loss. *J. Funct. Foods* **2018**, *42*, 262–270. [CrossRef] [PubMed]
22. Shen, C.L.; Smith, B.J.; Li, J.; Cao, J.J.; Song, X.; Newhardt, M.F.; Corry, K.A.; Tomison, M.D.; Tang, L.; Wang, J.S.; et al. Effect of Long-Term Green Tea Polyphenol Supplementation on Bone Architecture, Turnover, and Mechanical Properties in Middle-Aged Ovariectomized Rats. *Calcif. Tissue Int.* **2019**, *104*, 285–300. [CrossRef] [PubMed]
23. Singh, A.; Bodakhe, S.H. Resveratrol delay the cataract formation against naphthalene-induced experimental cataract in the albino rats. *J. Biochem. Mol. Toxicol.* **2020**, *34*, e22420. [CrossRef] [PubMed]
24. Rodríguez-Pérez, C.; García-Villanova, B.; Guerra-Hernández, E.; Verardo, V. Grape seeds proanthocyanidins: An overview of in vivo bioactivity in animal models. *Nutrients* **2019**, *11*, 2435.
25. Serrano, J.; Casanova-Martí, À.; Gual, A.; Pérez-Vendrell, A.M.; Blay, M.T.; Terra, X.; Ardévol, A.; Pinent, M. A specific dose of grape seed-derived proanthocyanidins to inhibit body weight gain limits food intake and increases energy expenditure in rats. *Eur. J. Nutr.* **2017**, *56*, 1629–1636. [CrossRef]
26. Gonzalez-Abuin, N.; Pinent, M.; Casanova-Marti, A.; Arola, L.L.; Blay, M.; Ardevol, A.; González-Abuín, N.; Pinent, M.; Casanova-Martí, A.; Arola, L.L.; et al. Procyanidins and their healthy protective effects against type 2 diabetes. *Curr. Med. Chem.* **2015**, *22*, 39–50. [CrossRef]
27. Quesada, H.; Pajuelo, D.; Fernández-Iglesias, A.; Díaz, S.; Ardevol, A.; Blay, M.; Salvadó, M.J.; Arola, L.; Blade, C. Proanthocyanidins modulate triglyceride secretion by repressing the expression of long chain acyl-CoA synthetases in Caco2 intestinal cells. *Food Chem.* **2011**, *129*, 1490–1494. [CrossRef]
28. Li, Y.; Bao, L.; Zhang, Z.; Dai, X.; Ding, Y.; Jiang, Y.; Li, Y. Effects of grape seed proanthocyanidin extract on renal injury in type 2 diabetic rats. *Mol. Med. Rep.* **2015**, *11*, 645–652.

29. Ma, J.; Fang, B.; Zeng, F.; Pang, H.; Ma, C.; Xia, J. Grape seed proanthocyanidins extract inhibits pancreatic cancer cell growth through down-regulation of miR-27a expression. *J. Cent. South Univ. Med. Sci.* **2015**, *40*, 46–52.
30. Serrano, J.; Casanova-Martí, À.; Gil-Cardoso, K.; Blay, M.T.; Terra, X.; Pinent, M.; Ardévol, A. Acutely administered grape-seed proanthocyanidin extract acts as a satiating agent. *Food Funct.* **2016**, *7*, 483–490. [CrossRef]
31. Gil-Cardoso, K.; Ginés, I.; Pinent, M.; Ardévol, A.; Blay, M.; Terra, X. The co-administration of proanthocyanidins and an obesogenic diet prevents the increase in intestinal permeability and metabolic endotoxemia derived to the diet. *J. Nutr. Biochem.* **2018**, *62*, 35–42. [CrossRef] [PubMed]
32. Ginés, I.; Gil-Cardoso, K.; Terra, X.; Blay, M.; Pérez-Vendrell, A.M.; Pinent, M.; Ardévol, A. Grape Seed Proanthocyanidins Target the Enteroendocrine System in Cafeteria-Diet-Fed Rats. *Mol. Nutr. Food Res.* **2019**, *63*, 1800912. [CrossRef] [PubMed]
33. Ginés, I.; Gil-Cardoso, K.; Serrano, J.; Casanova-Martí, À.; Blay, M.; Pinent, M.; Ardévol, A.; Terra, X. Effects of an Intermittent Grape-Seed Proanthocyanidin (GSPE) Treatment on a Cafeteria Diet Obesogenic Challenge in Rats. *Nutrients* **2018**, *10*, 315. [CrossRef] [PubMed]
34. Ginés, I.; Gil-cardoso, K.; Serrano, J.; Casanova-marti, À.; Lobato, M.; Terra, X.; Blay, M.T.; Ard, A. Proanthocyanidins Limit Adipose Accrual Induced by a Cafeteria Diet, Several Weeks after the End of the Treatment. *Genes* **2019**, *10*, 598. [CrossRef] [PubMed]
35. Mitchell, S.J.; Madrigal-Matute, J.; Scheibye-Knudsen, M.; Fang, E.; Aon, M.; González-reyes, J.A.; Cortassa, S.; Kaushik, S.; Gonzalez-Freire, M.; Patel, B.; et al. Effects of sex, strain, and energy intake on hallmarks of aging in mice. *Cell Metab.* **2016**, *23*, 1093–1112. [CrossRef]
36. López-Otín, C.; Blasco, M.A.; Partridge, L.; Serrano, M.; Kroemer, G. The hallmarks of aging. *Cell* **2013**, *153*, 1194. [CrossRef]
37. Ginés, I.; Gil-Cardoso, K.; D'addario, C.; Falconi, A.; Bellia, F.; Blay, M.T.; Terra, X.; Ardévol, A.; Pinent, M.; Beltrán-Debón, R. Long-lasting effects of gspe on ileal GLP-1R gene expression are associated with a hypomethylation of the GLP-1R promoter in female wistar rats. *Biomolecules* **2019**, *9*, 865. [CrossRef]
38. Foster, S.R.; Porrello, E.R.; Stefani, M.; Smith, N.J.; Molenaar, P.; Dos Remedios, C.G.; Thomas, W.G.; Ramialison, M. Cardiac gene expression data and in silico analysis provide novel insights into human and mouse taste receptor gene regulation. *Naunyn. Schmiedebergs. Arch. Pharmacol.* **2015**, *388*, 1009–1027. [CrossRef]
39. Barzilai, N.; Banerjee, S.; Hawkins, M.; Chen, W.; Rossetti, L. Caloric restriction reverses hepatic insulin resistance in aging rats by decreasing visceral fat. *J. Clin. Investig.* **1998**, *101*, 1353–1361. [CrossRef]
40. Margolis, L.M.; Rivas, D.A.; Ezzyat, Y.; Gaffney-Stomberg, E.; Young, A.J.; McClung, J.P.; Fielding, R.A.; Pasiakos, S.M. Calorie restricted high protein diets downregulate lipogenesis and lower intrahepatic triglyceride concentrations in male rats. *Nutrients* **2016**, *8*, 571. [CrossRef]
41. Shanik, M.H.; Xu, Y.; Skrha, J.; Dankner, R.; Zick, Y.; Roth, J. Insulin resistance and hyperinsulinemia: Is hyperinsulinemia the cart or the horse? *Diabetes Care* **2008**, *31* (Suppl. 2), S262–S268. [CrossRef] [PubMed]
42. Petersen, K.F.; Dufour, S.; Savage, D.B.; Bilz, S.; Solomon, G.; Yonemitsu, S.; Cline, G.W.; Befroy, D.; Zemany, L.; Kahn, B.B.; et al. The role of skeletal muscle insulin resistance in the pathogenesis of the metabolic syndrome. *Proc. Natl. Acad. Sci. USA* **2007**, *104*, 12587–12594. [CrossRef]
43. Salamanca, A.; Bárcena, B.; Arribas, C.; Fernández-Agulló, T.; Martínez, C.; Carrascosa, J.M.; Ros, M.; Andrés, A.; Gallardo, N. Aging impairs the hepatic subcellular distribution of ChREBP in response to fasting/feeding in rats: Implications on hepatic steatosis. *Exp. Gerontol.* **2015**, *69*, 9–19. [CrossRef] [PubMed]
44. Fernández, A.; Mazuecos, L.; Pintado, C.; Rubio, B.; López, V.; de Solís, A.J.; Rodríguez, M.; Andrés, A.; Gallardo, N. Effects of moderate chronic food restriction on the development of postprandial dyslipidemia with ageing. *Nutrients* **2019**, *11*, 1865.
45. Gebert, N.; Cheng, C.W.; Kirkpatrick, J.M.; Di Fraia, D.; Yun, J.; Schädel, P.; Pace, S.; Garside, G.B.; Werz, O.; Rudolph, K.L.; et al. Region-Specific Proteome Changes of the Intestinal Epithelium during Aging and Dietary Restriction. *Cell Rep.* **2020**, *31*, 107565. [CrossRef] [PubMed]
46. Brégère, C.; Rebrin, I.; Gallaher, T.K.; Sohal, R.S. Effects of age and calorie restriction on tryptophan nitration, protein content, and activity of succinyl-CoA:3-ketoacid CoA transferase in rat kidney mitochondria. *Free Radic. Biol. Med.* **2010**, *48*, 609–618. [CrossRef] [PubMed]

47. Soeters, M.R.; Sauerwein, H.P.; Faas, L.; Smeenge, M.; Duran, M.; Wanders, R.J.; Ruiter, A.F.; Ackermans, M.T.; Fliers, E.; Houten, S.M.; et al. Effects of Insulin on Ketogenesis Following Fasting in Lean and Obese Men. *Obesity* **2009**, *17*, 1326–1331. [CrossRef]
48. Kerndt, P.R.; Naughton, J.L.; Driscoll, C.E.; Loxterkamp, D.A. Fasting: The history, pathophysiology and complications. *West. J. Med.* **1982**, *137*, 379–399.
49. Panickar, K.S.; Jewell, D.E. The benefit of anti-inflammatory and renal-protective dietary ingredients on the biological processes of aging in the kidney. *Biology* **2018**, *7*, 45. [CrossRef]
50. Zhan, J.; Wang, K.; Zhang, C.C.; Zhang, C.C.; Li, Y.; Zhang, Y.; Chang, X.; Zhou, Q.; Yao, Y.; Liu, Y.; et al. GSPE inhibits HMGB1 release, attenuating renal IR-induced acute renal injury and chronic renal fibrosis. *Int. J. Mol. Sci.* **2016**, *17*, 1647. [CrossRef]
51. Rastogi, A.; Fonarow, G.C. The cardiorenal connection in heart failure. *Curr. Cardiol. Rep.* **2008**, *10*, 190–197. [CrossRef] [PubMed]
52. Maita, K.; Matsunuma, N.; Masuda, H.; Suzuki, Y. The age-related tumor incidence in Wistar-Imamichi rat. *Exp. Anim.* **1979**, *28*, 555–560. [CrossRef] [PubMed]
53. Dinicola, S.; Cucina, A.; Pasqualato, A.; D'Anselmi, F.; Proietti, S.; Lisi, E.; Pasqua, G.; Antonacci, D.; Bizzarri, M. Antiproliferative and apoptotic effects triggered by grape seed extract (GSE) versus epigallocatechin and procyanidins on colon cancer cell lines. *Int. J. Mol. Sci.* **2012**, *13*, 651–664. [CrossRef]
54. Yousef, M.I.; Khalil, D.K.A.M.; Abdou, H.M. Neuro- and nephroprotective effect of grape seed proanthocyanidin extract against carboplatin and thalidomide through modulation of inflammation, tumor suppressor protein p53, neurotransmitters, oxidative stress and histology. *Toxicol. Rep.* **2018**, *5*, 568–578. [CrossRef]
55. Guo, F.; Hu, Y.; Niu, Q.; Li, Y.; Ding, Y.; Ma, R.; Wang, X.; Li, S.; Xie, J. Grape Seed Proanthocyanidin Extract Inhibits Human Esophageal Squamous Cancerous Cell Line ECA109 via the NF-κB Signaling Pathway. *Mediators Inflamm.* **2018**, *2018*. [CrossRef]
56. Gil-cardoso, K.; Ginés, I.; Ardévol, A.; Blay, M.; Terra, X. Effects of flavonoids on intestinal inflammation, barrier integrity and changes in gut microbiota during diet-induced obesity. *Nutr. Res. Rev.* **2018**, *29*, 234–248. [CrossRef]
57. Spranger, I. Chemical characterization and antioxidant activities of oligomeric and polymeric procyanidin fractions from grape seeds. *Food Chem.* **2008**, *108*, 519–532. [CrossRef]

Publisher's Note: MDPI stays neutral with regard to jurisdictional claims in published maps and institutional affiliations.

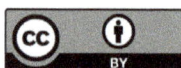

© 2020 by the authors. Licensee MDPI, Basel, Switzerland. This article is an open access article distributed under the terms and conditions of the Creative Commons Attribution (CC BY) license (http://creativecommons.org/licenses/by/4.0/).

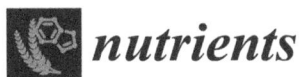

Article

Sixteen Weeks of Supplementation with a Nutritional Quantity of a Diversity of Polyphenols from Foodstuff Extracts Improves the Health-Related Quality of Life of Overweight and Obese Volunteers: A Randomized, Double-Blind, Parallel Clinical Trial

Cindy Romain [1], Linda H. Chung [2], Elena Marín-Cascales [2], Jacobo A. Rubio-Arias [2], Sylvie Gaillet [3], Caroline Laurent [3], Juana María Morillas-Ruiz [4], Alejandro Martínez-Rodriguez [2], Pedro Emilio Alcaraz [2] and Julien Cases [1],*

[1] Innovation and Scientific Affairs, Fytexia, 34350 Vendres, France; cromain@fytexia.com
[2] Research Center for High Performance Sport, Catholic University of Murcia, 30107 Murcia, Spain; lhchung@ucam.edu (L.H.C.); emarin@ucam.edu (E.M.-C.); jararias@ucam.edu (J.A.R.-A.); amrodriguez@ucam.edu (A.M.-R.); palcaraz@ucam.edu (P.E.A.)
[3] UMR 204 Nutripass, Research Institute for Development, University of Montpellier, 34095 Montpellier, France; sylvie.gaillet-foulon@univ-montp.fr (S.G.); caroline.laurent@univ-montp.fr (C.L.)
[4] Department of Food and Nutrition Technology, Catholic University of Murcia, 30107 Murcia, Spain; jmmorillas@ucam.edu
* Correspondence: jcases@fytexia.com; Tel.: +33-467-219-098

Citation: Romain, C.; Chung, L.H.; Marín-Cascales, E.; Rubio-Arias, J.A.; Gaillet, S.; Laurent, C.; Morillas-Ruiz, J.M.; Martínez-Rodriguez, A.; Alcaraz, P.E.; Cases, J. Sixteen Weeks of Supplementation with a Nutritional Quantity of a Diversity of Polyphenols from Foodstuff Extracts Improves the Health-Related Quality of Life of Overweight and Obese Volunteers: A Randomized, Double-Blind, Parallel Clinical Trial. Nutrients 2021, 13, 492. https://doi.org/10.3390/nu13020492

Academic Editors: Elena González-Burgo and Emad Al-Dujaili

Received: 14 December 2020
Accepted: 28 January 2021
Published: 2 February 2021

Publisher's Note: MDPI stays neutral with regard to jurisdictional claims in published maps and institutional affiliations.

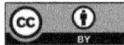

Copyright: © 2021 by the authors. Licensee MDPI, Basel, Switzerland. This article is an open access article distributed under the terms and conditions of the Creative Commons Attribution (CC BY) license (https://creativecommons.org/licenses/by/4.0/).

Abstract: Overweight and obesity adversely affect health-related quality of life (HRQOL) through day-to-day impairments of both mental and physical functioning. It is assumed that polyphenols within the Mediterranean diet may contribute to improving HRQOL. This investigation aimed at studying the effects of a polyphenol-rich ingredient on HRQOL in overweight and obese but otherwise healthy individuals. A randomized, double-blind, placebo-controlled study including 72 volunteers was conducted. Subjects were randomly assigned to receive for a 16-week period either 900 mg/day of the supplement or a placebo. Dietary recommendations were individually determined and intakes were recorded. Daily physical mobility was also monitored. Improvement of HRQOL was set as the primary outcome and assessed at baseline and at the end of the investigation using the Short-Form 36 (SF-36) health survey. Body composition was analyzed using dual-energy X-ray absorptiometry (DXA). Physical activity was calculated using the International Physical Activity Questionnaire (IPAQ). After 16 weeks, despite there being no adherence to the Mediterranean Diet Serving Score (MDSS), supplemented individuals experienced significant HRQOL improvement (+5.3%; $p = 0.001$), including enhanced perceived physical (+11.2%; $p = 0.002$) and mental health (+4.1%; $p = 0.021$) components, with bodily pain, vitality, and general health being the greatest contributors. Body fat mass significantly decreased (-1.2 kg; $p = 0.033$), mainly within the trunk area (-1.0 kg; $p = 0.002$). Engagement in physical activity significantly increased (+1308 Met-min (Metabolic Equivalent Task minutes)/week; $p = 0.050$). Hence, chronic supplementation with nutritional diversity and dosing of a Mediterranean diet-inspired, polyphenol-rich ingredient resulted in significant amelioration in both perceived physical and mental health, concomitant with the improvement of body composition, in healthy subjects with excessive adiposity.

Keywords: health-related quality of life; vitality; body composition; phenolic compounds; Mediterranean diet

1. Introduction

The World Health Organization (WHO) defines quality of life (QOL) as "an individual's perception of their position in life in the context of culture and value systems in which they live, and in relation to their goals, expectations, standards, and concerns" [1]. Such conception of QOL is subjective, multidimensional, and encompasses a broad range of life domains, among which health is one of the most important determinants.

In addition to being an objective medical evaluation, the health-related quality of life (HRQOL), which typically combines physical, psychological, and social domains of health [2], is more recognized as a central outcome in healthcare strategies, highlighting the fact that health is deeply intertwined with a patient's perspective. Accordingly, the use of HRQOL assessment is particularly relevant and is increasingly widespread in clinical practices [3], predominantly for ageing populations and for the inherent expansion in the prevalence of non-communicable diseases (NCDs), which include cardiovascular diseases, diabetes mellitus, and hypertension. NCDs are currently the leading cause of mortality in the modern world, contributing to 38 million deaths each year [4]. According to WHO, the global burden of NCDs is imputable to ageing, rapid urbanization, and to globalization of unhealthy lifestyles.

Among modifiable risk factors, overweight and obesity are significant contributors to the high prevalence rate of NCDs, making them the priority target in various public health programs [5]. A major cause of overweight and obesity is the excessive accumulation of body fat due to an imbalance between energy consumption and expenditure, particularly in populations with sedentary behaviors. The accumulation of body fat, predominantly within the abdominal region, is clearly associated with a chronic low-grade inflammatory state and an impaired redox status [6], both being principal pathological pathways involved in the development of NCDs. It is noteworthy that such disorders are also identified as validated metabolic indicators of ageing [7], suggesting that overweight and obesity are conditions that could potentially accelerate ageing and exacerbate the risk of ageing-linked NCDs [8].

In addition to their role in the etiology of these common medical conditions, overweight and obesity have profound adverse physical, social, and psychological consequences that can negatively affect HRQOL and impair everyday life [9,10], which appears to be an increasingly important outcome for patients and clinicians, as well as for policymakers. As a result, QOL has become a valuable endpoint assessed in both epidemiological and interventional weight management studies in overweight and obese volunteers [11–13]. Measuring HRQOL is the subjective perception of one's health, where patients are asked to rate several aspects of their life. Numerous studies have demonstrated that self-rated health measures are important predictors of mortality in various populations [14].

The Short-Form 36 Health survey (SF-36), a commonly used measure in HRQOL research, is a generic methodology developed and validated in the Medical Outcomes Study [15] that assesses eight important HRQOL domains that encompass health-related social, physical, and mental dimensions. The reliability of this questionnaire has been validated both in a healthy population [16] and among people with chronic and acute health conditions, but also when comparing between different groups of patients [10]. Furthermore, several authors have demonstrated a negative correlation between BMI and SF-36 scores [17,18], and also an improvement of HRQOL correlated with weight loss in overweight people [13].

Among the dietary patterns, which are mostly studied for their health effects, it appears that adherence to the Mediterranean diet has been correlated to a lower risk for NCDs [19]; it is assumed that particular bioactive constituents of the Mediterranean diet, namely polyphenols, significantly contribute to the reported health-promoted effects [20]. Moreover, along with their widely studied antioxidant properties, recent studies demonstrate the modulatory effects of phenolic compounds on various cellular signaling pathways and responses, such as inflammation and energy metabolism [21,22], highlighting the complex mode of their individual mechanism of action in preventing NCDs [23]. Emerging large cohort studies that investigated the Mediterranean diet, specifically the regular consumption of a diversity of its main polyphenol content, have shown a positive correlation to HRQOL [24,25], suggesting that such bioactive constituents might be beneficial in improving overweight- and obesity-linked impaired HRQOL.

The aim of this clinical study was to investigate whether 16 weeks of supplementation with an accurately characterized ingredient formulated from extracts of certain fruits and vegetables commonly consumed within the Mediterranean diet could improve HRQOL in overweight and obese, but otherwise healthy, subjects.

2. Materials and Methods

2.1. Subjects

Ninety-two healthy overweight and obese subjects were recruited through advertisements in the region of Murcia in southern Spain. Both men and women between the ages of 25–55 years, being overweight to obese (BMI: 25–40 kg/m^2) but otherwise healthy, were included in the study. Subjects were excluded if they: had a metabolic or chronic disease; had an allergy to carrot, grape, grapefruit, green tea, caffeine, or to guarana; were involved at the time of recruitment or within the previous 6 months in a chronic supplementation program, engaged in smoking cessation, or had high alcohol consumption; were pregnant or were breastfeeding; were in menopause; were suffering depression; or were involved in physical activity more than twice a week.

The study was approved by the Universidad Católica San Antonio de Murcia (UCAM), Spain) Ethics Committee (approval N° 5551) and conducted per the guidelines laid out in the Declaration of Helsinki [26] and in compliance with Good Clinical Practices defined in the ICH Harmonized Tripartite Guideline [27]. All participants were informed about the study procedures and signed written informed consent before entering the study. This trial was registered at clinicaltrials.gov as NCT03423719.

2.2. Test Supplement

Fiit-ns®, developed by FYTEXIA (France), is principally obtained by alcohol and water extraction of grapefruit (*Citrus paradisi* Macfad), grape (*Vitis vinifera* L.), and guarana seed (*Paullinia cupana* Kunth); by water extraction of green tea (*Camellia sinensis* L. Kuntze) and black carrot (*Daucus carota* L.). Fiit-ns® provides bioactive compounds, specifically polyphenols from the flavonoid family, and natural components of the methylxanthine family to from an extract of guarana seeds, as well as vitamin B3. The placebo product was 100% maltodextrin, which is polyphenol-, methylxanthine- and vitamin B3-free. Both Fiit-ns® and placebo were supplied in 450 mg capsules of identical appearance and flavor.

The supplement was analyzed by means of high-performance liquid chromatography (HPLC). An Agilent HPLC 1260 apparatus (Agilent Technologies, Les Ulis, France) using software Openlab CDS Chemstation Edition (version 1.3.1) coupled with a diode array detector was used. Separations were carried out by means of a Zorbax Stablebond SB-C18 column (4.6 × 150 mm; 5 μm particle size). To detect different phenolic classes, two different analytical methods were adopted: one for bioflavonoids and caffeine and one for anthocyanins.

For flavonoids and caffeine, mobile phase A consisted of water, mobile phase B was acetic acid, and mobile phase C was 100% acetonitrile. The linear gradient program was used as follows: (a) 0 to 5 min 94% A and 6% B; (b) 5 to 10 min 82.4%A, 5.6% B, and 12% C; (c) 10 to 15 min 76.6% A, 5.4% B, and 18% C; (d) 15 to 25 min 67.9% A, 5.1% B, and 27% C; (e) 25 to 30 min 65% A, 5% B, and 30% C; (f) 30 to 35 100% C; (g) 35 to 40 min 100% C; (h) 40 to 45 min 64% A and 6% B. Monitoring was performed at 280 nm at a flow rate of 1 mL/min and injection volume of 25 μL. Flavanones, flavanols, and caffeine were respectively expressed as naringin, catechin, and caffeine.

Regarding anthocyanins, mobile phase A was water, mobile phase B consisted of formic acid, and mobile phase C was acetonitrile. The gradient program used is described as follows: (a) 0 to 5 min 84.18% A, 10% B, and 5.82% C; (b) 5 to 20 min 77.6% A, 10% B, and 12.4% C; (c) 20 to 35 min 68.2% A, 10% B, and 21.8% C; (d) 35 to 40 min 58.8% A, 10% B, and 31.2% C; (e) 40 to 45 min 44.7% A, 10% B, and 45.3% C; (f) 45 to 50 min 44.7% A, 10% B, and

45.3% C; (g) 50 to 60 min 40% A, 10% B, and 50% C; (h) 60 to 65 min 84.18% A, 10% B, and 5.82% C. Monitoring was performed at 520 nm at a flow rate of 0.8 mL/min and injection volume of 10 µL. Anthocyanins were expressed as cyanidin 3-O-glucoside equivalents.

Naringin, catechin, and caffeine standards were purchased from Sigma-Aldrich Co. (St. Louis, MO, USA) and cyanidin 3-O-glucoside standard was purchased from Extrasynthese (Genay, France).

2.3. Study Design and Interventions

The study was designed as a 16 week, randomized, double-blinded, placebo-controlled clinical trial. Eligible participants were randomized using a simple block randomization of 1:1 with an additional stratification for sex (40% minimum and 60% maximum each sex), with a separated randomization list using computer-generated random numbers. Allocation concealment was achieved with sealed opaque envelops. Once enrolled, subjects received either the supplement (n = 43) or a visually identical placebo (n = 49). They were instructed to take two capsules daily for 16 weeks, one in the morning at breakfast and one at lunchtime.

Throughout the course of the study, volunteers were instructed by a dietitian to consume a normal caloric and balanced diet corresponding to their individual needs by determining their specific resting energy expenditure (REE), calculated from the revised Harris–Benedict equation and adjusted per individual level of physical activity [28]. At baseline (W_1), volunteers performed a 24 h diet recall interview corresponding to the consumption of two days during the previous week and one day during the previous weekend, in order to evaluate their usual dietary habits. At the end of the studied period, the same interview was performed to check compliance with dietary instructions. A difference of $\pm 10\%$ between the reported and recommended intakes at the end of the study was considered as satisfactory. Moreover, general adherence to the Mediterranean dietary pattern was assessed using the Mediterranean Diet Serving Score (MDSS) [29]. This score ranges from 0 to 24, with an optimal cut-off point of 13.5, which discriminates adherent and non-adherent individuals.

Subjects were also encouraged to maintain their usual level of physical activity throughout the 16-week-long intervention period. The subjects were provided with a pedometer (HJ-321, Omron Healthcare), which was worn at the hip, to record the physical mobility as the number of daily steps. Subjects reported their daily level of activity in a diary.

Subjects reported to the UCAM Research Center for 5 visits: (i) pre-inclusion visit at week 0 (W_0) to verify the subject's eligibility, to assess anthropometrics, and to collect blood samples for the evaluation of safety parameters; (ii) baseline visit (W_1); (iii) follow-up visits (W_4, W_8, and W_{12}); and final visit (W_{16}). During each visit, subjects returned their physical activity diary and the unused investigational supplements and were questioned about possible occurrence of adverse events before they were provided with a new pill dispenser for the 4 following weeks.

2.4. Measurements

2.4.1. Health-Related Quality of Life

HRQOL was measured at baseline (W_1) and at the end of the intervention period (W_{16}) using the Spanish version of the 36-item Short Form (SF-36) health survey [30]. This generic instrument assesses participants' self-reported HRQOL across physical and mental components. Questions pertained to the individuals' typical day during the past four weeks and usual experiences. The 36 questions were distributed across eight subscales: physical function (PF), role-physical (RP) limitations caused by physical problems, bodily pain (BP), general health (GH) perception, vitality (VT), social functioning (SF), role-emotional (RE) limitations caused by emotional problems, and emotional well-being (EWB). The eight dimensions ranged in score from 0 to 100, with higher scores indicating better HRQOL.

The SF-36 also included one Physical Component Summary (PCS) score and one Mental Component Summary (MCS) score, as well as an overall score of quality of life.

2.4.2. Body Composition

At baseline (W_1) and at the end of the study period (W_{16}), body composition was assessed in the morning, with volunteers in a fasted state and wearing light clothing and no shoes.

Body weight (kg) was measured with calibrated weighing scales (TBF-300MA, Tanita Corporation, IL, USA). Waist circumference (cm) was measured at the narrowest point between the lowest rib and the iliac crest using a non-stretchable tape. The Index of Central Obesity (ICO) scores were calculated as the waist-to-height ratio.

Body fat mass was determined using a dual-energy X-ray absorptiometry (DXA) scan of the whole body (XR-46; Norland Corp., Fort Atkinson, WI, USA). Discrimination of whole-body fat mass (FM) and body trunk fat mass (TFM) was performed with a computerized software (Software Illuminatus DXA v.4.4.0, Visual MED, Inc., Charlotte, NC, USA and Norland CooperSurgical Company, Minneapolis, MN, USA) using standardized procedures.

2.4.3. Self-Reported Physical Activity

The self-reported International Physical Activity Questionnaire (IPAQ) instrument was used to determine global physical activity levels [31]. This self-administered, long-form questionnaire consisted of 27 items that covered four different domains of physical activity (working, transportation, housework, and gardening and leisure-time) that occurred during the previous seven days. The results are presented as an estimation of energy expenditure in metabolic equivalent minutes per week (Met-min/week), and a categorical score was calculated to classify volunteers as inactive, moderately, or highly active. Volunteers completed the IPAQ questionnaire in the presence of an investigator at W_1 and W_{16}.

2.4.4. Safety Parameters

Safety parameters were assessed before inclusion into the study (W_0) and at the end of the intervention period (W_{16}) in order to verify and confirm the healthiness of the volunteers. Safety parameters included liver function parameters (alanine transaminase (ALT), aspartate aminotransferase (AST), gamma-glutamyltransferase (GGT)), renal function parameters (urea, creatinine, sodium (Na), potassium (K)), and heart rate.

2.5. Statistical Analysis

Data sets were analyzed using XLSTAT-Biomed software (v. 2017.6 for Mac, Addinsoft, Paris, France). The data are expressed as the mean ± standard deviation (SD). At baseline, the distribution was considered normal. Changes within and between groups at W_1 and W_{16} were analyzed using paired and unpaired Student's *t*-test, respectively. To compare baseline differences between the SF-36 scales and population norms, one sample *t*-test was used. A minimum value of $p \leq 0.05$ was selected as the threshold for statistical significance.

The primary outcome addressed in this study was the difference in SF-36 total scores after the 16 week intervention period. The power calculation was based on the previous results of a pilot study conducted with Fiit-ns® [32] ($\alpha = 0.05$, power $(1-\beta) = 0.8$) and was performed based on an expected clinical difference in SF-36 total scores between W_1 and W_{16} within the supplemented group of a +5% benefit minimum to determine the targeted final sample size (*n* = 28 per group). Considering a drop-out rate of 20% and failure rate risk of 20%, inclusion of 92 subjects was recommended.

3. Results

3.1. Characterization of the Supplement

The total bioactive content corresponds to 29.27 g/100 g dry matter, with a total flavonoid content measured at 24.75 g/100 g. The flavanol content corresponded to 15.67 g/100 g and included catechin, epigallocatechin gallate, epicatechin, and epicatechin gallate, respectively, measured at 1.47, 9.55, 2.37, and 2.28 g/100 g. The flavanone content corresponded to 8.91 g /100 g, among which isonaringin, naringin, hesperidin, and neohesperidin contents were 0.54, 7.65, 0.03, and 0.13 g/100 g, respectively, whereas total unidentified flavanone was evaluated as the naringin equivalent at 0.56 g/100 g. The total anthocyanin content corresponded to 0.17 g/100 g as the kuromanin equivalent. The caffeine content was measured at 4.52 g/100 g and a third-party laboratory measured the vitamin B3 content at 2.02 g/100 g (Table 1).

Table 1. Characterization of phenolic compounds and caffeine present in the supplement.

Compound	Rt (min)	Λ Max (nm)	Content (mg/100 g) Mean	SD
Caffeine	13.5	273	4523.2	(450.4)
Catechin	9.0	278	1472.9	(85.1)
Epigallocatechin Gallate	11.9	274	9549.9	(282.9)
Epicatechin	12.8	280	2373.0	(416.6)
Epicatechin Gallate	15.8	278	2279.3	(372.9)
Flavanone-like 1	16.1	284/323	97.6	(27.7)
Isonaringin	18.6	284/330	540.8	(156.1)
Naringin	19.5	284/330	7646.9	(66.3)
Hesperidin	20.3	284/328	25.4	(24.3)
Neohesperidin	21.2	284/328	134.2	(86.8)
Flavanone-like 2	27.6	284/329	263.5	(4.0)
Flavanone-like 3	30.4	289/328	196.4	(15.3)
Cyanidin-3-xylosylglucosylgalactoside	6.2	516	9.5	(2.0)
Cyanidin-3-xylosylgalactoside	7.9	518	39.3	(7.4)
Cyanidin-3-sinapoylxylosylglucosylgalactoside	11.2	531	13.8	(1.5)
Cyanidin-3-feruloylxylosylglucosylgalactoside	12.4	528	106.1	(13.1)
Cyanidin-3-pcoumarylxylosylglucosylgalactoside	14.3	528	3.0	(1.6)

3.2. Baseline Characteristics

From the 92 individuals who were randomly allocated to either the supplement (n = 43) or the placebo (n = 49), 78 subjects completed the 16 week intervention (85% of the randomly assigned subjects); after having started the intervention, a total of 14 volunteers dropped out for personal reasons, including 6 within the supplemented group and 8 within the placebo group. Moreover, at the end of the study period, 6 subjects were excluded from final analysis because of protocol deviation, including 2 subjects within the supplemented group and 4 within the placebo group who either did not complete the SF-36 questionnaire or who were non-compliant with the protocol. Finally, 72 volunteers were included in the analysis, with 35 individuals in the supplemented and 37 individuals in the placebo group (Figure 1). Baseline data of the study population are presented in Table 2. The two groups were similar with respect to age, height, body weight, and SF-36 total scores. At baseline, the placebo group had a significantly higher average BMI compared with the supplemented group.

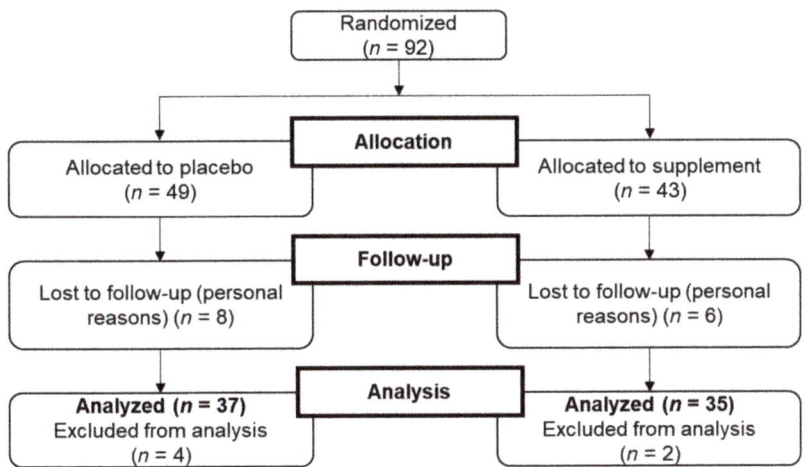

Figure 1. CONSORT (Consolidated Standards of Reporting Trials) flow diagram of study.

Table 2. Baseline characteristics of the study population.

Variable	Whole Population		Placebo Group		Supplemented Group	
Subjects, n (M/F)	72 (34/38)		37 (16/21)		35 (18/17)	
	Mean	SD	Mean	SD	Mean	SD
Age (years)	40	(6)	41	(6)	39	(7)
Height (meters)	1.69	(0.09)	1.68	(0.08)	1.70	(0.11)
Body weight (kg)	87.0	(12.6)	89.3	(12.2)	84.5	(12.6)
BMI (kg/m^2)	30.5	(3.5)	31.6	(4.0)	29.3 *	(2.5)
SF-36 score (points)	81.6	(9.2)	81.7	(8.2)	81.5	(10.3)

*—Significant at $p \leq 0.05$ level; M—male; F—female; BMI—Body mass index; SF-36—Short form 36 Health survey.

3.3. Health-Related Quality of Life

Regarding the whole population at baseline (Table 3), SF-36 subscales regarding vitality, emotional well-being, and mental component scores were significantly lower than the age-specific populations norms taken from the Spanish population reference values [33]. At W_1, placebo and supplemented groups exhibited similar SF-36 scores, including both individual domains and summary scores (Table 4). After 16 weeks of supplementation, the supplemented group experienced a significant +5.3% increase ($p = 0.001$) (Figure 2) in total SF-36 score, while no change was observed in the total score of the placebo group. The supplemented group showed statistically significant improvements in five out of eight domains of the health-related quality of life. Respective improvements were observed for the physical component summary (PCS; +11.2%, $p = 0.002$), including physical functioning (PF; +5.5%, $p = 0.006$), bodily pain (BP; +11.2%, $p = 0.028$), and general health (GH; +7.2%, $p = 0.010$), as well as for the mental component summary (MCS; +4.1%, $p = 0.021$), which included vitality (VT; +7.8%, $p = 0.006$) and emotional well-being (EWB; +5.2%, $p = 0.021$). No statistically significant changes were shown within the placebo group after the 16 week intervention.

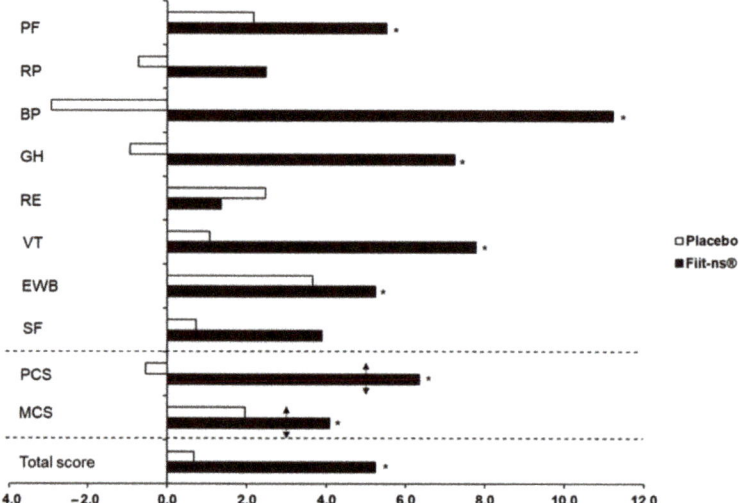

Figure 2. The percentage changes from baseline (W_1) to the end of the study (W_{16}) in individual SF-36 domains, as well as in the Physical Component Score (PCS), Mental Component Score (MCS), and total HRQOL score in placebo and in supplemented subjects. Arrows indicate clinically significant differences according to Samsa et al. [31]. Note: *—Indicates an intragroup difference between baseline (W_1) and end of the study (W_{16}) at $p \leq 0.05$ level. PF—physical functioning; RP—role physical; BP—bodily pain; GH—general health; RE—role emotional; VT—vitality; EWB—emotional well-being; SF—social functioning.

Table 3. Mean scores for SF-36 eight subscales at baseline in the study and in the Spanish population aged 25–54.

Scale	Baseline	Age Specific Population Norm [§]
Physical component score	83.8	83.0
Physical functioning	89.5	91.9
Role-physical	93.8	87.5
Bodily pain	79.0	82.6
General health	73.0	72.7
Mental component score	79.4 *	82.3
Role-emotional	92.4	91.3
Vitality	62.8 *	70.2
Emotional well-being	70.6 *	74.9
Social functioning	91.8	92.9

§—Combined score for men and women ages 25–54 as the age-specific population norm; *—a significant difference at baseline from the age-specific population norm for the scale at $p \leq 0.05$ level.

3.4. Body Composition

At baseline, all fat-mass-related variables (FM, TFM, Index of Central Obesity (ICO), and BMI) were significantly higher in the placebo group (Table 5). Such a discrepancy is explained by the higher number of obese individuals that completed the clinical investigation in the placebo group. After 16 weeks of supplementation, volunteers from the placebo group did not experience any significant changes in body composition. The supplemented group showed an improvement in anthropometrics after 16 weeks, with a statistically significant decrease in body weight by -1.3 kg ($p = 0.013$) and in BMI by -0.4 points ($p = 0.012$). Waist size significantly decreased by -1.1 cm ($p = 0.017$), consequently lowering the ICO by -1.3% ($p = 0.018$). Supplemented volunteers significantly lost -1.2 kg of FM ($p = 0.033$), of which -1.0 kg was fat lost only from the TFM ($p = 0.002$).

Table 4. Mean scores for SF-36 eight subscales, including both physical and mental components, and total health-related quality of life scores at baseline (W_1) and at the end of the study (W_{16}).

Scale	Placebo Group				Supplemented Group			
	W1		W16		W1		W16	
	Mean	SD	Mean	SD	Mean	SD	Mean	SD
SF-36 Total score	81.7	(8.2)	82.2	(8.2)	81.5	(10.3)	85.8 [a]*	(6.4)
Physical component score	84.3	(7.6)	83.8	(8.9)	83.4	(12.6)	88.7 [a]*	(7.6)
Physical functioning	88.6	(9.4)	90.6	(8.4)	90.4	(12.7)	95.4 [a]*	(7.0)
Role-physical	94.3	(7.3)	93.6	(8.1)	93.4	(11.6)	95.7	(6.6)
Bodily pain	80.7	(18.0)	78.3	(23.3)	77.1	(22.9)	85.8 *	(14.5)
General health	73.5	(13.3)	72.8	(11.7)	72.5	(16.0)	77.8 *	(13.7)
Mental component score	79.1	(10.8)	80.7	(10.5)	79.7	(10.7)	82.9 *	(8.0)
Role-emotional	91.2	(14.8)	93.5	(12.6)	93.6	(12.0)	94.9	(9.2)
Vitality	62.4	(11.1)	63.1	(12.2)	63.1	(13.4)	68.0 [a]*	(11.1)
Emotional well-being	70.9	(11.1)	73.5	(10.9)	70.3	(12.9)	73.9 *	(10.0)
Social functioning	91.9	(15.9)	92.6	(14.9)	91.8	(12.1)	95.4	(9.1)

*—An intragroup difference between baseline (W_1) and end of the study (W_{16}) at $p \leq 0.05$; [a]—an intergroup difference at the end of the study (W_{16}) at $p \leq 0.05$.

Table 5. Body weight, BMI, waist circumference, ICO, total body fat mass, and total trunk fat mass scores at baseline (W_1) and at the end of the study (W_{16}).

	Placebo Group				Supplemented Group			
	W1		W16		W1		W16	
	Mean	SD	Mean	SD	Mean	SD	Mean	SD
Body weight, kg	89.3	(12.2)	89.1	(12.5)	84.5	(12.6)	83.2 [b]*	(12.6)
BMI, kg/m^2	31.6	(4.0)	31.5	(3.9)	29.3 [a]	(2.5)	28.9 [b]*	(2.8)
Waist circumference, cm	94.2	(9.7)	94.6	(9.3)	90.7 [a]	(8.8)	89.6 [b]*	(9.3)
ICO	0.560	(0.05)	0.563	(0.05)	0.533 [a]	(0.04)	0.526 [b]*	(0.04)
Total body fat mass, kg	35.2	(10.4)	35.2	(10.8)	30.5 [a]	(7.4)	29.3 [b]*	(7.9)
Total trunk fat mass, kg	18.1	(5.4)	18.1	(5.9)	15.7 [a]	(4.1)	14.7 [b]*	(4.2)

*—An intragroup difference between baseline (W_1) and end of the study (W_{16}) at $p \leq 0.05$; [a,b]—intergroup differences at baseline (W_1) and at the end of the study (W_{16}) at $p \leq 0.05$.

3.5. Self-Reported Physical Activity and Average Daily Steps Recording

At baseline, both groups showed similar self-reported levels of physical activity. While it did not significantly change within the placebo population ($p = 0.280$), the supplemented subjects showed an increase of +1308 Met-min/week ($p = 0.05$) after 16 weeks of supplementation (Table 6). Regarding categorical scores at baseline, the rates of volunteers within each category (i.e., inactive, moderately active, and highly active) were similar between groups. After 16 weeks, the rates of inactive people remained the same in both groups; within the placebo group, the rate of highly active subjects decreased by −43%, while the rate of moderately active individuals increased by +14%. In contrast, within the supplemented population, the rate of moderately active subjects decreased by −14% but the number of highly active individuals increased by +43%. The number of average daily steps was significantly different at baseline between placebo and supplemented subjects ($p = 0.028$). The placebo group did not experience any significant change in average daily steps monitored after 16 weeks, while the supplemented subjects significantly decreased their average rate by −678 steps ($p = 0.019$) to reach a similar level to the placebo population.

Table 6. Mean total score for self-reported physical activity (IPAQ, International Physical Activity Questionnaire) and daily number of steps (pedometer) at baseline (W_1) and at the end of the study (W_{16}).

	Placebo Group				Supplemented Group			
	W1		W16		W1		W16	
	Mean	SD	Mean	SD	Mean	SD	Mean	SD
IPAQ score (Met-min/week)	4798	(4740)	4231	(4190)	4766	(4721)	6074 *	(6631)
Inactive (%)	15.2		15.2		12.5		12.5	
Moderately active (%)	63.6		72.7		65.6		56.3	
Highly active (%)	21.2		12.1		21.8		31.2	
	Mean	SD	Mean	SD	Mean	SD	Mean	SD
Daily steps	6770	(2239)	7186	(2679)	8169 [a]	(2797)	7491 *	(2964)

*—An intragroup difference between baseline (W_1) and end of the study (W_{16}) at $p \leq 0.05$; [a]—an intergroup difference at baseline (W_1) at $p \leq 0.05$. MET-min/week—Metabolic Equivalent Task minutes per week.

3.6. Recommended and Reported Dietary Intake

Recommended intake at baseline did not differ between the two groups ($p = 0.770$) (Table 7). When recommended intake was compared with reported intake at baseline, the differences were −13.7% and −7.8% for the placebo and supplemented groups, respectively. After 16 weeks, the differences between recommended and reported intake in both groups were lower than 10% (−8.8% and −9.0% for the placebo and for the supplemented groups, respectively). Mediterranean Diet Serving Scores (MDSS) were similar between both groups at 8.4 and 8.6 for placebo and supplemented populations, respectively, indicating a non-adherence to the Mediterranean diet pattern during the intervention period.

Table 7. Recommended and reported dietary intake at baseline (W_1) and at the end of the study (W_{16}).

	Placebo Group				Supplemented Group			
	W1		W16		W1		W16	
	Mean	SD	Mean	SD	Mean	SD	Mean	SD
Recommended intake (Kcal)	2074	(273)	2084	(281)	2096	(360)	2039	(342)
Reported intake (Kcal)	1789	(471)	1899 *	(502)	1933	(463)	1855	(392)
	Mean		SD		Mean		SD	
MDSS score	8.4		(3.7)		8.6		(4.2)	

*—An intragroup difference between baseline (W_1) and end of the study (W_{16}) at $p \leq 0.05$.

3.7. Safety

After 16 weeks, both liver and renal function parameters were within the healthy range in both groups, suggesting that no health impairment occurred throughout the course of the study. Moreover, heart rates stayed stable throughout the course of the study (Table 8). No adverse events or side effects linked to the supplement were reported during the course of the study.

Table 8. Clinical safety values at baseline (W_1) and at the end of the study (W_{16}).

Parameters (Normal Range)	Placebo Group				Supplemented Group			
	W1		W16		W1		W16	
	Mean	SD	Mean	SD	Mean	SD	Mean	SD
Liver function								
ALT (7–55 U/L)	21.4	(9.1)	21.0	(8.5)	25.0	(15.9)	25.1	(14.7)
AST (8–48 U/L)	20.2	(5.5)	20.1	(5.3)	22.4	(6.3)	23.3	(10.0)
GGT (6–48 U/L)	19.1	(11.7)	19.9	(11.9)	23.1	(13.4)	24.7	(14.0)
Kidney function								
Urea (15–46 mg/dL)	35.4	(9.1)	33.0	(7.7)	31.9	(7.8)	30.1	(7.4)
Creatinine (0.6–1.3 mg/dL)	0.79	(0.18)	0.74 *	(0.16)	0.74	(0.15)	0.76	(0.16)
Na (135–145 mmol/L)	141.2	(1.2)	141.2	(2.1)	141.7	(1.7)	141.1	(1.7)
K (3.6–5.2 mmol/L)	4.3	(0.3)	4.3	(0.2)	4.3	(0.2)	4.3	(0.3)
Heart rate (bpm)	71.8	(10.2)	72.1	(8.6)	71.3	(11.2)	70.4	(16.4)

*—An intragroup difference between baseline (W1) and end of the study (W_{16}) at $p \leq 0.05$.

4. Discussion

The main results of this study demonstrate that a 16-week-long supplementation period with an ingredient formulated from a blend of various botanical extracts, which are rich in a diversity of polyphenols and usually consumed as part of the typical Mediterranean diet, is associated with significant improvements of both the physical and mental components of the HRQOL in overweight and obese but otherwise healthy subjects of both sex.

At baseline, volunteers showed an impaired HRQOL, namely in vitality and emotional well-being subscales, for which values were below the Spanish age-specific population reference norms [33]. Although similar studies have previously reported impairment across all off the SF-36 subscales, most of them were conducted either with a population displaying a significantly higher grade of obesity or with an additional manifestation of comorbidities [10,17]. Here, baseline impairments observed for vitality and emotional well-being are in line with the work of Blissmer et al. [11], who found similar decrements in a highly comparable population of healthy overweight and moderately obese subjects, indicating higher feelings of tiredness and anxiety.

Following a 16 week intervention period associated with a normal caloric diet, both the physical and mental components of the HRQOL significantly improved in volunteers supplemented with the polyphenol-rich ingredient compared to the placebo group. Net improvements were shown by subjective ameliorations in bodily pain > general health > vitality > physical functioning > emotional well-being. It is noteworthy that after the 16-week-long period of supplementation, both the vitality and the emotional well-being values improved to achieve the level of the reference norms of the Spanish age-specific population. Improvements in these different subscales and in both the physical and mental component scores must be considered as clinically significant, as it has been stated that absolute differences of 3–5 points are clinically relevant [34].

In addition to these improvements, the 16 week chronic polyphenolic supplementation induced significant body weight loss, with an average difference between both groups of 1.1 kg. It is noteworthy that this decrease was essentially driven by an 86% fat mass reduction, for which 89% was located within the trunk area, pointing out a particularly beneficial effect on body composition. Such an improvement may, to some extent, positively impact the HRQOL. Indeed, some authors have demonstrated that weight loss was associated with improvement of both physical and mental health dimensions in several intervention trials [11,13,35–37]. Moreover, the amount of weight loss and the level of HRQOL improvement may be directly interconnected [37,38]. Nevertheless, here we did not demonstrate a significant correlation between weight or fat loss and HRQOL improvement, hypothesizing that weight loss could be an indirect consequence of HRQOL improvement, as it has been recently demonstrated with a bi-directional relationship between both parameters [39].

Moreover, catechins from green tea have previously been demonstrated to have antiobesity effects [40] through various mechanisms of action, such as the inhibition of pancreatic lipase [41], as well as through the regulation of obesity-related genes and proteins [42]. However, it is important to highlight that these interventional studies used significantly higher amounts of green tea catechins, whereas in the current supplement it only corresponded to one cup of green tea daily. Moreover, caffeine content and flavanones from grapefruit extract could also potentiate the decrease in body fat mass, as enhanced lipolysis leading to decreases in body weight and fat mass has previously been demonstrated in overweight and obese subjects supplemented with such kinds of bioactive compounds [43]. Accordingly, as each of the bioactive components in the supplement are present at lower levels compared to efficient dosages from the literature, it could be assumed that the beneficial observations for the supplement should be attributed to the whole formulation.

In parallel to body composition improvement, the level of physical activity, as assessed through the IPAQ questionnaire, significantly intensified ($p = 0.05$) after 16 weeks of supplementation. Thus, while 69% of volunteers from the supplemented group maintained their usual level of physical activity, 25% moved into a higher category compared with the placebo population, for which only 9% of volunteers improved their level of physical activity. Contradictorily, at the same time, the supplemented group showed a decrease in daily steps as assessed with a pedometer, while no change was observed in the placebo population. This discrepancy may be explained by the fact that pedometers are not suitable for the measurement of certain types of physical activity, such as swimming, cycling, or heavy lifting, which are otherwise assessed through the IPAQ questionnaire, making these both subjective and objective measurements, two complementary tools in physical activity assessment. As volunteers were encouraged to maintain their usual physical activity level throughout the course of the study, it can be hypothesized that the significantly higher physically active lifestyle reported within the supplemented group is not the result of conditioned mental engagement only. Indeed, the increase of HRQOL, and namely of the feeling of increased vitality, may explain such a rise in physical activity. A recent review that aimed at examining the link between physical activity and HRQOL concluded that there is a consistent cross-sectional association between physical activity level and HRQOL, namely in the vitality and in the physical functioning domains, however the finding could not confirm a causal relationship, i.e., "higher HRQOL leading to a higher level of physical activity, or vice versa, or mutual influence" [44]. Nevertheless, the engagement in a more active lifestyle within the supplemented population may also have a positive effect on body composition improvement, as discussed above.

Besides positive effects on body composition and engagement in physical activity, it appears that phenolic compounds may induce, through other various mechanisms, observable effects in terms of HRQOL improvement. Accordingly, adherence to a Mediterranean dietary pattern, characterized by wide consumption of fruits and vegetables, cereals, fish, olive oil, and red wine, has been directly associated with better QOL in an analysis including more than 11,000 participants that belonged to the SUN (Seguimiento University of Navarra) cohort [45,46]. While several nutrients and micronutrients may contribute to this effect, phenolic compounds have been suggested to be the main mediators; a large cross-sectional study demonstrated a direct relationship between the antioxidant contents of the Mediterranean diet, including the flavonoid content, and HRQOL [25]. In addition, in another recent study including more than 13,000 women, higher flavonoid intake at midlife was associated with increased odds of healthy ageing, based on higher survival at older ages free of chronic diseases and maintenance of midlife HRQOL (as assessed by the SF-36 survey) [47]. Here, despite the studied population being Spanish and particularly prone to complying with the Mediterranean diet, the MDSS did not demonstrate any significant adherence to this pattern in either groups, for whom the consumption of fruits and vegetables, the main sources of flavonoids, was below the recommendations of the last updated version of the Mediterranean Diet Pyramid [48]. Thus, it can be hypothesized that a regular basic diet has no or only a minor impact on HRQOL, since there were no improvements within the placebo population, whereas the supplemented subjects that covered the gap of phenolic micronutrients significantly improved their HRQOL.

Bioactive compounds occurring in the supplement may positively impact physiological functions related to both physical and mental health status—mainly vascular inflammation, coagulation factors, and endothelial function [25], which are all described to be impaired during overweight and obesity [49]. The aptitude of certain phenolic compounds in improving vascular health has been demonstrated both in vitro and in vivo [50]. Catechins from green tea positively impact vascular function through various complementary mechanisms linked to their antioxidative and anti-inflammatory properties, as well as to their capacity to activate endothelial NO synthase [51]. Similarly, grape polyphenols also demonstrated an aptitude to improving vascular impairments through similar molecular mechanisms [52], all contributing to a better peripheral and central blood flow, which in turn may positively affect physical and mental health status [53].

While modulation of both oxidative stress and inflammatory parameters, the main contributors in the improvement of vascular function and blood flow, has previously been demonstrated with the current supplement in a study involving obese subjects [32], specific mechanisms of flow-mediated dilation improvements and subsequent blood flow increase have not yet been investigated. Moreover, as the beneficial effect of the supplement on HRQOL has been demonstrated, further investigations will have to be conducted in attempts to confirm the causal relationship between the bioavailability and pharmacokinetics of the polyphenols metabolites and the mechanisms involved in improving vascular function.

Beyond the mentioned limitations, the results of the present study reveal the beneficial and systemic effects of phenolic compounds on subjective physical and mental symptoms linked to overweight and obesity. The study was designed to minimize bias, and thus individualized calorie intake recommendations and diet interviews, as well as monitoring of daily steps, were identified as possible confounding factors. Despite the studied population being recruited in a Mediterranean region, neither of the two groups adhered to the typical regional diet, which strengthens the hypothesis that phenolic compounds certainly contribute to subjective health, as previously proposed by others [25,47].

In conclusion, this study demonstrated that the 16-week-long consumption of an ingredient obtained from polyphenol-rich fruit and vegetable extracts associated with both caffein and vitamin B3 supports improvements in HRQOL, specifically in both mental and physical subjective feelings. In addition, the decrease in body fat mass and the significantly increased engagement in physical activity probably established a virtuous cycle between body composition, physical activity, and perceived HRQOL. The mechanisms of action likely involve improvements in vascular function via well-known antioxidative and anti-inflammatory properties of phenolic compounds. Such beneficial effects may be extended to other situations where HRQOL is impaired, particularly during the ageing process, where an imbalance of body composition and a loss of vitality and of physical functioning associated with a more sedentary lifestyle are commonly observed.

Author Contributions: Conceptualization, C.R. and J.C.; methodology, P.E.A. and L.H.C.; investigation, P.E.A., L.H.C., J.A.R.-A., E.M.-C., J.M.M.-R., and A.M.-R.; writing—original draft preparation, C.R.; writing—review and editing, C.R., J.C., P.E.A., L.H.C., J.A.R.-A., E.M.-C., J.M.M.-R., A.M.-R., S.G. and C.L. All authors have read and agreed to the published version of the manuscript.

Funding: This research received no external funding.

Institutional Review Board Statement: The study was conducted according to the guidelines of the Declaration of Helsinki, and approved by the Institutional Review Board of Comite de etica de la UCAM (protocol code N° 5551 on 24 April 2015).

Informed Consent Statement: Informed consent was obtained from all subjects involved in the study.

Data Availability Statement: The data presented in this study are available on request from the corresponding author, due to privacy restriction.

Conflicts of Interest: Fytexia is involved in the research and development and marketing and sales of polyphenol extract-based ingredients for food and nutraceutical industries. Therefore, Fytexia has a commercial interest in this publication. UCAM and UMR 204 Nutripass were paid by Fytexia to perform and report the scientific work that formed the basis of this publication. Fytexia, UCAM, UMR 204 Nutripass, and all authors declare that the data in this report represent a true and faithful representation of the work that has been performed. The financial assistance of Fytexia is gratefully acknowledged.

References

1. Whoqol Group. The World Health Organization Quality of Life assessment (WHOQOL): Position paper from the World Health Organization. *Soc. Sci. Med.* **1995**, *41*, 1403–1409. [CrossRef]
2. Testa, M.; Simonson, D. Current concepts: Assessment of quality-of-life outcomes. *N. Eng. J. Med.* **1996**, *334*, 835–840. [CrossRef]
3. Fayers, P.M.; Machin, D. *Quality of Life: Assessment, Analysis and Interpretation*; John Wiley and Sons: Chichester, UK, 2000.
4. WHO. Noncommunicable diseases. World Health Organization. Available online: http://www.who.int/mediacentre/factsheets/fs355/en/ (accessed on 7 March 2018).
5. Gortmaker, S.L.; Swinburn, B.A.; Levy, D.; Carter, R.; Mabry, P.L.; Finegood, D.T.; Huang, T.; Marsh, T.; Moodie, M.L. Changing the future of obesity: Science, policy, and action. *Lancet* **2011**, *378*, 838–847. [CrossRef]
6. Fernández-Sánchez, A.; Madrigal-Santillán, E.O.; Bautista, M.; Esquivel-Soto, J.; Morales-González, Á.; Esquivel-Chirino, C.; Durante-Montiel, I.; Sánchez-Rivera, G.; Valadez-Vega, C.; Morales-González, J.A. Inflammation, Oxidative Stress, and Obesity. *Int. J. Mol. Sci.* **2011**, *12*, 3117–3132. [CrossRef]
7. Rahman, I.; Bagchi, D. *Inflammation, Advancing Age and Nutrition*; Rahman, I., Bagchi, D., Eds.; Academic Press: London, UK, 2013.
8. Ahima, R.S. Connecting obesity, aging and diabetes. *Nat. Med.* **2009**, *15*, 996–997. [CrossRef]
9. Fontaine, K.R.; Barofsky, I. Obesity and health-related quality of life. *Obes. Rev.* **2001**, *2*, 173–182. [CrossRef] [PubMed]
10. Slagter, S.N.; Van Vliet-Ostaptchouk, J.V.; Van Beek, A.P.; Keers, J.C.; Lutgers, H.L.; Van Der Klauw, M.M.; Wolffenbuttel, B.H.R. Health-Related Quality of Life in Relation to Obesity Grade, Type 2 Diabetes, Metabolic Syndrome and Inflammation. *PLoS ONE* **2015**, *10*, 1–17. [CrossRef]
11. Blissmer, B.; Riebe, D.; Dye, G.; Ruggiero, L.; Greene, G.; Caldwell, M. Health-related quality of life following a clinical weight loss intervention among overweight and obese adults: Intervention and 24 month follow-up effects. *Health Qual. Life Outcomes* **2006**, *4*, 43. [CrossRef] [PubMed]
12. Ford, E.S.; Moriarty, D.G.; Zack, M.M.; Mokdad, A.H.; Chapman, D.P. Self-Reported Body Mass Index and Health-Related Quality of Life: Findings from the Behavioral Risk Factor Surveillance System. *Obes. Res.* **2001**, *9*, 21–31. [CrossRef] [PubMed]
13. Fine, J.T.; Colditz, G.A.; Coakley, E.H.; Moseley, G.; Manson, J.E.; Willett, W.C.; Kawachi, I. A Prospective Study of Weight Change and Health-Related Quality of Life in Women. *JAMA* **1999**, *282*, 2136–2142. [CrossRef] [PubMed]
14. Idler, E.L.; Benyamini, Y. Self-Rated Health and Mortality: A Review of Twenty-Seven Community Studies. *J. Health Soc. Behav.* **1997**, *38*, 21–37. [CrossRef] [PubMed]
15. Ware, J.E.; Snow, K.K.; Kosinski, M.; Gandek, B. *SF-36 Health Survey Manual and Interpretation Guide*; Health Institute, New England Medical Center: Boston, MA, USA, 1993.
16. Obidoa, C.; Reisine, S.; Cherniack, M. How does the SF 36 perform in healthy populations? A structured review of longitudinal studies. *J. Soc. Behav. Health* **2010**, *4*, 30–48.
17. Doll, H.A.; Petersen, S.E.K.; Stewart-Brown, S.L. Obesity and Physical and Emotional Well-Being: Associations between Body Mass Index, Chronic Illness, and the Physical and Mental Components of the SF-36 Questionnaire. *Obes. Res.* **2000**, *8*, 160–170. [CrossRef] [PubMed]
18. Marchesini, G.; Solaroli, E.; Baraldi, L.; Natale, S.; Migliorini, S.; Visani, F.; Forlani, G.; Melchionda, N. Health-related quality of life in obesity: The role of eating behaviour. *Diabetes Nutr. Metab.* **2000**, *13*, 156–164.
19. Caretto, A.; Lagattolla, V. Non-Communicable Diseases and Adherence to Mediterranean Diet. *Endocrine, Metab. Immune Disord.–Drug Targets* **2015**, *15*, 10–17. [CrossRef]
20. Tresserra-Rimbau, A.; Rimm, E.B.; Medina-Remón, A.; Martínez-González, M.A.; López-Sabater, M.C.; Covas, M.I.; Corella, D.; Salas-Salvadó, J.; Gómez-Gracia, E.; Lapetra, J.; et al. Polyphenol intake and mortality risk: A re-analysis of the PREDIMED trial. *BMC Med.* **2014**, *12*, 77. [CrossRef]
21. Crozier, A.; Jaganath, I.B.; Clifford, M.N. Dietary phenolics: Chemistry, bioavailability and effects on health. *Nat. Prod. Rep.* **2009**, *26*, 1001–1043. [CrossRef]
22. Boccellino, M.; D'Angelo, S. Anti-obesity effects of polyphenol intake: Current status and future possibilities. *Int. J. Mol. Sci.* **2020**, *21*, 5642. [CrossRef]
23. Castro-Barquero, S.; Lamuela-Raventós, R.M.; Doménech, M.; Estruch, R. Relationship between Mediterranean dietary polyphenol intake and obesity. *Nutrients* **2018**, *10*, 1523. [CrossRef]
24. Veronese, N.; Stubbs, B.; Noale, M.; Solmi, M.; Luchini, C.; Maggi, S. Adherence to the Mediterranean diett is associated with better quality of life: Data from the Osteoarthritis Initiative. *Am. J. Clin. Nutr.* **2016**, *104*, 1403–1409. [CrossRef]

25. Bonaccio, M.; Di Castelnuovo, A.; Bonanni, A.; Costanzo, S.; De Lucia, F.; Pounis, G.; Zito, F.; Donati, M.B.; De Gaetano, G.; Iacoviello, L. Adherence to a Mediterranean diet is associated with a better health-related quality of life: A possible role of high dietary antioxidant content. *BMJ Open* **2013**, *3*, 1–11. [CrossRef] [PubMed]
26. World Health Organisation. Declaration of Helsinki World Medical Association Declaration of Helsinki Ethical Principles for Medical Research Involving Human Subjects. *J. Am. Med. Assoc.* **2013**, *310*, 2191–2194. [CrossRef] [PubMed]
27. Vijayananthan, A.; Nawawi, O. The importance of Good Clinical Practice guidelines and its role in clinical trials. *Biomed. Imaging Interv. J.* **2008**, *4*, e5. [CrossRef]
28. Roza, A.; Shizgal, H. The Harris Benedict energy requirements equation reevaluated: Resting and the body cell mass. *Am. J. Clin. Nutr.* **1984**, *40*, 168–182. [CrossRef] [PubMed]
29. Monteagudo, C.; Mariscal-Arcas, M.; Rivas, A.; Lorenzo-Tovar, M.L.; Tur, J.A.; Olea-Serrano, F. Proposal of a Mediterranean Diet Serving Score. *PLoS ONE* **2015**, *10*, e0128594. [CrossRef]
30. Vilagut, G.; Ferrer, M.; Rajmil, L.; Rebollo, P.; Permanyer-Miralda, G.; Quintana, J.M.; Santed, R.; Valderas, J.M.; Ribera, A.; Domingo-Salvany, A.; et al. The Spanish version of the Short Form 36 Health Survey: A decade of experience and new developments. *Gac. Sanit.* **2005**, *19*, 135–150. [CrossRef]
31. Craig, C.L.; Marshall, A.L.; Sjöström, M.; Bauman, A.E.; Booth, M.L.; Ainsworth, B.E.; Pratt, M.; Ekelund, U.; Yngve, A.; Sallis, J.F.; et al. International physical activity questionnaire: 12-Country reliability and validity. *Med. Sci. Sports Exerc.* **2003**, *35*, 1381–1395. [CrossRef]
32. Cases, J.; Romain, C.; Dallas, C.; Gerbi, A.; Cloarec, M. Regular consumption of Fiit-ns, a polyphenol extract from fruit and vegetables frequently consumed within the Mediterranean diet, improves metabolic ageing of obese volunteers: A randomized, double-blind, parallel trial. *Int. J. Food Sci. Nutr.* **2015**, *66*, 120–125. [CrossRef]
33. Alonso, J.; Regidor, E.; Barrio, G.; Prieto, L. Valores poblacionales de referencia de la versión española del Cuestionario de Salud SF 36. *Med. Clin.* **1998**, *36*, 1–10.
34. Samsa, G.; Edelman, D.; Rothman, M.L.; Williams, G.R.; Lipscomb, J.; Matchar, D. Determining clinically important differences in health status measures: A general approach with illustration to the Health Utilities Index Mark II. *Pharmacoeconomics* **1999**, *15*, 141–155. [CrossRef]
35. Rippe, J.M.; Price, J.M.; Hess, S.A.; Kline, G.; Demers, K.A.; Damitz, S.; Kreidieh, I.; Freedson, P. Improved psychological well-being, quality of life, and health practices in moderately overweight women participating in a 12-week structured weight loss program. *Obes. Res.* **1998**, *6*, 208–218. [CrossRef] [PubMed]
36. Kolotkin, R.L.; Fujioka, K.; Wolden, M.L.; Brett, J.H.; Bjorner, J.B. Improvements in health-related quality of life with liraglutide 3.0 mg compared with placebo in weight management. *Clin. Obes.* **2016**, *6*, 233–242. [CrossRef] [PubMed]
37. Ross, K.M.; Milsom, V.A.; Rickel, K.A.; DeBraganza, N.; Gibbons, L.M.; Murawski, M.E.; Perri, M.G. The contributions of weight loss and increased physical fitness to improvements in health-related quality of life. *Eat. Behav.* **2009**, *10*, 84–88. [CrossRef] [PubMed]
38. Samsa, G.P.; Kolotkin, R.L.; Williams, G.R.; Nguyen, M.H.; Mendel, C.M. Effect of moderate weight loss on health-related quality of life: An analysis of combined data from 4 randomized trials of sibutramine vs placebo. *Am. J. Manag. Care* **2001**, *7*, 875–883. [PubMed]
39. Cameron, A.J.; Magliano, D.; Dunstan, D.; Zimmet, P.; Hesketh, K.D.; Peeters, A.; E Shaw, J. A bi-directional relationship between obesity and health-related quality of life: Evidence from the longitudinal AusDiab study. *Int. J. Obes.* **2011**, *36*, 295–303. [CrossRef]
40. Suzuki, T.; Pervin, M.; Goto, S.; Isemura, M.; Nakamura, Y. Beneficial effects of tea and the green tea catechin epigallocatechin-3-gallate on obesity. *Molecules* **2016**, *21*, 1305. [CrossRef] [PubMed]
41. Grove, K.A.; Sae-Tan, S.; Kennett, M.J.; Lambert, J.D. (−)−Epigallocatechin-3-gallate Inhibits Pancreatic Lipase and Reduces Body Weight Gain in High Fat-Fed Obese Mice. *Obesity* **2012**, *20*, 2311–2313. [CrossRef]
42. Yang, C.S.; Zhang, J.; Zhang, L.; Huang, J.; Wang, Y. Mechanisms of body weight reduction and metabolic syndrome alleviation by tea. *Mol. Nutr. Food Res.* **2016**, *60*, 160–174. [CrossRef]
43. Dallas, C.; Gerbi, A.; Elbez, Y.; Caillard, P.; Zamaria, N.; Cloarec, M. Clinical Study to Assess the Efficacy and Safety of a Citrus Polyphenolic Extract of Red Orange, Grapefruit, and Orange (Sinetrol-XPur) on Weight Management and Metabolic Parameters in Healthy Overweight Individuals. *Phytother. Res.* **2014**, *28*, 212–218. [CrossRef]
44. Bize, R.; Johnson, J.A.; Plotnikoff, R.C. Physical activity level and health-related quality of life in the general adult population: A systematic review. *Prev. Med.* **2007**, *45*, 401–415. [CrossRef]
45. Ruano-Rodríguez, C.; Henriquez, P. (Patricia); Martinez-Gonzalez, M. (Miguel Ángel); Bes-Rastrollo, M. (Maira); Ruiz-Canela, M. (Miguel); Sanchez-Villegas, A. (Almudena) Empirically Derived Dietary Patterns and Health-Related Quality of Life in the SUN Project. *PLoS ONE* **2013**, *8*, 1–10. [CrossRef]
46. Sánchez, P.H.; Ruano, C.; De Irala, J.; Ruizcanela, M.; A Martínez-González, M.; Sanchezvillegas, A. Adherence to the Mediterranean diet and quality of life in the SUN Project. *Eur. J. Clin. Nutr.* **2012**, *66*, 360–368. [CrossRef] [PubMed]
47. Samieri, C.; Sun, Q.; Townsend, M.K.; Rimm, E.B.; Grodstein, F. Dietary flavonoid intake at midlife and healthy aging in women. *Am. J. Clin. Nutr.* **2014**, *100*, 1489–1497. [CrossRef] [PubMed]
48. Bach-Faig, A.; Berry, E.M.; Lairon, D.; Reguant, J.; Trichopoulou, A.; Dernini, S.; Medina, F.; Battino, M.; Belahsen, R.; Miranda, G.; et al. Mediterranean diet pyramid today. Science and cultural updates. *Public Health Nutr.* **2011**, *14*, 2274–2284. [CrossRef]

49. Perticone, F.; Ceravolo, R.; Candigliota, M.; Ventura, G.; Iacopino, S.; Sinopoli, F.; Mattioli, P.L. Obesity and body fat distribution induce endothelial dysfunction by oxidative stress: Protective effect of vitamin C. *Diabetes* **2001**, *50*, 159–165. [CrossRef]
50. De Pascual-Teresa, S.; Moreno, D.A.; García-Viguera, C. Flavanols and Anthocyanins in Cardiovascular Health: A Review of Current Evidence. *Int. J. Mol. Sci.* **2010**, *11*, 1679–1703. [CrossRef]
51. Moore, R.J.; Jackson, K.G.; Minihane, A.M. Green tea (Camellia sinensis) catechins and vascular function. *Br. J. Nutr.* **2009**, *102*, 1790–1802. [CrossRef]
52. Dohadwala, M.M.; A Vita, J. Grapes and Cardiovascular Disease. *J. Nutr.* **2009**, *139*, 1788S–1793S. [CrossRef]
53. Watson, R.R.; Preedy, V.R.; Zibadi, S. *Polyphenols in Human Health and Disease*; Elsevier: Sandiego, CA, USA, 2014; Volume 1.

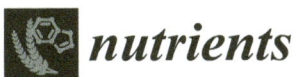

Article

Genetic Variation in the Bitter Receptors Responsible for Epicatechin Detection Are Associated with BMI in an Elderly Cohort

Alexandria Turner [1,*], Martin Veysey [2,3], Simon Keely [4,5], Christopher J. Scarlett [1], Mark Lucock [1] and Emma L. Beckett [1,5]

1. School of Environmental and Life Sciences, University of Newcastle, Ourimbah 2258, Australia; c.scarlett@newcastle.edu.au (C.J.S.); mark.lucock@newcastle.edu.au (M.L.); emma.beckett@newcastle.edu.au (E.L.B.)
2. School of Medicine and Public Health, University of Newcastle, Ourimbah 2258, Australia; martin.veysey@hyms.ac.uk
3. Hull York Medical School, University of Hull, Hull HU6 7RX, UK
4. School of Biomedical Sciences and Pharmacy, University of Newcastle, Callaghan 2308, Australia; simon.keely@newcastle.edu.au
5. Hunter Medical Research Institute, New Lambton Heights 2305, Australia
* Correspondence: alexandria.turner@uon.edu.au; Tel.: +(02)-4348-4158

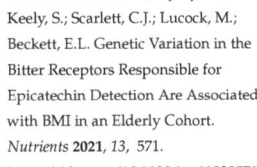

Citation: Turner, A.; Veysey, M.; Keely, S.; Scarlett, C.J.; Lucock, M.; Beckett, E.L. Genetic Variation in the Bitter Receptors Responsible for Epicatechin Detection Are Associated with BMI in an Elderly Cohort. *Nutrients* 2021, 13, 571. https://doi.org/10.3390/nu13020571

Academic Editor: Elena González-Burgos
Received: 8 January 2021
Accepted: 7 February 2021
Published: 9 February 2021

Publisher's Note: MDPI stays neutral with regard to jurisdictional claims in published maps and institutional affiliations.

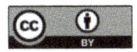

Copyright: © 2021 by the authors. Licensee MDPI, Basel, Switzerland. This article is an open access article distributed under the terms and conditions of the Creative Commons Attribution (CC BY) license (https://creativecommons.org/licenses/by/4.0/).

Abstract: Globally, more than one-third of adults are overweight. Overweight and obesity are complex and multifaceted conditions, associated with an increased risk of chronic illness and early mortality. While there are known risk factors, these alone do not fully explain the varying outcomes between individuals. Recently, taste receptors have been proposed to have a role in the risk for obesity. These receptors are expressed throughout the gastrointestinal tract. In this system, they may be involved in modulating dietary intake and metabolic processes. The taste 2 family of receptors (T2Rs) detects bitter compounds. Receptors T2R4 and T2R5 detect (-)-epicatechin (epicatechin), an antioxidant polyphenol, which may have protective effects against obesity. However, the potential role for taste receptors in this association has not been explored. This study assessed whether polymorphisms in *TAS2R4* (rs2233998 and rs2234001) and *TAS2R5* (rs2227264) were associated with body mass index (BMI). Genotyping (Taqman qPCR assays) was performed on DNA extracted from blood samples (n = 563) from an elderly cohort. Homozygosity for the minor allele of all polymorphisms was significantly associated with a lower BMI in males. The *TAS2R4*-rs2233998 CC genotype, the *TAS2R4*-rs2234001 CC genotype and the *TAS2R5*-rs2227264 TT genotype were associated with lower BMI (2.1, 2.1 and 2.2 units; p = 0.002, 0.003 and 0.001, respectively). Epicatechin intake was not associated with BMI and genotype was not associated with epicatechin intake. This suggests that the association between *TAS2R* genotype and elevated BMI risk occurs through altered extra-oral responses and not directly via altered epicatechin intake.

Keywords: BMI; bitter; epicatechin; phenol; obesity; taste genetics; taste receptors

1. Introduction

Catechins are part of a large group of plant polyphenols with exceptional antioxidant properties [1]. Interestingly, these compounds may have protective properties against obesity. A catechin-rich grape seed extract has been reported to significantly reduce body weight in mice with high-fat diet-induced obesity [2], while green tea catechins have been shown to reduce BMI, body weight and waist circumference in humans [3]. For (-)-epicatechin specifically (referred to as epicatechin throughout), murine studies have shown that epicatechin administration can reverse the negative effects of maternal obesity [4]. In humans, it has been demonstrated that epicatechin administration before a meal increased satiety [5], and further that epicatechin improved post-prandial fat and carbohydrate metabolism [6]. Altogether, there is evidence to suggest that catechins, and specifically epicatechin, may be protective against obesity.

Globally, more than 39% of adults are overweight and more than 13% are obese [7–9]. However, in Australia, more than 67% of adults are overweight [7]. Interestingly, obesity rates are increasing regardless of geographic location or socioeconomic status [8]. Importantly, obesity in the elderly is associated with earlier mortality relating to comorbidities such as hypertension, diabetes and heart disease [10–12]. Obesity is a complex and multifaceted disease that is not fully understood. However, there have been advancements in the investigations into the genetics of obesity [13], in particular the potential role of taste genetics on dietary intake and metabolism. This study explores the relationship between taste genetics, body mass index (BMI) and epicatechin intake.

Bitter taste receptors (T2Rs) are a family of receptors responsible for the detection of bitter compounds and potential toxins. Humans have 25 functional T2Rs which, when combined, are capable of detecting hundreds of bitter compounds [14–16]. In the oral cavity, genetic variation in these receptors influences oral detection, food preference and intake [17–20]. Importantly, these receptors are also expressed throughout the gastrointestinal tract, where they are thought to be involved in the modulation of appetite and satiation [17,21,22], gut motility [21–23] and glucose homeostasis [24]. In addition, functional T2R variants are associated with obesity in a porcine model [25]. Overall, bitter taste genetics may be associated with obesity via the modulation of dietary intake and/or by the regulation of gastrointestinal hormones and gut function [26].

TAS2R38 is a widely studied taste gene responsible for the detection of the bitter compounds phenylthiocarbamide (PTC) and 6-n-propyl-2-thiouracil (PROP) [27]. These compounds are commonly used as tools to detect taste phenotype. Three single-nucleotide polymorphisms (SNPs) give rise to two common forms of the gene. These polymorphisms are part of a haploblock and result in the amino acid substitutions proline-alanine-valine (PAV; associated with tasting PTC and PROP) or alanine-valine-isoleucine (AVI; associated with not tasting PTC or PROP). From this, there are three genotypes associated with taste sensitivity. PAV homozygotes can detect and respond strongly to PTC and PROP and are classified as super-tasters, heterozygotes are classified as tasters and AVI homozygotes cannot detect these compounds and are classified as non-tasters. It is important to note that *TAS2R38* genotype alone does not determine the ability to taste PTC and PROP [28]. However, it is still used as a general marker of taste acuity [29].

The *TAS2R38* genotype associated with non-taster status has been linked to significantly higher BMIs and/or increased dietary intake [30–37]. However, some studies report no association [38–40] and others report inverse associations [41]. These results may also vary with age and sex [37,39,42]. For example, in a study of 381 females and 348 males, the *TAS2R38*-rs1726866 T allele (non-taster) was associated with eating disinhibition in adult women [17]. Conversely, a study in 81 children found a significant relationship between tasters and high BMI, but reported no differences in energy intake [41]. Another study in children ($n = 53$) which compared taster status to weight-for-height percentiles, found that taster females had a significantly higher weight for height compared to non-taster females and, contrastingly, that non-taster males had a higher weight for height than male tasters [42]. Furthermore, a study in 118 elderly Polish women found no significant correlation between *TAS2R38* genotype and BMI [39]. Importantly, the relationship between bitter sensitivity and BMI is known to vary with age [43]. In a cross-sectional study of 311 men and women, it was found that individuals under 65 with a higher BMI (>28) were less sensitive to bitter taste. However, in the over 65 group, overweight subjects were more sensitive to bitter taste [43]. Overall, bitter sensitivity, and the relationship between *TAS2R38* genotype and BMI may vary with age and sex.

A group of bitter receptors, T2R4, T2R5 and T2R39, detect epicatechin [44]. Therefore, we analysed three common *TAS2R* polymorphisms that result in functional receptor changes. TAS2R39 was not analysed due to very low polymorphism frequency in this gene [45]. Two common polymorphisms in the *TAS2R4* gene (rs2233998 and rs2234001) and one polymorphism in the *TAS2R5* gene (rs2227264) were assessed. These three SNPs are part of a haploblock on chromosome 7 and have previously been linked to perceived bitterness of coffee [46]. This study explores the multidirectional interactions between *TAS2R* genotype, epicatechin intake, and BMI together in an elderly cohort.

2. Materials and Methods

2.1. Subjects and Data Collection

This study was a secondary analysis of cross-sectional data from the Retirement Health and Lifestyle Study, which was conducted on the NSW Central Coast of Australia from 2010 to 2012 [47]. Participants over the age of 65 were randomly selected from the Wyong and Gosford local areas, resulting in a cohort of primarily Caucasian heritage. This cohort was selected for this analysis to investigate the long-term effects of genotypes that correspond to functionally compromised taste receptors on BMI and dietary intake. Following screening and withdrawals, there were a total of 649 participants who gave blood samples and completed food frequency questionnaires (FFQ).

Dietary information was collected using a self-reported FFQ, adapted from the validated Commonwealth Scientific and Industrial Research Organisation Human Nutrition FFQ [48]. The FFQ contained 225 food items across all food groups with questions about frequency of consumption. For this study, this number was converted into serves per day. Participants were excluded if their FFQ was deemed invalid based on extreme energy excess or deficit (>30,000 or <3000 kJ/day) this excludes participants suspected of severely under- or overestimating daily dietary intake [49,50]. Participants who reported >11 serves per day of the same food group [51], or >4 serves of the same fruit, or same nut, per day were excluded as this is not representative of the general population [52]. Following exclusions, there were a total of 563 participants eligible for this study.

All participants supplied written informed consent. Study approval was obtained from the University of Newcastle Human Research Ethics Committee (approval number H-2008-0431).

2.2. Blood Samples and BMI

Blood samples were collected in EDTA-lined tubes by a trained phlebotomist and stored at −20 °C prior to DNA extraction. BMI was calculated from participant's weight and height [weight (kg)/height (m^2)]. Weight was measured to the nearest 0.01 kg using digital scales (Wedderbum© UWPM150 Platform Scale). Height was measured using the stretch stature method [53] and recorded to the nearest 0.01 cm.

2.3. Genotyping

Participant DNA was extracted from frozen blood samples using the QIAGEN QIAmp DNA mini kit following the manufacturer's whole-blood protocol [54,55]. DNA samples were stored at 20 °C prior to genotyping. Genotyping was carried out via qPCR (QuantStudio 7 Flex Real-Time PCR) with TaqMan™ SNP Genotyping Assays (Applied Biosystems™, ThermoFisher Scientific, CA, USA) and TaqMan™ Genotyping Master Mix according to the TaqMan™ user guide [56,57]. Participants were included in this study only upon successful genotyping.

2.4. Epicatechin Intake

Daily epicatechin intake data were estimated from a polyphenol database [58] and the FFQs [52]. The Phenol Explorer database contains the average mg/100 g of epicatechin for a large variety of foods and beverages [58]. In this study, foods that contained over 0.1 mg/100 g epicatechin from the Phenol Explorer database [58] were considered high-epicatechin foods, and were used as an indicator of epicatechin intake. This approach was used to estimate relative intake as it is notably difficult to estimate actual intake amounts (mg/day) [59]. This is primarily due to bias in self-reported dietary data and large variation in reported concentrations of epicatechin within foods [58,59] (Table 1).

Table 1. Foods with high epicatechin content (≥0.1 mg/100 g; Phenol Explorer).

Groups	High-Epicatechin Foods	Average mg/100 g [58]	SD	Standard Serving Size [52]	Average mg/Serve
Tea	Tea [Green], infusion	7.9	13.7	200 mL	15.9
	Tea [Black], infusion	3.9	4.3	200 mL	7.9
Chocolate	Chocolate, dark	70.3	29.5	25 g	17.7
	Chocolate, milk	14.6	4.8	25 g	3.7
Wine	Wine [Red]	3.8	3.2	100 mL	3.8
	Wine [White]	1.0	1.4	100 mL	1.0
Fruits	Apple [Dessert], raw	8.4	3.7	150 g	12.6
	Peach, peeled	8.0	4.2	150 g	12.0
	Apple [Dessert], pure juice	7.8	7.7	150 g	11.6
	Grape [Black]	5.2	5.6	150 g	7.9
	Red raspberry, raw	5.1	3.7	150 g	7.6
	Apricot, raw	3.5	4.3	150 g	5.2
	Nectarine, peeled	3.0	1.1	150 g	4.5
	Plum, fresh	2.2	2.2	150 g	3.3
	Blueberry, raw	1.1	0	150 g	1.7
	Grape [Green]	0.5	0.5	150 g	0.7
	Avocado, raw	0.4	0.2	150 g	0.6
	Kiwi	0.3	0.2	150 g	0.4
	Banana, raw	0.1	0.1	150 g	0.2
Vegetables	Broad bean seed, raw	22.5	0	75 g	16.9
	Green bean, raw	0.7	2.7	75 g	0.5
Nuts	Lentils, whole, raw	0.1	0.3	75 g	0.1
	Cashew nut, raw	0.9	0	30 g	0.3
	Pecan nut	0.8	0	30 g	0.2
	Almond	0.6	0.4	30 g	0.2
	Hazelnut, raw	0.2	0	30 g	0.1

The food items that fit into an FFQ category, and also contained >0.01 mg/100 g epicatechin according to the Phenol Explorer database, were included in this study (Table 1). These foods included teas, chocolates, wines, many fruits, nuts and legumes (Table 1).

Due to the resolution of the FFQ, in this analysis, all teas, including black, green and herbal, were analysed as a group (i.e., total serves of tea per day). Additionally, all chocolate, including milk, dark, chocolate bars and chocolate biscuits were grouped together (i.e., total serves of chocolate products per day). FFQ data were available for individual wines, fruits, vegetables and nuts (i.e., serves per day of individual products).

2.5. Statistics

Statistical analyses were performed using JMP (version 14.2.0, SAS Institute Inc., Cary, NC, USA). The relationship between genotype and BMI was examined using standard least squares regression. All analyses were adjusted for age and sex, or adjusted for age and stratified by sex. BMI was reported as least squares means with 95% confidence intervals. Genotypes were combined to analyse presence vs. absence of the major allele according to the TOPMED database. Dunnett's post-hoc analysis was used to determine statistically significant differences between genotypes ($p < 0.05$). The relationship between energy intake and serves of high-epicatechin foods per day, and the relationship between BMI and serves of high-epicatechin foods per day was analysed using least squares regression. p-values and standardised beta values (β) were reported for correlation. Graphs were presented using Graphpad Prism (version 7.01, GraphPad Software, La Jolla, CA, USA).

3. Results

A total of 563 participants were included in this study following exclusions (Table 2). Of these, 254 were male and 309 were female. The average overall age was 77.4. In men, the average age was 77.4; and in women, the average age was 77.3 The average BMI for men was 28.5 and 28.6 for women, with an average of 28.5 overall. The average overall energy intake was 8223.5 kJ (8453.1–7993.9). There was a significant difference in average male daily energy intake (8656.2 kJ (8311.3–9001.1)) compared to females (7866.7 kJ (7563.1–8170.3)). The average number of serves of high-epicatechin foods per day was 5.2 for men, women and overall.

The genotype distributions are shown in Table 3. The *TAS2R4* rs2233998 polymorphism has a minor allele frequency (MAF) of 0.42. 21% of participants were homozygous for the minor allele (CC), 25% were homozygous for the major allele (TT) and 54% of participants were heterozygotes. In the rs2234001 polymorphism, 20% of participants were homozygous for the minor allele (CC; MAF = 0.48), 25% were homozygous for the major allele (GG) and 55% were heterozygotes. In the *TAS2R5* rs2227264 polymorphism, 21% of participants were homozygous for the minor allele (TT; MAF = 0.44), 27% of participants were homozygous for the major allele and 62% were heterozygotes.

Table 2. Participant characteristics reported as the mean (95% CI).

Characteristic	Male (*n* = 254)	Female (*n* = 309)	Total (*n* = 563)
Age	77.4 (76.6–78.3)	77.3 (76.6–78.2)	77.4 (76.8–78.0)
BMI	28.5 (27.9–29.1)	28.6 (28.0–29.2)	28.5 (28.1–29.0)
Daily energy intake (kJ)	* 8656.2 (8311.3–9001.1)	* 7866.7 (7563.1–8170.3)	8223.5 (8453.1–7993.9)
Serves of high-epicatechin foods per day **	5.2 (4.9–5.6)	5.2 (4.9–5.5)	5.2 (5.0–5.4)

** High-epicatechin foods are defined as having ≥ 0.1 mg/100 g (Phenol Explorer [58]); * significant difference in energy intake between males and females ($p = 0.0005$).

Table 3. *TAS2R* genotype distributions.

SNP	Genotype	n	%	MAF	HWE χ^2	HWE *p*
TAS2R4 (rs2233998)	CC	112	21%	0.42	3.8	0.05
	CT	287	54%	-		
	TT	131	25%	-		
TAS2R4 (rs2234001)	CC	108	20%	0.48	121.8	<0.0001
	CG	302	55%	-		
	GG	135	25%	-		
TAS2R5 (rs2227264)	TT	120	21%	0.44	0.8	0.4
	TG	291	62%	-		
	GG	151	27%	-		

SNP = single-nucleotide polymorphism; MAF = minor allele frequency; HWE = Hardy–Weinberg equilibrium.

Homozygosity of the minor allele was associated with significantly lower BMI in both *TAS2R4* polymorphisms (Figure 1). The *TAS2R4*-rs2233998 CC genotype was associated with an average BMI of 27.7 (95% CI [26.8, 28.6]) and the presence of the G allele was associated with significantly larger average BMI of 28.7 (95% CI [28.2, 29.2]; $p = 0.02$). The *TAS2R4*-rs2234001 CC genotype was similarly associated with a lower BMI (27.6 (95% CI [26.7, 28.5])) compared to the presence of the G allele (28.8 (95% CI [28.3, 29.2]); $p = 0.01$). The presence of the major allele in the *TAS2R5* polymorphism (rs2227264) was not associated with a significant difference in BMI in this cohort.

The relationship between BMI and TASR genotype was sex specific (Figure 2). For all three polymorphisms (rs2233998, rs2234001 and rs2227264), the presence of the major allele was associated with a significantly higher BMI than in males homozygous for the minor allele. The *TAS2R4*-rs2233998 CC genotype was associated with a BMI of 26.8 (25.6–28.0) and the presence of the G allele was associated with a significantly higher BMI (28.9 (28.3–29.6); $p = 0.002$). The *TAS2R4*-s2234001 CC genotype was associated with a BMI of 26.9 (25.7–28.1), whereas the presence of the G allele was associated with a significantly higher BMI of 29.0 (28.4–29.7; $p = 0.003$). Finally, the *TAS2R5*-rs2227264 TT genotype was associated with a BMI of 26.8 (25.7–28.0) compared to 29.0 (28.4–29.6; $p = 0.001$).

In females, there was no significant difference in BMI of individuals homozygous for the minor allele, compared to the presence of the major allele. Additionally, these results remained significant when adjusted for daily energy intake.

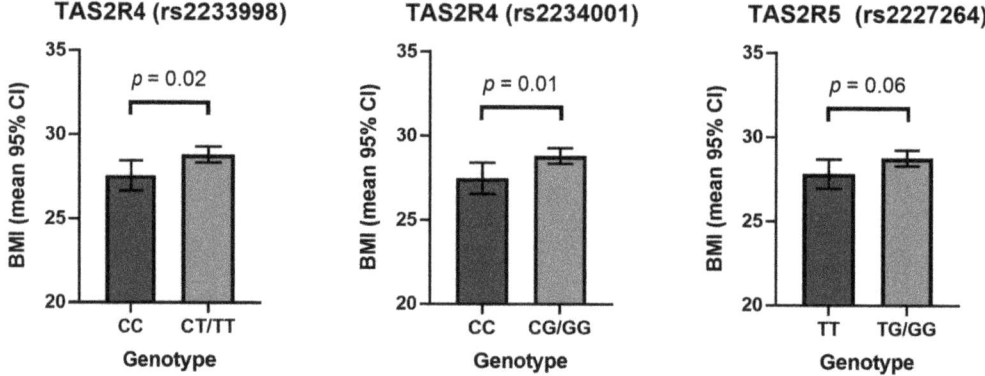

Figure 1. The relationship between *TAS2R* genotype and BMI. Data are presented as the mean BMI with 95% confidence intervals, adjusted for age and sex.

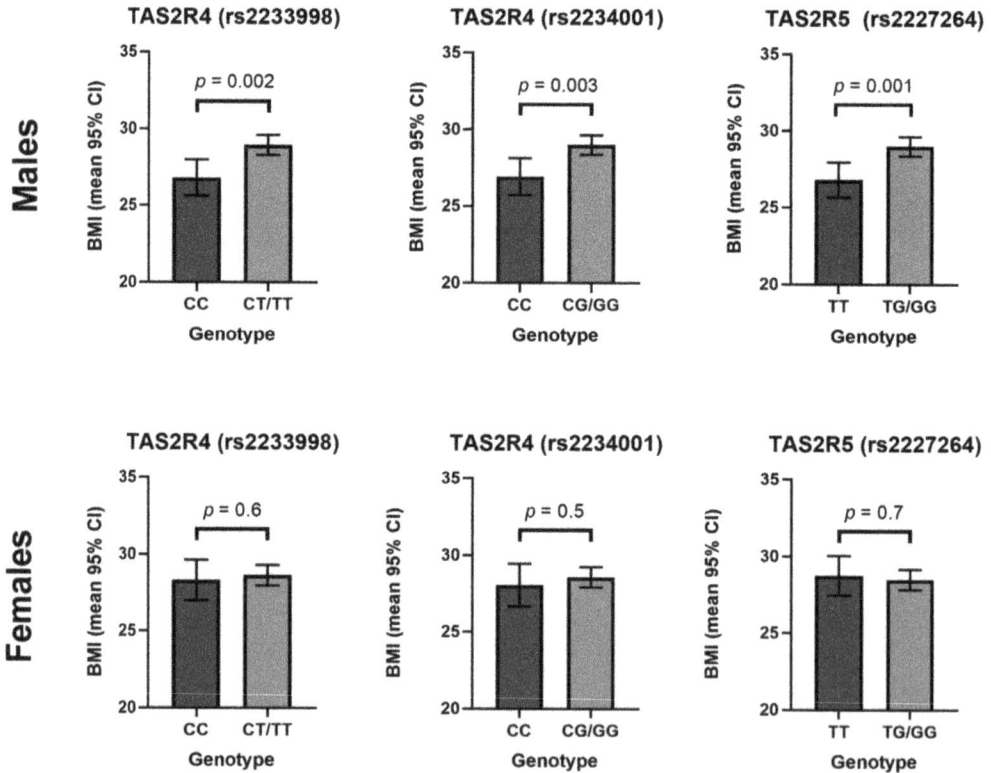

Figure 2. The relationship between *TAS2R* genotype and BMI by sex. Data are presented as the mean BMI with 95% confidence intervals, adjusted for age.

Due to the significant difference in energy intake between males and females (Table 2), the data were analysed for a relationship between *TAS2R* genotype and daily energy intake, this analysis was stratified by sex (Table 4). The presence of the major allele was not associated with a significant different energy intake compared to homozygosity for the minor allele in any of the three polymorphisms. When stratified by sex, there was also no significant differences between the genotypes analysed.

There was a significant correlation between increased daily energy intake and increased epicatechin intake ($p < 0.0001$; $\beta = 0.5$) (Figure 3A). There was no significant relationship between BMI and serves of high-epicatechin foods per day ($p = 0.2$; $\beta = -0.06$) (Figure 3B). Additionally, there was no significant association between dietary energy intake per day and BMI ($p = 0.5$; $\beta = -0.03$) in this cohort.

Table 4. Daily energy intake is not significantly associated with *TAS2R* genotype.

SNP	*TAS2R4* (rs2233998)			*TAS2R4* (rs2234001)			*TAS2R5* (rs2227264)		
	CC	CT/TT	*p*	CC	CG/GG	*p*	TT	TG/GG	*p*
Mean kJ/day (95% CI)	7934.5 (7428.0–8441.0)	8278.6 (8013.4–8543.7)	0.2	7905.2 (7386.8–8423.7)	8272.3 (8011.8–8532.8)	0.2	8056.8 (7564.0–8549.6)	8304.7 (8045.3–8564.2)	0.4
Male mean kJ/day (95% CI)	8530.8 (7777.1–9284.6)	8644.6 (8236.8–9052.4)	0.8	8552.8 (7794.8–9310.9)	8585.0 (8189.5–8980.6)	0.9	8574.6 (7834.9–9314.3)	8686.0 (8288.6–9083.4)	0.8
Female mean kJ/day (95% CI)	7350.2 (6660.4–8039.9)	7902 (7554.9–8249.3)	0.1	7282.3 (6565.9–7998.7)	7943.7 (7598.9–8288.4)	0.1	7561.5 (6896.1–8226.9)	7914.7 (7573.4–8256.0)	0.4

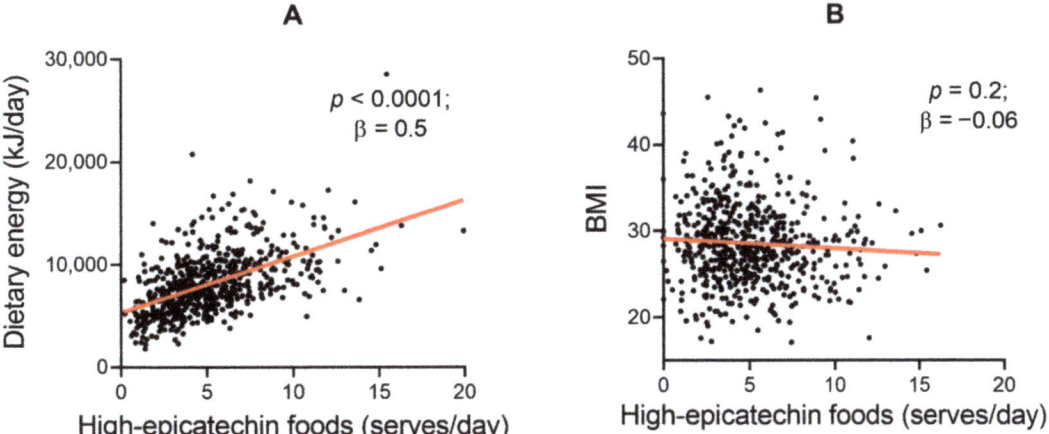

Figure 3. Epicatechin intake is significantly associated with dietary energy intake (A), but is not associated with BMI (B). Standardised β and p values reported for correlation.

There was no significant association between *TAS2R* genotype and the average number of serves of high-epicatechin foods (Table 5). However, there was consistently higher epicatechin intake observed in males homozygous for the minor allele of all three polymorphisms (compared to male carriers of the major allele and both female groups). Interestingly, these are the same groups associated with significantly lower BMIs in Figure 2.

Table 5. TAS2R genotype does not significantly affect the average number of serves of high-epicatechin foods per day.

SNP	TAS2R4 (rs2233998)		p	TAS2R4 (rs2234001)		p	TAS2R5 (rs2227264)		p
	CC	CT/TT		CC	CG/GG		TT	TG/GG	
Mean (95% CI)	5.3 (4.8–5.7)	5.2 (4.9–5.4)	0.7	5.3 (4.8–5.8)	5.2 4.9–5.4)	0.8	5.4 (4.9–5.9)	5.2 (4.9–5.5)	0.5
Male mean (95% CI)	5.5 (4.8–6.3)	5.1 (4.7–5.5)	0.3	5.4 (4.7–6.1)	5.1 (4.7–5.5)	0.5	5.6 (4.8–6.3)	5.2 (4.8–5.6)	0.4
Female mean (95% CI)	5.0 (4.2–5.7)	5.2 (4.8–5.6)	0.6	5.1 (4.4–5.8)	5.2 (4.9–5.6)	0.7	5.2 (4.5–5.9)	5.2 (4.9–5.6)	1.0

4. Discussion

The secondary analysis presented here identifies potential associations between common *TAS2R4* polymorphisms and BMI. Homozygosity for the minor alleles of *TAS2R4*-rs2233998 and *TAS2R4*-rs2234001 was associated with significantly lower BMI compared to carriers of the major allele in this cohort. The three *TAS2R*SNPs analysed in this study (*TAS2R4*-rs2233998, *TAS2R4*-rs2234001 and *TAS2R5*-rs2227264) are part of a haploblock on chromosome 7 [46]. Therefore, it was expected that the SNPs assessed may be associated with the same parameter (BMI). Importantly, the association between *TAS2R4* genotypes (*TAS2R4*-rs2233998, *TAS2R4*-rs2234001) and BMI could not be explained in this cohort by daily energy intake or by daily epicatechin intake. The lack of association between energy intake and BMI suggests *TAS2R4* genotypes do not modulate food intake. Alternatively, functional *TAS2R4* polymorphisms may affect the extra-oral roles of taste receptors in energy metabolism [26].

Importantly, this study highlights a previously unexplored potential relationship between *TAS2R4* and *TAS2R5* genotypes and BMI. In males, homozygosity for the minor allele of all three polymorphisms corresponded to a lower BMI (>2 BMI units) in each instance, this equates to several kilograms of weight difference, depending on height. The risk for conditions associated with higher BMI such as hypertension, diabetes and cardiovascular disease increases with increased BMI [8,9,60]. For example, each one-unit increase in BMI is significantly associated with a 4% risk of ischemic stroke and a 6% increase in risk of hemorrhagic stroke [61]. Additionally, in adolescent men ($n = 37674$), risk for diabetes increases by 9.8% and risk for heart disease increases by 12% per one BMI unit increase [62]. The effects of increased BMI is particularly pronounced in the elderly where overweight and obese individuals experience earlier mortality than their normal weight counterparts [10–12]. Overall, this study provides insight into the genetic risk factors for obesity in the elderly.

A potential role for other extra-oral bitter receptors genotypes in predicting BMI has previously been suggested [35,41]. A Korean study ($n = 3567$) identified that the *TAS2R38*-rs10246939 TT genotype (associated phenotypically with non-tasting) was associated with a significantly higher BMI in females. However, there was no association between genotype and energy intake, suggesting another biological mechanism [35]. Additionally, a study in children ($n = 81$) which found a significant association between tasters and high BMI, found no complementary relationship between taster status and energy intake [41]. When taken together with the results presented here, a potential role for extra-oral T2Rs in predicting BMI, without modulating energy intake is suggested.

The extra-oral roles of T2R activation on appetite and gut motility may be a potential explanatory factor for these observations. Treatment with bitter taste receptor agonists has been shown to alter satiation, food intake and gastric emptying. Intra-gastric administration of 1 μmol/kg of the bitter taste receptor agonist, denatonium benzoate, significantly increased satiation in healthy volunteers ($n = 13$) [21]. Furthermore, a study in 16 women that examined the effects of chewing and then expectorating either a bitter bar or a pleasant-tasting bar determined that gastric emptying was significantly delayed in response to the bitter-tasting bar [23]. In animal and cell models, it has been identified that intestinal taste receptors modulate the secretion of gastrointestinal hormones GLP-1, GIP, ghrelin, CCK and PYY [21–24,26,63,64] involved in appetite, digestion and glucose homeostasis [21,22,24,63–65]. Therefore, functional extra-oral receptor changes related to *TAS2R* genotype may influence the secretion of gastrointestinal hormones in response to bitter agonists and impact obesity risk. However, additional studies are needed to determine the causative mechanism(s).

Although there was no association between epicatechin intake and BMI in this cohort, the administration of epicatechin (detected by T2R4 and T2R5) has previously been associated with improved cardiometabolic function [6,66]. A study in 20 adults found that following 1 mg/kg epicatechin ingestion, lipid oxidation was significantly increased in overweight subjects and post-prandial triglyceridemia decreased in normal and overweight subjects [6]. Another small study (12 males) reported significantly improved vascular function following 1–2 mg/kg body weight oral dose of epicatechin [66]. However, results from the present study suggest that nutritive doses of epicatechin did not have an effect on BMI in elderly subjects. Similarly, a previous study identified that a nutritive dose of 25 mg/day had no effect on cardiometabolic factors (blood pressure, glucose, insulin, insulin resistance, triglycerides, or total LDL, or HDL cholesterol) [67].

Interestingly, the number of serves of high-epicatechin foods per day was associated with increased daily energy intake in this study. It may be that higher epicatechin intake in this study is simply a function of higher overall food intake. By contrast, it has previously been demonstrated in humans that epicatechin administration before a meal increased satiety [5]. Additionally, while *TAS2R38* genotypes have previously been associated with altered oral detection, food preference and intake [17–20], there was no significant association between *TAS2R4* and *TAS2R5* genotypes and epicatechin intake in this study. This suggests that these polymorphisms are not altering oral detection and modulating intake of epicatechin containing foods. However, functional receptor changes associated with these *TAS2R* polymorphisms may alter extra-oral metabolic responses to epicatechin.

Associations between *TAS2R38* genotypes and BMI and associated taster status and BMI have previously been reported [30–37,41]. However, this study is unique in examining the relationship between *TAS2R4* and *TAS2R5* genotypes and BMI and supports a role for *TAS2R* genotypes in predicting BMI in males. The association between homozygosity for the minor alleles of *TAS2R4*-rs2233998, *TAS2R4*-rs2234001 and *TAS2R5*-rs2227264 and lower BMI appears to be specific to males in this cohort. Sex specificity has been previously identified between *TAS2R* genotypes and a variety of outcomes, including dietary intake [17,68], BMI, [35,42] and thyroid function, which effects metabolism [69]. The sex specificity of the observed results may be explained by potential interactions between sex hormones and taste signalling, other genes located on sex chromosomes, or social determinants of food choice that are gender specific. Further studies are needed to understand these relationships. Altogether, this study provides further evidence of a potential sex dimorphism in the relationship between *TAS2R4* and *TAS2R5* genotypes and BMI in elderly subjects.

It is important to note that the identified relationship between *TAS2R38* and BMI may also vary with age. This study found no significant association between *TAS2R4* or *TAS2R5* genotypes and BMI in elderly women, while other studies in children [32,41] and adults [30,31,33–35] report potential links between *TAS2R38* genotype and BMI, and a previous study in elderly women found no significant association between *TAS2R38* genotype and BMI [39]. It is well-documented that taste loss occurs during ageing [70,71]. Therefore, further studies are needed in children and adults to determine whether the relationship between *TAS2R4* and *TAS2R5* genotypes and BMI is age specific as well as sex specific.

The use of an elderly cohort means that these results may be specific to elderly and not necessarily applicable to younger populations. However, this cohort was useful in studying the long-term effects of *TAS2R* genotypes on BMI. Another limitation of this study included estimations of energy intake and epicatechin intake. Dietary intake estimations are limited by low-accuracy and subject bias of food frequency questionnaires [72]. Additionally, it is important to note that epicatechin intake is hard to quantify due to the high variability of food composition [59] and the large variation in reported concentrations of epicatechin within foods [58].

Overall, we propose that *TAS2R* genotypes, resulting in functional receptor changes, may alter metabolic hormone secretion in a sex-specific manner, with downstream effects on BMI. Additional studies in larger and more diverse age groups are needed to establish this potential association between *TAS2R* genotype(s) and BMI. Importantly, if these relationships are established, they may be used to predict obesity risk, and potentially combat conditions associated with a larger BMI in the form of personalised nutrition therapies. Ultimately, this study provides initial insight into the complex relationship between taste genetics and BMI and the potential roles for extra-oral T2Rs in obesity risk.

Author Contributions: Conceptualization, A.T. and E.L.B.; writing—original draft preparation, A.T., E.L.B. and S.K.; writing—review and editing, C.J.S., M.L. and M.V. All authors have read and agreed to the published version of the manuscript.

Funding: A.T. is supported by a Commonwealth Government of Australia 2018 Research Training Scholarship. E.L.B. is supported by an NHMRC Early Career Fellowship.

Institutional Review Board Statement: This study was conducted according to the guidelines of the Declaration of Helsinki, and approved by the Human Research Ethics Committee of University of Newcastle (approval number H-2008-0431).

Informed Consent Statement: Informed consent was obtained from all subjects involved in this study.

Data Availability Statement: The data presented in this study are available on request from the corresponding author. The data are not publicly available due to ethical reasons.

Conflicts of Interest: The authors declare no conflict of interest.

References

1. Grzesik, M.; Naparlo, K.; Bartosz, G.; Sadowska-Bartosz, I. Antioxidant properties of catechins: Comparison with other antioxidants. *Food Chem.* **2018**, *241*, 480–492. [CrossRef]
2. Ohyama, K.; Furuta, C.; Nogusa, Y.; Nomura, K.; Miwa, T.; Suzuki, K. Catechin-Rich Grape Seed Extract Supplementation Attenuates Diet-Induced Obesity in C57BL/6J Mice. *Ann. Nutr. Metab.* **2011**, *58*, 250–258. [CrossRef] [PubMed]
3. Phung, O.J.; Baker, W.L.; Matthews, L.J.; Lanosa, M.; Thorne, A.; Coleman, C.I. Effect of green tea catechins with or without caffeine on anthropometric measures: A systematic review and meta-analysis. *Am. J. Clin. Nutr.* **2009**, *91*, 73–81. [CrossRef]
4. De Los Santos, S.; Reyes-Castro, L.A.; Coral-Vazquez, R.M.; Mendez, J.P.; Leal-Garcia, M.; Zambrano, E.; Canto, P. (-)-Epicatechin reduces adiposity in male offspring of obese rats. *J. Dev. Orig. Health Dis.* **2020**, *11*, 37–43. [CrossRef] [PubMed]
5. Greenberg, J.A.; O'Donnell, R.; Shurpin, M.; Kordunova, D. Epicatechin, procyanidins, cocoa, and appetite: A randomized controlled trial. *Am. J. Clin. Nutr.* **2016**, *104*, 613–619. [CrossRef]
6. Gutiérrez-Salmeán, G.; Ortiz-Vilchis, P.; Vacaseydel, C.M.; Rubio-Gayosso, I.; Meaney, E.; Villarreal, F.; Ramírez-Sánchez, I.; Ceballos, G. Acute effects of an oral supplement of (-)-epicatechin on postprandial fat and carbohydrate metabolism in normal and overweight subjects. *Food Funct.* **2014**, *5*, 521–527. [CrossRef] [PubMed]
7. World Health Organization. Prevalence of overweight among adults, BMI $\geq$ 25 (crude estimate) (%). Available online: https://www.who.int/data/gho/data/indicators/indicator-details/GHO/prevalence-of-overweight-among-adults-bmi-greaterequal-25-(crude-estimate)-(-) (accessed on 12 November 2020).
8. Chooi, Y.C.; Ding, C.; Magkos, F. The epidemiology of obesity. *Metabolism* **2019**, *92*, 6–10. [CrossRef]
9. Collaborators, G.B.D.O.; Afshin, A.; Forouzanfar, M.H.; Reitsma, M.B.; Sur, P.; Estep, K.; Lee, A.; Marczak, L.; Mokdad, A.H.; Moradi-Lakeh, M.; et al. Health Effects of Overweight and Obesity in 195 Countries over 25 Years. *N. Engl. J. Med.* **2017**, *377*, 13–27. [CrossRef]
10. Osher, E.; Stern, N. Obesity in Elderly Subjects: In Sheep's Clothing Perhaps, but still a Wolf! *Diabetes Care* **2009**, *32*, S398–S402. [CrossRef]
11. Adams, K.F.; Schatzkin, A.; Harris, T.B.; Kipnis, V.; Mouw, T.; Ballard-Barbash, R.; Hollenbeck, A.; Leitzmann, M.F. Overweight, obesity, and mortality in a large prospective cohort of persons 50 to 71 years old. *N. Engl. J. Med.* **2006**, *355*, 763–778. [CrossRef]
12. Rillamas-Sun, E.; LaCroix, A.Z.; Waring, M.E.; Kroenke, C.H.; LaMonte, M.J.; Vitolins, M.Z.; Seguin, R.; Bell, C.L.; Gass, M.; Manini, T.M.; et al. Obesity and late-age survival without major disease or disability in older women. *JAMA Intern. Med.* **2014**, *174*, 98–106. [CrossRef]
13. Goodarzi, M.O. Genetics of obesity: What genetic association studies have taught us about the biology of obesity and its complications. *Lancet Diabetes Endocrinol.* **2018**, *6*, 223–236. [CrossRef]
14. Go, Y.; Satta, Y.; Takenaka, O.; Takahata, N. Lineage-specific loss of function of bitter taste receptor genes in humans and nonhuman primates. *Genetics* **2005**, *170*, 313–326. [CrossRef]
15. Meyerhof, W.; Batram, C.; Kuhn, C.; Brockhoff, A.; Chudoba, E.; Bufe, B.; Appendino, G.; Behrens, M. The molecular receptive ranges of human *TAS2R* bitter taste receptors. *Chem. Senses* **2010**, *35*, 157–170. [CrossRef]

16. Shi, P.; Zhang, J.; Yang, H.; Zhang, Y.-P. Adaptive Diversification of Bitter Taste Receptor Genes in Mammalian Evolution. *Mol. Biol. Evol.* **2003**, *20*, 805–814. [CrossRef]
17. Dotson, C.D.; Shaw, H.L.; Mitchell, B.D.; Munger, S.D.; Steinle, N.I. Variation in the gene *TAS2R38* is associated with the eating behavior disinhibition in Old Order Amish women. *Appetite* **2010**, *54*, 93–99. [CrossRef] [PubMed]
18. Choi, J.H.; Lee, J.; Yang, S.; Kim, J. Genetic variations in taste perception modify alcohol drinking behavior in Koreans. *Appetite* **2017**, *113*, 178–186. [CrossRef] [PubMed]
19. Diószegi, J.; Llanaj, E.; Ádány, R. Genetic Background of Taste Perception, Taste Preferences, and Its Nutritional Implications: A Systematic Review. *Front. Genet.* **2019**, *10*, 1272. [CrossRef]
20. Perna, S.; Riva, A.; Nicosanti, G.; Carrai, M.; Barale, R.; Vigo, B.; Allegrini, P.; Rondanelli, M. Association of the bitter taste receptor gene *TAS2R38* (polymorphism RS713598) with sensory responsiveness, food preferences, biochemical parameters and body-composition markers. A cross-sectional study in Italy. *Int. J. Food Sci. Nutr.* **2018**, *69*, 245–252. [CrossRef]
21. Avau, B.; Rotondo, A.; Thijs, T.; Andrews, C.N.; Janssen, P.; Tack, J.; Depoortere, I. Targeting extra-oral bitter taste receptors modulates gastrointestinal motility with effects on satiation. *Sci. Rep.* **2015**, *5*, 15985. [CrossRef]
22. Janssen, S.; Laermans, J.; Verhulst, P.J.; Thijs, T.; Tack, J.; Depoortere, I. Bitter taste receptors and α-gustducin regulate the secretion of ghrelin with functional effects on food intake and gastric emptying. *Proc. Natl. Acad. Sci. USA* **2011**, *108*, 2094–2099. [CrossRef]
23. Wicks, D.; Wright, J.; Rayment, P.; Spiller, R. Impact of bitter taste on gastric motility. *Eur. J. Gastroenterol. Hepatol.* **2005**, *17*, 961–965. [CrossRef]
24. Dotson, C.D.; Zhang, L.; Xu, H.; Shin, Y.K.; Vigues, S.; Ott, S.H.; Elson, A.E.; Choi, H.J.; Shaw, H.; Egan, J.M.; et al. Bitter taste receptors influence glucose homeostasis. *PLoS ONE* **2008**, *3*, e3974. [CrossRef]
25. Cirera, S.; Clop, A.; Jacobsen, M.J.; Guerin, M.; Lesnik, P.; Jorgensen, C.B.; Fredholm, M.; Karlskov-Mortensen, P. A targeted genotyping approach enhances identification of variants in taste receptor and appetite/reward genes of potential functional importance for obesity-related porcine traits. *Anim. Genet.* **2018**, *49*, 110–118. [CrossRef] [PubMed]
26. Turner, A.; Veysey, M.; Keely, S.; Scarlett, C.; Lucock, M.; Beckett, E.L. Interactions between Bitter Taste, Diet and Dysbiosis: Consequences for Appetite and Obesity. *Nutrients* **2018**, *10*, 1336. [CrossRef]
27. Kim, U.K.; Jorgenson, E.; Coon, H.; Leppert, M.; Risch, N.; Drayna, D. Positional cloning of the human quantitative trait locus underlying taste sensitivity to phenylthiocarbamide. *Science (N.Y.)* **2003**, *299*, 1221–1225. [CrossRef] [PubMed]
28. Hayes, J.E.; Bartoshuk, L.M.; Kidd, J.R.; Duffy, V.B. Supertasting and PROP Bitterness Depends on More Than the *TAS2R38* Gene. *Chem. Senses* **2008**, *33*, 255–265. [CrossRef] [PubMed]
29. Tepper, B.J.; White, E.A.; Koelliker, Y.; Lanzara, C.; d'Adamo, P.; Gasparini, P. Genetic variation in taste sensitivity to 6-n-propylthiouracil and its relationship to taste perception and food selection. *Ann. N Y Acad. Sci.* **2009**, *1170*, 126–139. [CrossRef]
30. Tepper, B.J.; Ullrich, N.V. Influence of genetic taste sensitivity to 6-n-propylthiouracil (PROP), dietary restraint and disinhibition on body mass index in middle-aged women. *Physiol. Behav.* **2002**, *75*, 305–312. [CrossRef]
31. Choi, S.E.; Chan, J. Relationship of 6-n-propylthiouracil taste intensity and chili pepper use with body mass index, energy intake, and fat intake within an ethnically diverse population. *J. Acad. Nutr. Dietetics* **2015**, *115*, 389–396. [CrossRef] [PubMed]
32. Keller, K.L.; Adise, S. Variation in the Ability to Taste Bitter Thiourea Compounds: Implications for Food Acceptance, Dietary Intake, and Obesity Risk in Children. *Ann. Rev. Nutr.* **2016**, *36*, 157–182. [CrossRef]
33. Duffy, V.B. Associations between oral sensation, dietary behaviors and risk of cardiovascular disease (CVD). *Appetite* **2004**, *43*, 5–9. [CrossRef] [PubMed]
34. Ortega, F.J.; Aguera, Z.; Sabater, M.; Moreno-Navarrete, J.M.; Alonso-Ledesma, I.; Xifra, G.; Botas, P.; Delgado, E.; Jimenez-Murcia, S.; Fernandez-Garcia, J.C.; et al. Genetic variations of the bitter taste receptor *TAS2R38* are associated with obesity and impact on single immune traits. *Mol. Nutr. Food Res.* **2016**, *60*, 1673–1683. [CrossRef] [PubMed]
35. Choi, J.-H. Variation in the *TAS2R38* Bitterness Receptor Gene Was Associated with Food Consumption and Obesity Risk in Koreans. *Nutrients* **2019**, *11*, 1973. [CrossRef]
36. Tepper, B.J.; Koelliker, Y.; Zhao, L.; Ullrich, N.V.; Lanzara, C.; D'Adamo, P.; Ferrara, A.; Ulivi, S.; Esposito, L.; Gasparini, P. Variation in the Bitter-taste Receptor Gene *TAS2R38*, and Adiposity in a Genetically Isolated Population in Southern Italy. *Obesity* **2008**, *16*, 2289–2295. [CrossRef]
37. Keller, K.L.; Reid, A.; MacDougall, M.C.; Cassano, H.; Song, J.L.; Deng, L.; Lanzano, P.; Chung, W.K.; Kissileff, H.R. Sex Differences in the Effects of Inherited Bitter Thiourea Sensitivity on Body Weight in 4–6-Year-Old Children. *Obesity* **2010**, *18*, 1194–1200. [CrossRef]
38. Goldstein, G.L.; Daun, H.; Tepper, B.J. Influence of PROP taster status and maternal variables on energy intake and body weight of pre-adolescents. *Physiol. Behav.* **2007**, *90*, 809–817. [CrossRef] [PubMed]
39. Mikolajczyk-Stecyna, J.; Malinowska, A.M.; Chmurzynska, A. *TAS2R38* and CA6 genetic polymorphisms, frequency of bitter food intake, and blood biomarkers among elderly woman. *Appetite* **2017**, *116*, 57–64. [CrossRef]
40. Pawellek, I.; Grote, V.; Rzehak, P.; Xhonneux, A.; Verduci, E.; Stolarczyk, A.; Closa-Monasterolo, R.; Reischl, E.; Koletzko, B. Association of *TAS2R38* variants with sweet food intake in children aged 1-6 years. *Appetite* **2016**, *107*, 126–134. [CrossRef] [PubMed]
41. Lumeng, J.C.; Cardinal, T.M.; Sitto, J.R.; Kannan, S. Ability to taste 6-n-propylthiouracil and BMI in low-income preschool-aged children. *Obesity* **2008**, *16*, 1522–1528. [CrossRef]

42. Keller, K.L.; Tepper, B.J. Inherited Taste Sensitivity to 6-n-Propylthiouracil in Diet and Body Weight in Children. *Obesity Res.* **2004**, *12*, 904–912. [CrossRef] [PubMed]
43. Simchen, U.; Koebnick, C.; Hoyer, S.; Issanchou, S.; Zunft, H.J. Odour and taste sensitivity is associated with body weight and extent of misreporting of body weight. *European J. Clin. Nutr.* **2006**, *60*, 698–705. [CrossRef] [PubMed]
44. Soares, S.; Kohl, S.; Thalmann, S.; Mateus, N.; Meyerhof, W.; De Freitas, V. Different Phenolic Compounds Activate Distinct Human Bitter Taste Receptors. *J. Agric. Food Chem.* **2013**, *61*, 1525–1533. [CrossRef]
45. Roudnitzky, N.; Behrens, M.; Engel, A.; Kohl, S.; Thalmann, S.; Hübner, S.; Lossow, K.; Wooding, S.P.; Meyerhof, W. Receptor Polymorphism and Genomic Structure Interact to Shape Bitter Taste Perception. *PLoS Genet.* **2015**, *11*, e1005530. [CrossRef]
46. Hayes, J.E.; Wallace, M.R.; Knopik, V.S.; Herbstman, D.M.; Bartoshuk, L.M.; Duffy, V.B. Allelic Variation in *TAS2R* Bitter Receptor Genes Associates with Variation in Sensations from and Ingestive Behaviors toward Common Bitter Beverages in Adults. *Chem. Senses* **2010**, *36*, 311–319. [CrossRef]
47. Ferguson, J.J.A.; Veysey, M.; Lucock, M.; Niblett, S.; King, K.; MacDonald-Wicks, L.; Garg, M.L. Association between omega-3 index and blood lipids in older Australians. *J. Nutr. Biochem.* **2016**, *27*, 233–240. [CrossRef] [PubMed]
48. Lassale, C.; Guilbert, C.; Keogh, J.; Syrette, J.; Lange, K.; Cox, D.N. Estimating food intakes in Australia: Validation of the Commonwealth Scientific and Industrial Research Organisation (CSIRO) food frequency questionnaire against weighed dietary intakes. *J. Hum. Nutr. Diet. Off. J. Br. Diet. Assoc.* **2009**, *22*, 559–566. [CrossRef]
49. Ward, S.J.; Coates, A.M.; Hill, A.M. Application of an Australian Dietary Guideline Index to Weighed Food Records. *Nutrients* **2019**, *11*, 1286. [CrossRef]
50. Willett, W. *Nutritional Epidemiology*; Oxford University Press: Oxford, UK, 2012.
51. Beckett, E.L.; Martin, C.; Boyd, L.; Porter, T.; King, K.; Niblett, S.; Yates, Z.; Veysey, M.; Lucock, M. Reduced plasma homocysteine levels in elderly Australians following mandatory folic acid fortification – A comparison of two cross-sectional cohorts. *J. Nutr. Intermed. Metab.* **2017**, *8*, 14–20. [CrossRef]
52. Australian Bureau of Statistics. Australian Health Survey: Consumption of Food Groups from the Australian Dietary Guidelines. Available online: https://www.abs.gov.au/ausstats/abs@.nsf/Lookup/by%20Subject/4364.0.55.012~{}2011-12~{}Main%20Features~{}Key%20Findings~{}1 (accessed on 16 July 2020).
53. Marfell-Jones, M.; Stewart, T.O.A.; Carter, L. *International Standards for Anthropometric Assessment*; International Society for the Advancement of Kinanthropometry: Potchefstroom, South Africa, 2006.
54. Beckett, E.L.; Duesing, K.; Martin, C.; Jones, P.; Furst, J.; King, K.; Niblett, S.; Yates, Z.; Veysey, M.; Lucock, M. Relationship between methylation status of vitamin D-related genes, vitamin D levels, and methyl-donor biochemistry. *J. Nutr. Intermed. Metab.* **2016**, *6*, 8–15. [CrossRef]
55. QIAGEN. QIAamp®DNA Mini and Blood Mini Handbook. Available online: https://www.qiagen.com/au/resources/resourcedetail?id=62a200d6-faf4-469b-b50f-2b59cf738962&lang=en (accessed on 23 April 2020).
56. Thermo Fisher Scientific Inc. TaqMan®SNP Genotyping Assays USER GUIDE. Available online: https://assets.thermofisher.com/TFS-Assets/LSG/manuals/MAN0009593_TaqManSNP_UG.pdf (accessed on 23 April 2020).
57. Ferraris, C.; Turner, A.; Kaur, K.; Piper, J.; Veysey, M.; Lucock, M.; Beckett, E.L. Salt Taste Genotype, Dietary Habits and Biomarkers of Health: No Associations in an Elderly Cohort. *Nutrients* **2020**, *12*, 1056. [CrossRef] [PubMed]
58. Neveu, V.; Perez-Jiménez, J.; Vos, F.; Crespy, V.; du Chaffaut, L.; Mennen, L.; Knox, C.; Eisner, R.; Cruz, J.; Wishart, D.; et al. Phenol-Explorer: An online comprehensive database on polyphenol contents in foods. *Database* **2010**, *2010*. [CrossRef] [PubMed]
59. Kuhnle, G.G.C. Nutrition epidemiology of flavan-3-ols: The known unknowns. *Mol. Asp. Med.* **2018**, *61*, 2–11. [CrossRef]
60. Kivimaki, M.; Kuosma, E.; Ferrie, J.E.; Luukkonen, R.; Nyberg, S.T.; Alfredsson, L.; Batty, G.D.; Brunner, E.J.; Fransson, E.; Goldberg, M.; et al. Overweight, obesity, and risk of cardiometabolic multimorbidity: Pooled analysis of individual-level data for 120,813 adults from 16 cohort studies from the USA and Europe. *Lancet Public Health* **2017**, *2*, e277–e285. [CrossRef]
61. Akil, L.; Ahmad, H.A. Relationships between obesity and cardiovascular diseases in four southern states and Colorado. *J. Health Care Poor Underserved* **2011**, *22*, 61–72. [CrossRef]
62. Tirosh, A.; Shai, I.; Afek, A.; Dubnov-Raz, G.; Ayalon, N.; Gordon, B.; Derazne, E.; Tzur, D.; Shamis, A.; Vinker, S.; et al. Adolescent BMI trajectory and risk of diabetes versus coronary disease. *N. Engl. J. Med.* **2011**, *364*, 1315–1325. [CrossRef]
63. Jeon, T.-I.; Zhu, B.; Larson, J.L.; Osborne, T.F. SREBP-2 regulates gut peptide secretion through intestinal bitter taste receptor signaling in mice. *J. Clin. Investig.* **2008**, *118*, 3693–3700. [CrossRef]
64. Monica, C.; Chen, S.; Wu, V.; Joseph, R.; Reeve, J.; Rozengurt, E. Bitter stimuli induce Ca^{2+} signaling and CCK release in enteroendocrine STC-1 cells: Role of L-type voltage-sensitive Ca^{2+} channels. *Am. J. Physiol. Cell Physiol.* **2006**, *291*, C726–C739. [CrossRef]
65. Depoortere, I. Taste receptors of the gut: Emerging roles in health and disease. *Gut* **2014**, *63*, 179–190. [CrossRef]
66. Schroeter, H.; Heiss, C.; Balzer, J.; Kleinbongard, P.; Keen, C.L.; Hollenberg, N.K.; Sies, H.; Kwik-Uribe, C.; Schmitz, H.H.; Kelm, M. (−)-Epicatechin mediates beneficial effects of flavanol-rich cocoa on vascular function in humans. *Proc. Natl. Acad. Sci. USA* **2006**, *103*, 1024–1029. [CrossRef] [PubMed]
67. Kirch, N.; Berk, L.; Liegl, Y.; Adelsbach, M.; Zimmermann, B.F.; Stehle, P.; Stoffel-Wagner, B.; Ludwig, N.; Schieber, A.; Helfrich, H.-P.; et al. A nutritive dose of pure (−)-epicatechin does not beneficially affect increased cardiometabolic risk factors in overweight-to-obese adults—a randomized, placebo-controlled, double-blind crossover study. *Am. J. Clin. Nutr.* **2018**, *107*, 948–956. [CrossRef] [PubMed]

68. Beckett, E.L.; Duesing, K.; Boyd, L.; Yates, Z.; Veysey, M.; Lucock, M. A potential sex dimorphism in the relationship between bitter taste and alcohol consumption. *Food Funct.* **2017**, *8*, 1116–1123. [CrossRef]
69. Choi, J.-H.; Lee, J.; Yang, S.; Lee, E.K.; Hwangbo, Y.; Kim, J. Genetic variations in TAS2R3 and *TAS2R4* bitterness receptors modify papillary carcinoma risk and thyroid function in Korean females. *Sci. Rep.* **2018**, *8*, 15004. [CrossRef]
70. Boyce, J.M.; Shone, G.R. Effects of ageing on smell and taste. *Postgrad. Med. J.* **2006**, *82*, 239–241. [CrossRef]
71. Sergi, G.; Bano, G.; Pizzato, S.; Veronese, N.; Manzato, E. Taste loss in the elderly: Possible implications for dietary habits. *Crit. Rev. Food Sci. Nutr.* **2017**, *57*, 3684–3689. [CrossRef] [PubMed]
72. Shim, J.-S.; Oh, K.; Kim, H.C. Dietary assessment methods in epidemiologic studies. *Epidemiol. Health* **2014**, *36*, e2014009. [CrossRef] [PubMed]

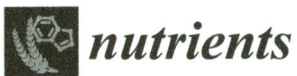

Review

Immunomodulatory Effects of Dietary Polyphenols

Hira Shakoor [1], Jack Feehan [2,3], Vasso Apostolopoulos [2], Carine Platat [1], Ayesha Salem Al Dhaheri [1], Habiba I. Ali [1], Leila Cheikh Ismail [4,5], Marijan Bosevski [6] and Lily Stojanovska [1,2,*]

[1] Department of Nutrition and Health, College of Medicine and Health Sciences, United Arab Emirates University, Al Ain 15551, United Arab Emirates; 201890012@uaeu.ac.ae (H.S.); PlatatCarine@uaeu.ac.ae (C.P.); ayesha_aldhaheri@uaeu.ac.ae (A.S.A.D.); habali@uaeu.ac.ae (H.I.A.)

[2] Institute for Health and Sport, Victoria University, Melbourne 3011, Australia; jfeehan@student.unimelb.edu.au (J.F.); vasso.apostolopoulos@vu.edu.au (V.A.)

[3] Department of Medicine-Western Health, The University of Melbourne, Melbourne 3000, Australia

[4] Clinical Nutrition and Dietetics Department, College of Health Sciences, Research Institute of Medical and Health Sciences (RIMHS), University of Sharjah, Sharjah 27272, United Arab Emirates; lcheikhismail@sharjah.ac.ae

[5] Nuffield Department of Women's & Reproductive Health, University of Oxford, Oxford OX1 2JD, UK

[6] St. Cyril and Methodius Faculty of Medicine, University Cardiology Clinic, 1000 Skopje, North Macedonia; marijanbosevski@yahoo.com

* Correspondence: lily.stojanovska@uaeu.ac.ae

Citation: Shakoor, H.; Feehan, J.; Apostolopoulos, V.; Platat, C.; Al Dhaheri, A.S.; Ali, H.I.; Ismail, L.C.; Bosevski, M.; Stojanovska, L. Immunomodulatory Effects of Dietary Polyphenols. *Nutrients* **2021**, *13*, 728. https://doi.org/10.3390/nu13030728

Academic Editor: Elena González-Burgos

Received: 29 January 2021
Accepted: 19 February 2021
Published: 25 February 2021

Publisher's Note: MDPI stays neutral with regard to jurisdictional claims in published maps and institutional affiliations.

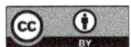

Copyright: © 2021 by the authors. Licensee MDPI, Basel, Switzerland. This article is an open access article distributed under the terms and conditions of the Creative Commons Attribution (CC BY) license (https:// creativecommons.org/licenses/by/ 4.0/).

Abstract: Functional and nutraceutical foods provide an alternative way to improve immune function to aid in the management of various diseases. Traditionally, many medicinal products have been derived from natural compounds with healing properties. With the development of research into nutraceuticals, it is becoming apparent that many of the beneficial properties of these compounds are at least partly due to the presence of polyphenols. There is evidence that dietary polyphenols can influence dendritic cells, have an immunomodulatory effect on macrophages, increase proliferation of B cells, T cells and suppress Type 1 T helper (Th1), Th2, Th17 and Th9 cells. Polyphenols reduce inflammation by suppressing the pro-inflammatory cytokines in inflammatory bowel disease by inducing Treg cells in the intestine, inhibition of tumor necrosis factor-alpha (TNF-α) and induction of apoptosis, decreasing DNA damage. Polyphenols have a potential role in prevention/treatment of auto-immune diseases like type 1 diabetes, rheumatoid arthritis and multiple sclerosis by regulating signaling pathways, suppressing inflammation and limiting demyelination. In addition, polyphenols cause immunomodulatory effects against allergic reaction and autoimmune disease by inhibition of autoimmune T cell proliferation and downregulation of pro-inflammatory cytokines (interleukin-6 (IL-6), IL-1, interferon-γ (IFN-γ)). Herein, we summarize the immunomodulatory effects of polyphenols and the underlying mechanisms involved in the stimulation of immune responses.

Keywords: polyphenols; immunomodulation; pro-inflammatory cytokines; anti-inflammatory cytokines

1. Introduction

With advancing knowledge of the importance of adequate nutrition, and increased public health awareness about diet, there is growing attention on the health benefits of natural products including those that are rich in polyphenols. Polyphenols are the most extensive group of non-energetic secondary metabolites and are produced by plants in response to stress [1] (Figure 1). Polyphenols have been called 'lifespan essentials' due to their significant impact on health [2]. There are as many as 8000 different polyphenols which are divided into different classes based on their chemical structure. Despite the different classifications, all polyphenols have the key structural features of an aromatic ring and at least one hydroxyl group [3,4]. Dietary polyphenols are abundant in plant-based foods such as fruits, vegetables, dry legumes, cereals, olives, cocoa, tea, coffee and wine [5].

Some common dietary polyphenols include the lignins present in nuts and whole-grain cereals; pro-anthocyanidins in grapes, pine bark and cocoa; anthocyanins/anthocyanidins in brightly colored fruits and vegetables like berries; isoflavones in soybeans; catechins in green tea, grapes and wine; tannins in tea and nuts; quercetin in grapes and onion; resveratrol in wines and naringenin/hesperidin in citrus fruits [6].

Research into the beneficial health effects of polyphenols has increased considerably over the last two decades [7]. Polyphenols have shown anti-inflammatory, antimicrobial, antioxidant, anticarcinogenic, antiadipogenic, antidiabetic and neuroprotective effects [8–12]. Polyphenols may also counteract cytotoxicity and apoptosis due to their immunomodulatory properties [13] and regulate innate and adaptive immunity. Polyphenols have also been shown to reduce oxidative stress and inflammation [14], modulate immune cells, regulate gut microbiota composition and immunity (Figure 1). Through this regulation of the immune system, polyphenols could beneficially impact a number of chronic diseases [15]. Herein, we discuss the immunomodulatory effect of polyphenols and the resulting effects on different chronic diseases, including inflammatory bowel disease, atopic eczema or dermatitis, allergic asthma, rhinitis, type 1 diabetes, multiple sclerosis and rheumatoid arthritis.

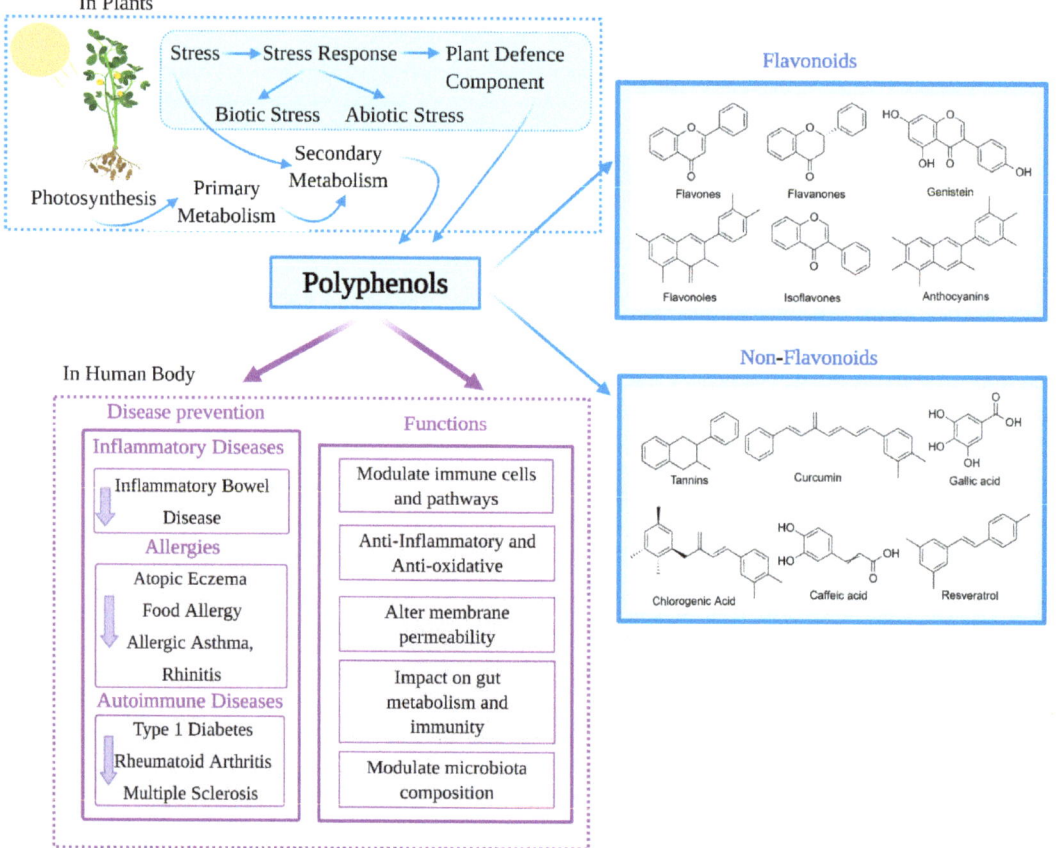

Figure 1. Classification and health benefits of polyphenols.

2. Methods

Extraction of current and relevant data was performed using the electronic databases, Science Direct, PubMed, Springer and Google Scholar. Searches were conducted in two sections. The first part aimed to identify evidence on the effect of polyphenols on the immune system and immune cells. Search terms used were 'Polyphenols' OR 'Phytochemicals' OR 'Phenolic' AND 'Immunity' OR 'Immune system' OR 'Immune function' AND 'Immune cells' OR 'Dendritic cells' OR 'Macrophages' OR 'Monocytes' OR 'Neutrophils' OR 'Natural Killer cells' OR 'B cells' OR 'T cells' OR 'T helper cells. The second part aimed to identify evidence on the impact of polyphenols in chronic inflammatory and auto-immune diseases. Additional search terms included 'Inflammatory diseases' OR 'Inflammatory Bowel Disease' AND 'Allergy' OR 'Atopic Eczema' OR 'Dermatitis' OR 'Food Allergy' OR 'Rhinitis' OR 'Asthma' AND 'Autoimmune Disease' OR 'Type-1 diabetes' OR 'Rheumatoid arthritis' OR 'Multiple sclerosis'. Articles published in English were included. The titles and abstracts were scanned to exclude any irrelevant studies. A total of 167 papers that focused only on the immunomodulatory effect of polyphenols on health were screened and articles containing relevant data were reviewed.

3. Immune Modulation of Polyphenols to Immune Cells

The immune system as a whole consists of innate and adaptive immunity, each with different roles and functions [16]. The innate immune system is the first line of defense, and protects against foreign antigens through the skin, pulmonary system, and gut epithelial cells, forming a barrier between the organism and its environment [17]. The innate system is broadly divided into cellular and non-cellular systems. The cellular system consists of several cell subsets, including dendritic cells (DCs), monocytes, macrophages, granulocytes and natural killer (NK) cells. The non-cellular system is very diverse, ranging from simple mucus barriers to complex protein pathways, such as the complement cascade, however all function to prevent pathogen entry, and facilitate pathogen destruction by phagocytosis [18]. The adaptive immune system comprises T and B cells. B cells secrete antibodies, whilst T cells are involved in the production of cytokines, direct cytotoxic destruction of infected or malignant tissue, and activation of other immune cells [16]. Polyphenols modulate immune responses in both the innate and adaptive systems, having both stimulatory and inhibitory effects in different areas [19] (Figure 2).

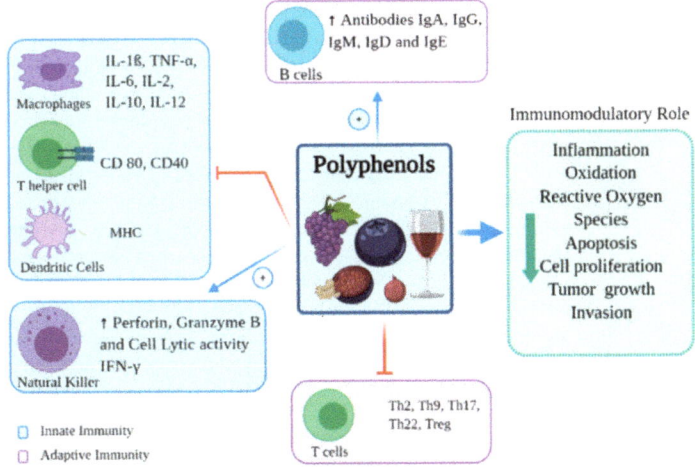

Figure 2. Immunomodulatory effects of polyphenols on immune cells.

3.1. Effects of Polyphenols on Dendritic Cells

DCs are the most potent antigen-presenting cells which act to prime the adaptive immune system to recognize foreign antigens, and so are vital in the initiation and regulation of the adaptive immune response [20]. It has been shown that polyphenols can influence the differentiation of DCs [21]. In fact, resveratrol has been identified as affecting human DC differentiation from monocytes, with a strong potential for regulatory action [22]. Likewise, epigallocatechin gallate (EGCG) induces apoptosis and affects the phenotype of developing DCs. Molecules that are essential for antigen presentation by DCs such as CD83, CD80, CD11c, and major histocompatibility complex (MHC) class II, are downregulated by EGCG, suggesting an immunosuppressive action [23]. Other polyphenols, including EGCG, curcumin, quercetin, apigenin, silibinin, and blackberry polyphenols cause inhibition of murine bone marrow-derived DC maturation and expression of MHC molecules, reducing antigen uptake and decreasing secretion of the pro-inflammatory cytokines interleukin-1 (IL-1), IL-2, IL-6, IL-12 [24–27]. A study in an animal model showed that administration of fisetin (50 mg/kg) decreased DC migration and DC allo-stimulatory capacity [28]. Similarly, in vitro resveratrol has an inhibitory effect on DC maturation [29].

3.2. Effects of Polyphenols on Monocytes and Macrophages

Macrophages are phagocytes that ingest pathogens and dead cells, which differentiate from the transitory monocyte. Like DCs, macrophages can also function as antigen-presenting cells (albeit with less potent activity) being able to activate naïve T cells into effector T cells in the presence of an antigen [19]. Macrophages play an important role in inflammation, host defense, and tissue repair [30,31]. Importantly, macrophages also play a pathogenic role in various chronic diseases including asthma, inflammatory bowel disease, atherosclerosis and rheumatoid arthritis [31–33]. Macrophages are classically considered in two categories, known as polarization: the classical inflammatory M1 and immunosuppressive/anabolic M2 phenotypes. Initiation of M1 differentiation is by interferon-γ (IFN-γ) stimulation and the activation of toll-like receptors (TLRs) by bacterial lipopolysaccharides (LPS); while M2 polarization is triggered by IL-4 [34]. It has been shown that polyphenolic cocoa extract suppressed M1 mediated inflammation and drove M2 polarization of activated macrophages [35]. Polyphenol-rich green tea has anti-tumor effects secondary to the activation of macrophages and NK cells [36]. Inonotus sanghuang, a plant known for its medicinal value, rich in rutin, quercetin, quercitrin, isorhamnetin and chlorogenic acid, has been shown to reduce inflammation by modulating the interaction between macrophages and adipocytes. It was suggested that in this way it may improve insulin resistance and metabolic syndrome [37]. Moreover, Overman et al. reported that grape powder extract decreased LPS-stimulated inflammation in macrophages and reduce insulin resistance [38].

Monocytes and macrophages play a fundamental role in the progression of atherosclerosis [35]. Increased oxidative stress causes low-density lipoprotein oxidation (oxLDL), with the resulting lipoproteins engulfed by macrophages resulting in the formation of foam cells. This process triggers an inflammatory response in the neighboring endothelial cells which secrete pro-inflammatory cytokines and chemokines [39–41]. When monocytes migrate towards the intima, they transform into macrophages on stimulation by macrophage colony-stimulating factor, increasing the expression of scavenger receptors outside the cell [39,40]. Polyphenols are known to regulate this interplay between immune and vascular endothelial function. Evidence has shown that polyphenols reduce atherosclerotic progression by increasing high-density lipoprotein (HDL) levels and decrease LDL accumulation in macrophages, reducing foam cell formation [3,42].

3.3. Effects of Polyphenols on Natural Killer Cells

NK cells are a subset of lymphocytes, but are part of the innate immune response, with the function of eliminating infected or malignant cells [19]. NK cells have a strong cytolytic function and a considerable role in immune regulation [43]. NK cells are activated by CD4+ T cell secretion of IL-2 and IFN-γ [44]. Once activated NK cells secrete perforin and granzyme B, which induce apoptosis and necrosis in target cells. Polyphenols have immunomodulatory effects on NK cells, increasing their number and activity. Green tea catechin metabolites increase NK cell cytotoxicity [45] and quercetin enhances NK cell lytic activity [46] in animal models. In a clinical trial, healthy participant prescribed a diet low in polyphenols and supplemented with juices rich in polyphenols increased lymphocyte proliferative responsiveness, IL-2 secretion and lytic activity by NK cells [47]. Berries rich in flavonoids and pro-anthocyanidins have a cancer-preventive effect but are also involved in the modulation of NK cells [48]. A study in marathon runners noted that daily consumption of 250 g of blueberries for six weeks resulted in doubled NK cell counts [49]. Evidence showed that purple sweet potato leaves that are rich in flavonoids enhanced the lytic activity of NK cells in 16 healthy participants [50].

3.4. Effects of Polyphenols on T and B Cells

T and B cells are the principal components of the adaptive immune system. B cells secrete antibodies known as immunoglobulins (Igs), which bind to antigens and underpin hypersensitivity reactions and antimicrobial immune responses. When B cells are activated to a specific antigen, they differentiate into plasma cells and produce Immunoglobulin (Ig)A, IgG, IgM, IgD and IgE [19]. Polyphenols have been suggested to modulate the function of B cells; however, this has been poorly described, and further research is required. In an in vitro study it was noted that green tea polyphenols and EGCG decreased the production of IgE in a dose and time-dependent manner [51], and another study showed that polyphenols inhibit the proliferation of CD19+ cells and reduce IgG production [52]. It was noted that administration of green tea extract to mice for 6 weeks reduced the production antigen-specific IgE by enhancing CD4+ CD25+ regulatory T cells (Treg) in the spleen, resulting in reduction of allergic response [53].

T cells are divided into three major types: cytotoxic T cells, T helper (Th) cells and the Treg cells depending upon expression of the CD4 or CD8 molecules. CD4+ T cells are helper T cells that assist and control immune cell activity and activation. CD8+ cytotoxic T cells act to directly lyse and destroy malignant, senescent or infected cells [19]. Polyphenols have been associated with the modulation of enzymatic signaling, via the inhibition of the serine-threonine and tyrosine-protein kinase pathways. These enzymes are primarily linked with B cell activation and T cell proliferation as well as the production of cytokines by activated monocytes [3]. Treg play a crucial role in immunity tolerance and control of auto-immunity [54]. A study on mice showed that regular treatment of EGCG for a week increased the frequency of Treg cells in the spleen, pancreatic lymph nodes and mesenteric lymph nodes. The Treg cells obtained from the treated group could suppress cytotoxic T cell function, reducing proliferation and IFN-γ production [54]. In addition, EGC-M5 (a major metabolite of EGCG) at a dosage of 10 mg/kg of body weight were provided to rats for 14 days and caused upregulation of CD4+ T cell activity and cytotoxic activity of NK cells [45].

3.5. Effects of Polyphenols on T Cell Differentiation

CD4+ T helper cells differentiate into T helper (Th)1, Th2, Th9, Th17, Th22, depending upon the cytokine environment [55]. Th1 cells are involved in cell-mediated immunity and are produced in the presence of IL-12, whilst Th2 cells are critical for humoral immunity and differentiate in the presence of IL-4 and IL-13 [56]. Th17 cells secrete IL-17, IL-22, and chemokine ligands 20 (CCL20) [57] and have been shown to have a role in the progression and pathogenesis of chronic inflammatory diseases like rheumatoid arthritis, multiple sclerosis, psoriasis, atopic dermatitis, and asthma [56,58]. Th22 cells produce IL-22, a cytokine responsible for maintaining the epithelial barrier and skin integrity [57]. In mice, polyphenols like apigenin and chrysin suppresses serum IgE induced by ovalbumin immunization by downregulating Th2 responses [59]. Similarly, tea polyphenols, such as EGCG, reduce Th1 differentiation and numbers of Th17 and Th9 cells [60], as well as resveratrol by decreasing Th17 cell numbers in an inflammatory arthritis model in rodents [61]. Grape seed pro-anthocyanidin extract also showed anti-arthritic properties and upregulated the number of Tregs and maintained the balance between Th17/Treg, attenuating inflammation [62].

3.6. Effects of Polyphenols in Inflammation

The inflammatory response of the innate immune system is a vital part of the defense against microbial infection. However despite its vital role in promoting the immune response, its timely resolution is equally important [63]. Chronic inflammation is a key cause of a number of life-threatening diseases [64]. A study on pomegranate peel polyphenols (PPPs) and its specific components such as punicalagin (PC) and ellagic acid (EA) showed a reduction in pro-inflammatory cytokines TNF-α, IL-1β and IL-6 and downregulation other inflammatory mediators including nitric oxide (NO) and prostaglandin E2 (PGE$_2$) by decreasing inducible nitric oxide synthase (iNOS) and cyclooxygenase-2 (COX-2) expression [65]. Similarly, PPPs, PC, and EA have shown inhibitory effects on LPS-induced production of intracellular reactive oxygen species (ROS) and suppression of TLR4 at both the mRNA and protein levels, all of which have major mechanistic roles in inflammation [66]. In addition, grape seed extract, has been shown to decrease pro-inflammatory cytokine, ROS and superoxide production whilst elevating antioxidant enzyme gene expression and secretion of anti-inflammatory mediators [67,68]. Green tea polyphenols also reduce the production of inflammatory cytokines (TNF-α, IL-6, IL-1β), and inhibit the TLR4 signaling pathway [69]. The immunomodulatory effects of polyphenols are summarized in Table 1.

Table 1. The immunomodulatory effects of polyphenols.

Polyphenols	Signaling Pathways	Immunomodulatory Responses
Curcumin [70,71]	Suppress NF-κB	↓ Bcl-2 in PHA-activated Tcells Suppress maturation of DCs Inhibit IL-12, IL-8 ↑ IL-4
Resveratrol, Quercetin, Silibinin [72]	Altering PI3K/Akt	↓IL-6 and IL-1
Genistein [71,73]	Activate AMPK Inhibit ROS/Akt/NF-κB	↓ IL-1β, IL-6, IL-8 ↓COX-2
EGCG [74]	Suppress NF-κB and MAPK	Inhibit Th1 and Th17 differentiation ↓ Transcription factors (STAT1 and T-bet for Th1, and STAT3 and RORγt for Th17) ↑ T-reg in lymphoid tissues and central nervous system
Proanthocyanidins Procyanidins [75,76]	Suppress NF-κB and MAPK	↓TNF-α, IL-1β Inhibit iNOS and COX-2
Caffeic acid [77–79]	Suppress p38 MAPK, JNK1/2 and NF-κB	↓ IL-1β, IL-6, TNF-α ↓ Monocyte chemoattractant protein (MCP)-1 Inhibit xanthine oxidase and COX

PHA: Phytohemagglutinin, DC: Dendritic cell, IL: Interleukin, COX: Cyclooxygenase, Th: T helper, STAT: Signal transducer and activator of transcription, NF-κB: Nuclear factor kappa-B, ROS: Reactive oxygen species, TNF-α: Tumor necrosis factor-alpha, MCP: Monocyte chemoattractant protein, iNOS: Inducible nitric oxide synthase, PI3K/Akt: Phosphatidylinositol 3-kinase/protein kinase B, AMPK: Adenosine monophosphate-activated protein kinase, MAPK: Mitogen-Activated Protein Kinase.

4. Immune Modulation of Polyphenols to Prevent and Control Chronic Diseases

Dietary polyphenols have preventive and therapeutic potential for a number of chronic diseases whose development involves dysregulation of the immune function.

4.1. Polyphenols and Inflammatory Bowel Disease

The intestinal epithelium is generally in a state of low-grade inflammation, due to microbial, chemical and mechanical stimuli that maintain a moderate inflammatory response [80]. Generally, it is controllable, but if inflammation exceeds the normal limit due to disease, it can disrupt epithelial tissues and impede intestinal dysfunction. These uncontrollable inflammatory conditions are known collectively as inflammatory bowel disease (IBD), comprised of two specific pathologies; Crohn's disease and ulcerative colitis [81]. Globally, the annual incidence of IBD is approximately 396 cases per 100,000 persons per year [82]. There is evidence to suggest polyphenol supplementation could play a role in managing IBD. The proposed mechanism by which this occurs is through polyphenol modulation of pattern recognition receptors (PRRs), such as the TLRs and nucleotide-binding oligomerization domain proteins, which are highly expressed in intestinal epithelial and immune cells. PRRs activate immune responses against pathogens through recognition of related molecular structures [83], and polyphenols are known to be able to modulate the expression of PRRs and their associated inflammatory response in the intestine [80]. Activation of PRRs induces inflammation by increasing cytokine secretion and cyclooxygenase-2 expression. Polyphenols like curcumin and isothiocyanate inhibit TLR4 dimerization, an essential step for TLR4 activation [84,85]. Resveratrol also interferes with TLR4 signal transduction by inhibiting TANK binding kinase 1 which regulates the downstream pathways that result in cytokine production [86]. In addition, resveratrol acts as anti-inflammatory agent in intestinal mucosa [87]. Polyphenols are also known to modulate key inflammatory genes, such as cyclooxygenase-2 and the inflammatory cytokines, further implying potential for an anti-inflammatory effect in IBD [88,89]. It has also been shown that flavonoids are able to regulate the activity of Treg cells in the intestine, downregulating the expression of inflammatory cytokines, and consequently suppressing inflammation [90,91]. Polyphenols are also able to influence the gut microbiota as a probiotic. Green tea polyphenols promote the growth of beneficial microbiota like *Bifidobacterium* and *Lactobacillus* and suppress pathogenic bacteria, such as, *E Coli* and *Salmonella* [12,92]. This supports the maintenance of intestinal homeostasis and reduces inflammation [93]. Grape seed and green tea polyphenols also have potential to prevent or delay the progression of IBD [68,94,95]. Pomegranate polyphenols also provide protective effects against IBD by modulating the intestinal inflammatory response reducing expression of various pro-inflammatory cytokines, such as iNOS, COX-2, PGE2, as well as regulating the composition of the luminal microbiota [96]. A recent study reported that dietary polyphenols from mango (gallotannins and gallic acid) improved the symptoms of IBD. This study included 10 subjects who received 200–400 g/day of mango pulp for 8 weeks. A significant reduction was observed in a factors related to neutrophil-induced inflammation like IL-8, growth-regulated oncogene and granulocyte macrophage colony-stimulating factor by 16.2%, 25.0% and 28.6%, respectively [97]. Another study showed that Bronze tomatoes, which are rich in anthocyanins, flavonols, and stilbenoids, had a significant impact in alleviating the symptoms of IBD in mice [98]. Taken together, this suggests that polyphenols can help in the prevention and treatment of IBD by reducing pro-inflammatory cytokines, regulating the activity of Treg cells and promoting the growth of beneficial microbiota in the intestine.

4.2. Polyphenols and Allergies

The prevalence of allergic disorders has been increasing dramatically with competing environmental, genetic, diet and hygiene factors likely to underlie their advance [99,100]. Allergic reactions result from a hyper-reaction of the immune response against allergens such as those in the environment (dust, grass pollen) or food (milk, fish, eggs, nuts and wheat) [101]. Due to their growing incidence, there is significant attention on interventions to assist in their management, and polyphenols have been proposed as viable solutions [101] (Table 2). Certain polyphenols influence allergic responses at two critical stages: (1) allergic sensitization and (2) re-exposure to the allergen. During the sensitization phase, polyphenols such as caffeic and ferulic acid bind with allergenic proteins, forming insoluble complexes and rendering them non-reactive [101]. Additionally, flavonoids directly affect antigen presentation by DCs by either inhibiting cell surface expression of MHC-II and co-stimulatory molecules (CD80, CD86), leading to ineffective antigen presentation, or by inhibiting cytokine production [102,103]. Polyphenols like catechins and their derivatives inhibit Th2 cytokine production [104,105] as well as T cell activation and proliferation [106,107]. Recruitment of B cells to sites of allergic inflammation and their production of IgE have also been shown to be inhibited by polyphenols [59,108,109]. Of interest, the interaction between polyphenols and proteins results in the modulation of allergic sensitization and their direct effect on mast cells hence inhibiting the release of allergic mediators and eventually decreasing the symptoms of allergy [101]. In addition, polyphenols such as caffeic, ferulic, and chlorogenic acids can bind irreversibly with the peanut allergens, Ara h1 and Ara h2, reducing their allergenicity [110]. In mice, administration of polyphenol-enriched areca nut extracts suppressed the level of ovalbumin (OVA)-specific IgE, the expression of IL-4, downregulating Th2 driven immunity and enhancing the activity of myeloid-derived suppressor cells, attenuating allergic responses [111]. In another study, 30 female mice treated with cranberry and blueberry polyphenol complexed peanut protein for 6 weeks, had reduced expression of CD63 and decreased plasma IgE levels [112]. Evidence has also shown that polyphenol-rich cranberry extracts interact with wheat gliadins forming insoluble complexes in a mouse model, which decreased wheat gliadin immunogenicity and allergenicity [113]. Furthermore, polyphenolic ellagic acid effectively binds with allergenic proteins within the food matrix [114,115]. Punicalagin (a polyphenol derived from pomegranate), rutin and phloridzin increased the growth of beneficial bacteria species such as *Bifidobacterium* and *Lactobacillus* which are known to have beneficial impacts in food allergies [116,117]. Oral administration of a polyphenol-rich grape skin extract that had been fermented with *Lactobacillus Plantarum* had an inhibitory effect on allergic responses when compared to a non-fermented extract [118].

Table 2. Effect of dietary polyphenols on allergic reaction.

Dietary Polyphenols	Treatment and Duration	Results
Atopic Eczema or Dermatitis		
Quercetin (pure isolated polyphenols)	15 human subjects with contact dermatitis. Quercetin applied topically for five days	No change as compared to the control [119]
Cocoa flavanols (catechin, epicatechin, procyanidins) at a lower dose of 27 mg or a higher dose of 329 mg	Ten healthy women consumed a low and high dose.	The higher dose of cocoa drink reduced water loss and improved the blood circulation in the skin [120]
Water extract of whey powder dodder rich in quercetin	Randomized control trial (RCT) study recruited 52 subjects atopic dermatitis recruited for 30 days	Quercetin reduces allergy and inhibits the secretion of the mast cell. Elevate skin moisture and elasticity [121]
Apple condensed tannins (ACT) at a dose of 10 mg/kg	Apple polyphenols were investigated in subjects with atopic eczema for 8 weeks.	Reduced inflammation and itching in disease subjects compared with the control group. ACT has an anti-allergic effect [122]
Food Allergy		
Polyphenol enriched extracts or purified epicatechin (1, 0.3 and 0.01%)	Female BALB/c mice treated with polyphenols for 8 days	Epicatechin exhibited a significant anti-allergic effect [123]
Polyphenol-enriched apple extract (>40%)	BALB/c mice treated with an apple extract for 7 weeks	Reduce allergenicity by protein–polyphenol interaction, decrease intestinal mast cell protease and pro-inflammatory genes, diminished cytokine secretion. [105]
Cocoa diet with 0.2% polyphenols	Rats received either a cocoa diet or a standard diet for 4 weeks	Cocoa diet decreased total serum immunoglobulin (Ig)E, Tumor necrosis factor (TNF)-α and interleukin (IL)-10 secretion. No effect on IL-4 synthesis [124]

Table 2. Cont.

Dietary Polyphenols	Treatment and Duration	Results
Asthma and Rhinitis		
Drinks containing apple polyphenols at low and high dose (50 mg and 100 mg)	33 subjects having moderate or severe persistent allergic rhinitis treated with apple polyphenols for 4 weeks	Improve sneezing attacks nasal discharger and swelling of the nasal turbinate in the low-dose group and high dose group [125]
100 mg pycnogenol mixture of water-soluble bioflavonoids	76 patients with asthma	Decrease by 15.2% of the specific IgE, whereas IgG1 and IgG4 remained unchanged. Reduced the need for medication [126]
500 mg/day Apple condensed tannins (ACT) and polyphenols	A double-blind comparative study on 36 subjects with rhinitis for 12 weeks	Significant improvement in sneezing scores and nasal discharge inhibited in perennial rhinitis due in the group taking polyphenols treatment [127]

4.3. Polyphenols in Atopic Eczema or Dermatitis

Atopic eczema and dermatitis are allergic skin disorders that primarily occur during early infanthood (3–4 months of age) and continue to develop until 2 years of age [128]. They cause dryness of skin, itching, inflammation and erythema (redness). Polyphenols have anti-inflammatory properties that can alleviate this allergic inflammation. Green tea extracts (catechins, epicatechin, epigallocatechin gallate and their derivatives) protect against cutaneous inflammation [129]. Similarly, EGCG suppresses the secretion of the pro-inflammatory cytokine IL-2 in vitro, an important mediator in allergic dermatological conditions [130]. Polyphenols have also been shown to improve the characteristic itching and pruritis associated with these conditions. Oat-derived polyphenol avenanthramide was shown to reduce the characteristics of pruritis and itching associated with dermatological conditions [131]. The effect of polyphenols on keratinocytes and immune cells was also analyzed in vitro and shown to reduce nuclear factor κB (NF-κB) activation, TNF-α and IL-8 [132]. Likewise, quercetin and luteolin also inhibit skin itching and flush reaction [133]. By suppressing pro-inflammatory cytokines, polyphenols can reduce the symptoms and occurrence of allergic skin disorders.

4.4. Polyphenols in Allergic Asthma and Rhinitis

Asthma, an allergic inflammatory lung disease characterized by increased leukocyte infiltration into the airways, most notably granulocytes, resulting in decreased respiratory function. Often the inflammation can cause bronchoconstriction, airway hyperresponsiveness (AHR) and increased mucus production [134]. In the airways, exposure to an allergen such as pollen produces a Th2-dominated response by recruiting and activating inflammatory cells and upregulating IL-4, IL-13, and IL-5 [135]. In an animal model of asthma, it was shown that resveratrol had a suppressive effect on asthmatic parameters as it inhibited the production of Th-2 cytokines like IL-4 and IL-5 in the plasma and bronchoalveolar lavage fluid, and caused suppression of airway hyperresponsiveness, eosinophilia, and hypersecretion of mucus [136]. Moreover, quercetin is known to ameliorate the pathogenic process of asthma by decreasing IL-4 and IFN-γ synthesis and by regulating Th1/Th2 balance [137]. Recent evidence showed that the administration of polyphenol-rich ethanolic extract of *Boehmeria nivea* (caffeic acid, catechin, epicatechin, β-sissterol, rutin, luteolin-7-glucoside, naringin, hesperidin, chlorogenic acid, and tangeretin) reduces allergic response in mice by suppressing mast cell mediated inflammation, decreasing TNF-α, IL-1β, IL-6, Th2, extracellular-signal-regulated kinase (ERK) and Mitogen-Activated Protein Kinase (MAPK) expression [138]. In murine asthma models, it was found that sesamin (rich in flavonoids) reduced allergic inflammation induce by asthma and airway hyperresponsiveness (AHR), making them an effective adjunct for the treatment of asthma [139].

5. Immune Modulation of Polyphenols in Autoimmunity

The immune system protects against foreign substances, but it is also responsible for self-tolerance, by which host tissues are protected from immunological action. Dysfunction can lead to loss of this immune tolerance and disturbed homeostasis, resulting in autoimmune disease [140]. The prevalence of autoimmune diseases is about 5%, and approximately 80 types of autoimmune diseases have been described [141]. Several factors lead to the development of autoimmune diseases, including genetic, epigenetic, environmental, nutritional and microbiotic diseases. Polyphenols have been shown to have a beneficial role in some common autoimmune diseases.

5.1. Polyphenols and Type-1 Diabetes

Type-1 diabetes is a multifactorial disease linked to a combination of genetic and environmental factors. It is characterized by the autoimmune destruction of pancreatic β cells, resulting in severe insulin deficiency and resultant hyperglycemia [142]. Polyphenols help in the regulation of pancreatic β-cells, type-1 diabetes and complications associated with type-1 diabetes [143]. Polyphenols involved in activation of the phosphatidylinositol 3-kinase/protein kinase B (PI3K/Akt) signaling pathway, thus helping to reduce the progression of type-1 diabetes [140]. It was shown that pomegranate peel extract inhibited immune cell infiltration into pancreatic islets and interferes with IL-17 and IFN-γ synthesis in gut-associated lymphoid tissue in type-1 diabetes [144]. A study in mice with type-1 diabetes quercetin treatment modulated Th1/Th2 balance and had glucose-lowering potential [145]. In addition, butein (a plant polyphenol) was able to prevent cytokine-induced β-cell damage by inhibiting NO production, iNOS expression, NF-κB translocation and glucose-stimulated insulin secretion which, prevented the progression of type-1 diabetes in rats [146]. Similarly, *Broussonetia kazinoki* polyphenols have been shown to have therapeutic potential in the prevention of cytokine-induced β-cell damage and reduce/delay the extent of pancreatic β-cell damage in type-1 diabetes [147]. Consequently, polyphenols may play a role in modulating key signaling pathways, T helper cell response and reducing cytokine induced β-cell damage, which may aid in the management of type-1 diabetes.

5.2. Polyphenols and Rheumatoid Arthritis

Rheumatoid arthritis, is a systemic autoimmune disease, characterized by erosive and symmetric synovitis, particularly in the peripheral joints. Degradation of cartilage and bone erosion leads to the eventual destruction of a joint [148]. In developed countries, rheumatoid arthritis affects about 0.5–1% of the population and women are at three times greater risk [149]. While the reason for the development of this disease is still unknown, genetics is thought to play an important role. Polyphenols may also have an impact in the management of rheumatoid arthritis. For instance, curcumin, a potent anti-inflammatory agent, decreases IL-1β, induces IL-6 and vascular endothelial growth factor by rheumatoid arthritis-fibroblast-like synoviocytes [150]. In addition, curcumin also induces apoptosis of rheumatoid arthritis-fibroblast-like synoviocytes, which are typically resistant to apoptotic signaling, by upregulating pro-apoptotic proteins, such as Bax, and downregulating the anti-apoptotic protein Bcl-2 [151]. In addition, resveratrol has both protective and therapeutic effects in inflammatory arthritis, by inhibiting the function of Th-17, B-cells and MAPK signaling pathways [61,152]. A clinical trial reported that a 1 g capsule of resveratrol for 3 months decreased the swelling and tenderness of joints by regulating pro-inflammatory cytokines [153]. Moreover, EGCG suppresses osteoclast differentiation and decreases clinical symptoms in an animal model of rheumatoid arthritis [154]. Grape polyphenols have shown immuno-regulatory effects, establishing a balance between Th17 and Treg cells and inhibiting TNFα in rheumatoid arthritis, hence mitigating inflammation, oxidative stress and rheumatoid arthritis associated symptoms [155–157]. Administration of extra virgin olive oil polyphenol extract (100 and 200 mg/kg body weight) to arthritic mice decreased the pro-inflammatory cytokines, PGE2, COX-2, and microsomal prostaglandin E synthase-1 as well as NF-κB translocation, resulting in decreased progression of the joint disease [158].

Evidence showed that quercetin supplements (500 mg/day) for 8 weeks resulted in a significant reduction of morning stiffness, morning pain, and after-activity pain [159]. Therefore, polyphenols may improve the quality of life of patients with rheumatoid arthritis.

5.3. Polyphenols and Multiple Sclerosis

Multiple sclerosis, is a chronic neurological autoimmune disorder characterized by the breakdown of the myelin sheath, alongside dysfunction of the blood–brain barrier, perivascular inflammation, as well as damaged axons and oligodendrocytes-all of which lead to progressive nervous system damage and clinical disability [140]. Polyphenols may play a role in the prevention and treatment of multiple sclerosis [160]. Quercetin exerts an immunomodulatory effect aiding in the treatment of multiple sclerosis by inhibiting proliferation of autoimmune T-cells, and the expression of TNF-α by mononuclear cells in vitro [161,162]. It has also been shown to reduce peripheral blood mononuclear cell proliferation [163]. The polyphenolic flavones apigenin and luteolin have a robust inhibitory potential on T-cell proliferation while also reducing IFN-γ production [162]. Strikingly, flavonoids have been shown to limit demyelination in multiple sclerosis and so may confer neuroprotective benefits [164]. In a mouse model, resveratrol prevented neuronal loss, and delayed the onset of autoimmune encephalomyelitis suggesting that resveratrol could play an immunomodulatory role in managing multiple sclerosis [165]. Similarly, administration of resveratrol (250 mg/kg/day) for 3 weeks showed therapeutic potential as an adjunct in the treatment of multiple sclerosis by improving motor coordination and balance, mitochondrial function, reducing oxidative stress, and inhibiting NF-κB signaling [166]. In a study of 66 patients with multiple sclerosis who were treated with grape seed capsules for one month it was found that the capsules positively impacted physical and mental functioning, improving quality of life [167]. Given this, polyphenols may have therapeutic potential as an adjunct treatment in multiple sclerosis patients.

6. Conclusions

Polyphenols are promising candidates for novel adjunct therapeutic approaches. They can modulate multiple immune system processes and reduce the burden of various diseases such as IBD, allergies and autoimmune disorders. In addition to their demonstrated antioxidant qualities, polyphenols have broad health-promoting effects, due to their ability to modulate inflammation and immune responses. They improve the interplay between immune cells and decrease expression of pro-inflammatory cytokines. Further research is required to clinically validate the therapeutic potential of polyphenols on immunomodulation as well as to explore their interaction with gut microbiota.

Author Contributions: Conceptualization, L.S. and C.P.; formal analysis, H.S.; investigation, H.S.; writing—original draft preparation, H.S. and J.F.; writing—review and editing, J.F., V.A., H.I.A., A.S.A.D., L.C.I., M.B. and L.S.; visualization, H.S.; supervision, L.S. and C.P.; All authors have read and agreed to the published version of the manuscript.

Funding: This research received no external funding.

Data Availability Statement: Not applicable.

Acknowledgments: H.S., L.S., H.I.A, A.S.A.D. and C.P. would like to acknowledge the Department of Nutrition and Health, United Arab Emirates University for their ongoing support. L.C. thanks the College of Heatlh Sciences and RIMHS University of Sharjah for their support and M.B. acknowledges the St. Ciril and Methodius Faculty of Medicine University of Cardiology clinic for their research support. J.F. would like to acknowledge the Australian Government for the support for an RTP training scholarship and the University of Melbourne Stipend. J.F. and V.A. would like to thank the Immunology and Translational Research Group within the Institute for Health and Sport, Victoria University Australia, for their support.

Conflicts of Interest: The authors declare no conflict of interest.

References

1. Swallah, M.S.; Sun, H.; Affoh, R.; Fu, H.; Yu, H. Antioxidant potential overviews of secondary metabolites (polyphenols) in fruits. *Int. J. Food Sci.* **2020**, *2020*, 9081686.
2. Chandrasekara, A.; Shahidi, F. Content of insoluble bound phenolics in millets and their contribution to antioxidant capacity. *J. Agric. Food Chem.* **2010**, *58*, 6706–6714.
3. Santhakumar, A.B.; Battino, M.; Alvarez-Suarez, J.M. Dietary polyphenols: Structures, bioavailability and protective effects against atherosclerosis. *Food Chem. Toxicol.* **2018**, *113*, 49–65.
4. Yamagata, K.; Tagami, M.; Yamori, Y. Dietary polyphenols regulate endothelial function and prevent cardiovascular disease. *Nutrition* **2015**, *31*, 28–37.
5. Cardona, F.; Andrés-Lacueva, C.; Tulipani, S.; Tinahones, F.J.; Queipo-Ortuño, M.I. Benefits of polyphenols on gut microbiota and implications in human health. *J. Nutr. Biochem.* **2013**, *24*, 1415–1422.
6. Martin, K.R.; Appel, C.L. Polyphenols as dietary supplements: A double-edged sword. *Nutr. Diet. Suppl.* **2009**, *2*, 1–12.
7. Quiñones, M.; Miguel, M.; Aleixandre, A. Beneficial effects of polyphenols on cardiovascular disease. *Pharmacol. Res.* **2013**, *68*, 125–131.
8. Cassidy, A.; O'Reilly, É.J.; Kay, C.; Sampson, L.; Franz, M.; Forman, J.P.; Curhan, G.; Rimm, E.B. Habitual intake of flavonoid subclasses and incident hypertension in adults. *Am. J. Clin. Nutr.* **2011**, *93*, 338–347.
9. Chiva-Blanch, G.; Urpi-Sarda, M.; Ros, E.; Valderas-Martinez, P.; Casas, R.; Arranz, S.; Guillén, M.; Lamuela-Raventós, R.M.; Llorach, R.; Andres-Lacueva, C. Effects of red wine polyphenols and alcohol on glucose metabolism and the lipid profile: A randomized clinical trial. *Clin. Nutr.* **2013**, *32*, 200–206.
10. Hanhineva, K.; Törrönen, R.; Bondia-Pons, I.; Pekkinen, J.; Kolehmainen, M.; Mykkänen, H.; Poutanen, K. Impact of dietary polyphenols on carbohydrate metabolism. *Int. J. Mol. Sci.* **2010**, *11*, 1365–1402.
11. Hooper, L.; Kay, C.; Abdelhamid, A.; Kroon, P.A.; Cohn, J.S.; Rimm, E.B.; Cassidy, A. Effects of chocolate, cocoa, and flavan-3-ols on cardiovascular health: A systematic review and meta-analysis of randomized trials. *Am. J. Clin. Nutr.* **2012**, *95*, 740–751.
12. Ahtesh, F.B.; Stojanovska, L.; Feehan, J.; de Courten, M.P.; Flavel, M.; Kitchen, B.; Apostolopoulos, V. Polyphenol Rich Sugar Cane Extract Inhibits Bacterial Growth. *Prilozi* **2020**, *41*, 49–57.
13. Scalbert, A.; Manach, C.; Morand, C.; Rémésy, C.; Jiménez, L. Dietary polyphenols and the prevention of diseases. *Crit. Rev. Food Sci. Nutr.* **2005**, *45*, 287–306.
14. Hussain, T.; Tan, B.; Yin, Y.; Blachier, F.; Tossou, M.C.B.; Rahu, N. Oxidative stress and inflammation: What polyphenols can do for us? *Oxidative Med. Cell. Longev.* **2016**, *2016*, 7432797.
15. Wolowczuk, I.; Verwaerde, C.; Viltart, O.; Delanoye, A.; Delacre, M.; Pot, B.; Grangette, C. Feeding our immune system: Impact on metabolism. *Clin. Dev. Immunol.* **2008**, *2008*, 639803.
16. Medzhitov, R.; Janeway, C. Innate immunity. *N. Engl. J. Med.* **2000**, *343*, 338–344.
17. Beutler, B. Innate immunity: An overview. *Mol. Immunol.* **2004**, *40*, 845–859.
18. Clark, R.; Kupper, T. Old meets new: The interaction between innate and adaptive immunity. *J. Investig. Dermatol.* **2005**, *125*, 629–637.
19. Hachimura, S.; Totsuka, M.; Hosono, A. Immunomodulation by food: Impact on gut immunity and immune cell function. *Biosci. Biotechnol. Biochem.* **2018**, *82*, 584–599.
20. Buckwalter, M.R.; Albert, M.L. Orchestration of the immune response by dendritic cells. *Curr. Biol.* **2009**, *19*, R355–R361.
21. del Cornò, M.; Scazzocchio, B.; Masella, R.; Gessani, S. Regulation of dendritic cell function by dietary polyphenols. *Crit. Rev. Food Sci. Nutr.* **2016**, *56*, 737–747.
22. Švajger, U.; Obermajer, N.; Jeras, M. Dendritic cells treated with resveratrol during differentiation from monocytes gain substantial tolerogenic properties upon activation. *Immunology* **2010**, *129*, 525–535.
23. Yoneyama, S.; Kawai, K.; Tsuno, N.H.; Okaji, Y.; Asakage, M.; Tsuchiya, T.; Yamada, J.; Sunami, E.; Osada, T.; Kitayama, J. Epigallocatechin gallate affects human dendritic cell differentiation and maturation. *J. Allergy Clin. Immunol.* **2008**, *121*, 209–214.
24. Lee, J.S.; Kim, S.G.; Kim, H.K.; Lee, T.H.; Jeong, Y.I.; Lee, C.M.; Yoon, M.S.; Na, Y.J.; Suh, D.S.; Park, N.C. Silibinin polarizes Th1/Th2 immune responses through the inhibition of immunostimulatory function of dendritic cells. *J. Cell. Physiol.* **2007**, *210*, 385–397.
25. Huang, R.-Y.; Yu, Y.-L.; Cheng, W.-C.; OuYang, C.-N.; Fu, E.; Chu, C.-L. Immunosuppressive effect of quercetin on dendritic cell activation and function. *J. Immunol.* **2010**, *184*, 6815–6821.
26. Yoon, M.-S.; Lee, J.S.; Choi, B.-M.; Jeong, Y.-I.; Lee, C.-M.; Park, J.-H.; Moon, Y.; Sung, S.-C.; Lee, S.K.; Chang, Y.H. Apigenin inhibits immunostimulatory function of dendritic cells: Implication of immunotherapeutic adjuvant. *Mol. Pharmacol.* **2006**, *70*, 1033–1044.
27. Gupta, S.C.; Tyagi, A.K.; Deshmukh-Taskar, P.; Hinojosa, M.; Prasad, S.; Aggarwal, B.B. Downregulation of tumor necrosis factor and other proinflammatory biomarkers by polyphenols. *Arch. Biochem. Biophys.* **2014**, *559*, 91–99.
28. Liu, S.-H.; Lin, C.-H.; Hung, S.-K.; Chou, J.-H.; Chi, C.-W.; Fu, S.-L. Fisetin inhibits lipopolysaccharide-induced macrophage activation and dendritic cell maturation. *J. Agric. Food Chem.* **2010**, *58*, 10831–10839.
29. Buttari, B.; Profumo, E.; Facchiano, F.; Ozturk, E.I.; Segoni, L.; Saso, L.; Riganò, R. Resveratrol prevents dendritic cell maturation in response to advanced glycation end products. *Oxidative Med. Cell. Longev.* **2013**, *2013*, 574029.

30. Bottazzi, B.; Doni, A.; Garlanda, C.; Mantovani, A. An integrated view of humoral innate immunity: Pentraxins as a paradigm. *Annu. Rev. Immunol.* **2009**, *28*, 157–183.
31. Murray, P.J.; Wynn, T.A. Protective and pathogenic functions of macrophage subsets. *Nat. Rev. Immunol.* **2011**, *11*, 723–737.
32. Hansson, G.K.; Hermansson, A. The immune system in atherosclerosis. *Nat. Immunol.* **2011**, *12*, 204.
33. Kamada, N.; Hisamatsu, T.; Okamoto, S.; Chinen, H.; Kobayashi, T.; Sato, T.; Sakuraba, A.; Kitazume, M.T.; Sugita, A.; Koganei, K. Unique CD14+ intestinal macrophages contribute to the pathogenesis of Crohn disease via IL-23/IFN-γ axis. *J. Clin. Investig.* **2008**, *118*, 2269–2280.
34. Sica, A.; Mantovani, A. Macrophage plasticity and polarization: In vivo veritas. *J. Clin. Investig.* **2012**, *122*, 787–795.
35. Dugo, L.; Belluomo, M.G.; Fanali, C.; Russo, M.; Cacciola, F.; Maccarrone, M.; Sardanelli, A.M. Effect of cocoa polyphenolic extract on macrophage polarization from proinflammatory M1 to anti-inflammatory M2 state. *Oxidative Med. Cell. Longev.* **2017**, *2017*, 6293740.
36. Park, H.-R.; Hwang, D.; Suh, H.-J.; Yu, K.-W.; Kim, T.Y.; Shin, K.-S. Antitumor and antimetastatic activities of rhamnogalacturonan-II-type polysaccharide isolated from mature leaves of green tea via activation of macrophages and natural killer cells. *Int. J. Biol. Macromol.* **2017**, *99*, 179–186.
37. Zhang, M.; Xie, Y.; Su, X.; Liu, K.; Zhang, Y.; Pang, W.; Wang, J. Inonotus sanghuang polyphenols attenuate inflammatory response via modulating the crosstalk between macrophages and adipocytes. *Front. Immunol.* **2019**, *10*, 286.
38. Overman, A.; Bumrungpert, A.; Kennedy, A.; Martinez, K.; Chuang, C.C.; West, T.; Dawson, B.; Jia, W.; McIntosh, M. Polyphenol-rich grape powder extract (GPE) attenuates inflammation in human macrophages and in human adipocytes exposed to macrophage-conditioned media. *Int. J. Obes.* **2010**, *34*, 800–808.
39. McLaren, J.E.; Michael, D.R.; Ashlin, T.G.; Ramji, D.P. Cytokines, macrophage lipid metabolism and foam cells: Implications for cardiovascular disease therapy. *Prog. Lipid Res.* **2011**, *50*, 331–347.
40. Moss, J.W.E.; Ramji, D.P. Nutraceutical therapies for atherosclerosis. *Nat. Rev. Cardiol.* **2016**, *13*, 513.
41. Ramji, D.P.; Davies, T.S. Cytokines in atherosclerosis: Key players in all stages of disease and promising therapeutic targets. *Cytokine Growth Factor Rev.* **2015**, *26*, 673–685.
42. Sevov, M.; Elfineh, L.; Cavelier, L.B. Resveratrol regulates the expression of LXR-α in human macrophages. *Biochem. Biophys. Res. Commun.* **2006**, *348*, 1047–1054.
43. Ruggeri, L.; Capanni, M.; Urbani, E.; Perruccio, K.; Shlomchik, W.D.; Tosti, A.; Posati, S.; Rogaia, D.; Frassoni, F.; Aversa, F. Effectiveness of donor natural killer cell alloreactivity in mismatched hematopoietic transplants. *Science* **2002**, *295*, 2097–2100.
44. Hu, J.-Y.; Zhang, J.; Cui, J.-L.; Liang, X.-Y.; Lu, R.; Du, G.-F.; Xu, X.-Y.; Zhou, G. Increasing CCL5/CCR5 on CD4+ T cells in peripheral blood of oral lichen planus. *Cytokine* **2013**, *62*, 141–145.
45. Kim, Y.H.; Won, Y.-S.; Yang, X.; Kumazoe, M.; Yamashita, S.; Hara, A.; Takagaki, A.; Goto, K.; Nanjo, F.; Tachibana, H. Green tea catechin metabolites exert immunoregulatory effects on CD4+ T cell and natural killer cell activities. *J. Agric. Food Chem.* **2016**, *64*, 3591–3597.
46. Exon, J.H.; Magnuson, B.A.; South, E.H.; Hendrix, K. Dietary quercetin, immune functions and colonic carcinogenesis in rats. *Immunopharmacol. Immunotoxicol.* **1998**, *20*, 173–190.
47. Bub, A.; Watzl, B.; Blockhaus, M.; Briviba, K.; Liegibel, U.; Müller, H.; Pool-Zobel, B.L.; Rechkemmer, G. Fruit juice consumption modulates antioxidative status, immune status and DNA damage. *J. Nutr. Biochem.* **2003**, *14*, 90–98.
48. McAnulty, L.S.; Nieman, D.C.; Dumke, C.L.; Shooter, L.A.; Henson, D.A.; Utter, A.C.; Milne, G.; McAnulty, S.R. Effect of blueberry ingestion on natural killer cell counts, oxidative stress, and inflammation prior to and after 2.5 h of running. *Appl. Physiol. Nutr. Metab.* **2011**, *36*, 976–984.
49. McAnulty, L.S.; Collier, S.R.; Landram, M.J.; Whittaker, D.S.; Isaacs, S.E.; Klemka, J.M.; Cheek, S.L.; Arms, J.C.; McAnulty, S.R. Six weeks daily ingestion of whole blueberry powder increases natural killer cell counts and reduces arterial stiffness in sedentary males and females. *Nutr. Res.* **2014**, *34*, 577–584.
50. Chen, C.-M.; Li, S.-C.; Lin, Y.-L.; Hsu, C.-Y.; Shieh, M.-J.; Liu, J.-F. Consumption of purple sweet potato leaves modulates human immune response: T-lymphocyte functions, lytic activity of natural killer cell and antibody production. *World J. Gastroenterol. WJG* **2005**, *11*, 5777.
51. Hassanain, E.; Silverberg, J.I.; Norowitz, K.B.; Chice, S.; Bluth, M.H.; Brody, N.; Joks, R.; Durkin, H.G.; Smith-Norowitz, T.A. Green tea (Camelia sinensis) suppresses B cell production of IgE without inducing apoptosis. *Ann. Clin. Lab. Sci.* **2010**, *40*, 135–143.
52. Sanbongi, C.; Suzuki, N.; Sakane, T. Polyphenols in chocolate, which have antioxidant activity, modulate immune functions in humansin vitro. *Cell. Immunol.* **1997**, *177*, 129–136.
53. Kuo, C.-L.; Chen, T.-S.; Liou, S.-Y.; Hsieh, C.-C. Immunomodulatory effects of EGCG fraction of green tea extract in innate and adaptive immunity via T regulatory cells in murine model. *Immunopharmacol. Immunotoxicol.* **2014**, *36*, 364–370.
54. Wong, C.P.; Nguyen, L.P.; Noh, S.K.; Bray, T.M.; Bruno, R.S.; Ho, E. Induction of regulatory T cells by green tea polyphenol EGCG. *Immunol. Lett.* **2011**, *139*, 7–13.
55. Gorenec, L.; Lepej, S.Z.; Grgic, I.; Planinic, A.; Bes, J.I.; Vince, A.; Begovac, J. The comparison of Th1, Th2, Th9, Th17 and Th22 cytokine profiles in acute and chronic HIV-1 infection. *Microb. Pathog.* **2016**, *97*, 125–130.
56. Louten, J.; Boniface, K.; de Waal Malefyt, R. Development and function of TH17 cells in health and disease. *J. Allergy Clin. Immunol.* **2009**, *123*, 1004–1011.

57. Cavani, A.; Pennino, D.; Eyerich, K. Th17 and Th22 in Skin Allergy. In *New Trends in Allergy and Atopic Eczema*; Karger Publishers: Basel, Switzerland, 2012; Volume 96, pp. 39–44.
58. Zheng, Y.; Danilenko, D.M.; Valdez, P.; Kasman, I.; Eastham-Anderson, J.; Wu, J.; Ouyang, W. Interleukin-22, a TH 17 cytokine, mediates IL-23-induced dermal inflammation and acanthosis. *Nature* **2007**, *445*, 648–651.
59. Yano, S.; Umeda, D.; Yamashita, T.; Ninomiya, Y.; Sumida, M.; Fujimura, Y.; Yamada, K.; Tachibana, H. Dietary flavones suppresses IgE and Th2 cytokines in OVA-immunized BALB/c mice. *Eur. J. Nutr.* **2007**, *46*, 257–263.
60. Wang, J.; Pae, M.; Meydani, S.N.; Wu, D. Green tea epigallocatechin-3-gallate modulates differentiation of naïve CD4+ T cells into specific lineage effector cells. *J. Mol. Med.* **2013**, *91*, 485–495.
61. Xuzhu, G.; Komai-Koma, M.; Leung, B.P.; Howe, H.S.; McSharry, C.; McInnes, I.B.; Xu, D. Resveratrol modulates murine collagen-induced arthritis by inhibiting Th17 and B-cell function. *Ann. Rheum. Dis.* **2012**, *71*, 129–135.
62. Ahmad, S.F.; Zoheir, K.M.A.; Abdel-Hamied, H.E.; Ashour, A.E.; Bakheet, S.A.; Attia, S.M.; Abd-Allah, A.R.A. Grape seed proanthocyanidin extract has potent anti-arthritic effects on collagen-induced arthritis by modifying the T cell balance. *Int. Immunopharmacol.* **2013**, *17*, 79–87.
63. Zhang, H.; Tsao, R. Dietary polyphenols, oxidative stress and antioxidant and anti-inflammatory effects. *Curr. Opin. Food Sci.* **2016**, *8*, 33–42.
64. Dandona, P.; Aljada, A.; Chaudhuri, A.; Mohanty, P.; Garg, R. Metabolic syndrome: A comprehensive perspective based on interactions between obesity, diabetes, and inflammation. *Circulation* **2005**, *111*, 1448–1454.
65. Du, L.; Li, J.; Zhang, X.; Wang, L.; Zhang, W. Pomegranate peel polyphenols inhibits inflammation in LPS-induced RAW264. 7 macrophages via the suppression of MAPKs activation. *J. Funct. Foods* **2018**, *43*, 62–69.
66. Du, L.; Li, J.; Zhang, X.; Wang, L.; Zhang, W.; Yang, M.; Hou, C. Pomegranate peel polyphenols inhibits inflammation in LPS-induced RAW264. 7 macrophages via the suppression of TLR4/NF-κB pathway activation. *Food Nutr. Res.* **2019**, *63*. [CrossRef]
67. Nallathambi, R.; Poulev, A.; Zuk, J.B.; Raskin, I. Proanthocyanidin-Rich Grape Seed Extract Reduces Inflammation and Oxidative Stress and Restores Tight Junction Barrier Function in Caco-2 Colon Cells. *Nutrients* **2020**, *12*, 1623.
68. Wang, Y.; Wang, Y.; Shen, W.; Wang, Y.; Cao, Y.; Nuerbulati, N.; Chen, W.; Lu, G.; Xiao, W.; Qi, R. Grape Seed Polyphenols Ameliorated Dextran Sulfate Sodium-Induced Colitis via Suppression of Inflammation and Apoptosis. *Pharmacology* **2020**, *105*, 9–18.
69. Li, Y.; Rahman, S.U.; Huang, Y.; Zhang, Y.; Ming, P.; Zhu, L.; Chu, X.; Li, J.; Feng, S.; Wang, X. Green tea polyphenols decrease weight gain, ameliorate alteration of gut microbiota, and mitigate intestinal inflammation in canines with high-fat-diet-induced obesity. *J. Nutr. Biochem.* **2020**, *78*, 108324.
70. Abdollahi, E.; Momtazi, A.A.; Johnston, T.P.; Sahebkar, A. Therapeutic effects of curcumin in inflammatory and immune-mediated diseases: A nature-made jack-of-all-trades? *J. Cell. Physiol.* **2018**, *233*, 830–848.
71. Zheng, M.; Zhang, Q.; Joe, Y.; Lee, B.H.; Kwon, K.B.; Ryter, S.W.; Chung, H.T. Curcumin induces apoptotic cell death of activated human CD4+ T cells via increasing endoplasmic reticulum stress and mitochondrial dysfunction. *Int. Immunopharmacol.* **2013**, *15*, 517–523.
72. Busch, F.; Mobasheri, A.; Shayan, P.; Lueders, C.; Stahlmann, R.; Shakibaei, M. Resveratrol modulates interleukin-1β-induced phosphatidylinositol 3-kinase and nuclear factor κB signaling pathways in human tenocytes. *J. Biol. Chem.* **2012**, *287*, 38050–38063.
73. Venkatachalam, K.; Mummidi, S.; Cortez, D.M.; Prabhu, S.D.; Valente, A.J.; Chandrasekar, B. Resveratrol inhibits high glucose-induced PI3K/Akt/ERK-dependent interleukin-17 expression in primary mouse cardiac fibroblasts. *Am. J. Physiol. Heart Circ. Physiol.* **2008**, *294*, H2078–H2087.
74. Wu, D.; Wang, J.; Pae, M.; Meydani, S.N. Green tea EGCG, T cells, and T cell-mediated autoimmune diseases. *Mol. Asp. Med.* **2012**, *33*, 107–118.
75. Bak, M.-J.; Truong, V.L.; Kang, H.-S.; Jun, M.; Jeong, W.-S. Anti-inflammatory effect of procyanidins from wild grape (Vitis amurensis) seeds in LPS-induced RAW 264.7 cells. *Oxidative Med. Cell. Longev.* **2013**, *2013*, 409321.
76. Chu, H.; Tang, Q.; Huang, H.; Hao, W.; Wei, X. Grape-seed proanthocyanidins inhibit the lipopolysaccharide-induced inflammatory mediator expression in RAW264. 7 macrophages by suppressing MAPK and NF-κb signal pathways. *Environ. Toxicol. Pharmacol.* **2016**, *41*, 159–166.
77. Armutcu, F.; Akyol, S.; Ustunsoy, S.; Turan, F.F. Therapeutic potential of caffeic acid phenethyl ester and its anti-inflammatory and immunomodulatory effects. *Exp. Ther. Med.* **2015**, *9*, 1582–1588.
78. Juman, S.; Yasui, N.; Ikeda, K.; Ueda, A.; Sakanaka, M.; Negishi, H.; Miki, T. Caffeic acid phenethyl ester suppresses the production of pro-inflammatory cytokines in hypertrophic adipocytes through lipopolysaccharide-stimulated macrophages. *Biol. Pharm. Bull.* **2012**, *35*, 1941–1946.
79. Zhang, M.; Zhou, J.; Wang, L.; Li, B.; Guo, J.; Guan, X.; Han, Q.; Zhang, H. Caffeic acid reduces cutaneous tumor necrosis factor alpha (TNF-α), IL-6 and IL-1β levels and ameliorates skin edema in acute and chronic model of cutaneous inflammation in mice. *Biol. Pharm. Bull.* **2014**, *37*, 347–354.
80. Shimizu, M. Multifunctions of dietary polyphenols in the regulation of intestinal inflammation. *J. Food Drug Anal.* **2017**, *25*, 93–99.
81. Singh, D.; Srivastava, S.; Pradhan, M.; Kanwar, J.R.; Singh, M.R. Inflammatory bowel disease: Pathogenesis, causative factors, issues, drug treatment strategies, and delivery approaches. *Crit. Rev. Ther. Drug Carr. Syst.* **2015**, *32*, 181–214.

82. Center for Disease Control and Prevention. Inflammatory Bowel Disease. 2012. Available online: https://www.cdc.gov/ibd/data-statistics.htm (accessed on 10 December 2020).
83. Fukata, M.; Arditi, M. The role of pattern recognition receptors in intestinal inflammation. *Mucosal Immunol.* **2013**, *6*, 451–463.
84. Huang, S.; Zhao, L.; Kim, K.; Lee, D.S.; Hwang, D.H. Inhibition of Nod2 signaling and target gene expression by curcumin. *Mol. Pharmacol.* **2008**, *74*, 274–281.
85. Shibata, T.; Nakashima, F.; Honda, K.; Lu, Y.-J.; Kondo, T.; Ushida, Y.; Aizawa, K.; Suganuma, H.; Oe, S.; Tanaka, H. Toll-like receptors as a target of food-derived anti-inflammatory compounds. *J. Biol. Chem.* **2014**, *289*, 32757–32772.
86. Youn, H.S.; Lee, J.Y.; Fitzgerald, K.A.; Young, H.A.; Akira, S.; Hwang, D.H. Specific inhibition of MyD88-independent signaling pathways of TLR3 and TLR4 by resveratrol: Molecular targets are TBK1 and RIP1 in TRIF complex. *J. Immunol.* **2005**, *175*, 3339–3346.
87. Nunes, S.; Danesi, F.; Del Rio, D.; Silva, P. Resveratrol and inflammatory bowel disease: The evidence so far. *Nutr. Res. Rev.* **2018**, *31*, 85–97.
88. Kostyuk, V.A.; Potapovich, A.I.; Suhan, T.O.; de Luca, C.; Korkina, L.G. Antioxidant and signal modulation properties of plant polyphenols in controlling vascular inflammation. *Eur. J. Pharmacol.* **2011**, *658*, 248–256.
89. Mackenzie, G.G.; Delfino, J.M.; Keen, C.L.; Fraga, C.G.; Oteiza, P.I. Dimeric procyanidins are inhibitors of NF-κB–DNA binding. *Biochem. Pharmacol.* **2009**, *78*, 1252–1262.
90. Wang, H.-K.; Yeh, C.-H.; Iwamoto, T.; Satsu, H.; Shimizu, M.; Totsuka, M. Dietary flavonoid naringenin induces regulatory T cells via an aryl hydrocarbon receptor mediated pathway. *J. Agric. Food Chem.* **2012**, *60*, 2171–2178.
91. Josefowicz, S.Z.; Lu, L.-F.; Rudensky, A.Y. Regulatory T cells: Mechanisms of differentiation and function. *Annu. Rev. Immunol.* **2012**, *30*, 531–564.
92. Lee, H.C.; Jenner, A.M.; Low, C.S.; Lee, Y.K. Effect of tea phenolics and their aromatic fecal bacterial metabolites on intestinal microbiota. *Res. Microbiol.* **2006**, *157*, 876–884.
93. Magrone, T.; Jirillo, E. The interplay between the gut immune system and microbiota in health and disease: Nutraceutical intervention for restoring intestinal homeostasis. *Curr. Pharm. Des.* **2013**, *19*, 1329–1342.
94. Rahman, S.U.; Li, Y.; Huang, Y.; Zhu, L.; Feng, S.; Wu, J.; Wang, X. Treatment of inflammatory bowel disease via green tea polyphenols: Possible application and protective approaches. *Inflammopharmacology* **2018**, *26*, 319–330.
95. Barbalho, S.M.; Bosso, H.; Salzedas-Pescinini, L.M.; de Alvares Goulart, R. Green tea: A possibility in the therapeutic approach of inflammatory bowel diseases?: Green tea and inflammatory bowel diseases. *Complementary Ther. Med.* **2019**, *43*, 148–153.
96. Hollebeeck, S.; Larondelle, Y.; Schneider, Y.-J.; During, A. The use of pomegranate (Punica granatum l.) phenolic compounds as potential natural prevention against IBDs. *Inflamm. Bowel Dis. Adv. Pathog. Manag. Intech-Publ. Belg.* **2012**, 275–300. [CrossRef]
97. Kim, H.; Venancio, V.P.; Fang, C.; Dupont, A.W.; Talcott, S.T.; Mertens-Talcott, S.U. Mango (Mangifera indica L.) polyphenols reduce IL-8, GRO, and GM-SCF plasma levels and increase Lactobacillus species in a pilot study in patients with inflammatory bowel disease. *Nutr. Res.* **2020**, *75*, 85–94.
98. Scarano, A.; Butelli, E.; De Santis, S.; Cavalcanti, E.; Hill, L.; De Angelis, M.; Giovinazzo, G.; Chieppa, M.; Martin, C.; Santino, A. Combined dietary anthocyanins, flavonols, and stilbenoids alleviate inflammatory bowel disease symptoms in mice. *Front. Nutr.* **2018**, *4*, 75.
99. Devereux, G. The increase in the prevalence of asthma and allergy: Food for thought. *Nat. Rev. Immunol.* **2006**, *6*, 869–874.
100. Tai, A.; Volkmer, R.; Burton, A. Prevalence of asthma symptoms and atopic disorders in preschool children and the trend over a decade. *J. Asthma* **2009**, *46*, 343–346.
101. Singh, A.; Holvoet, S.; Mercenier, A. Dietary polyphenols in the prevention and treatment of allergic diseases. *Clin. Exp. Allergy* **2011**, *41*, 1346–1359.
102. Gong, J.; Chen, S.-S. Polyphenolic antioxidants inhibit peptide presentation by antigen-presenting cells. *Int. Immunopharmacol.* **2003**, *3*, 1841–1852.
103. Kim, J.-Y.; Kina, T.; Iwanaga, Y.; Noguchi, H.; Matsumura, K.; Hyon, S.-H. Tea polyphenol inhibits allostimulation in mixed lymphocyte culture. *Cell Transplant.* **2007**, *16*, 75–83.
104. Iwamura, C.; Shinoda, K.; Yoshimura, M.; Watanabe, Y.; Obata, A.; Nakayama, T. Naringenin chalcone suppresses allergic asthma by inhibiting the type-2 function of CD4 T cells. *Allergol. Int.* **2010**, *59*, 67–73.
105. Zuercher, A.W.; Holvoet, S.; Weiss, M.; Mercenier, A. Polyphenol-enriched apple extract attenuates food allergy in mice. *Clin. Exp. Allergy* **2010**, *40*, 942–950.
106. Aires, V.; Adote, S.; Hirchami, A.; Moutairou, K.; Boustani, E.-S.E.; Khan, N.A. Modulation of intracellular calcium concentrations and T cell activation by prickly pear polyphenols. *Mol. Cell. Biochem.* **2004**, *260*, 103–110.
107. Schoene, N.W.; Kelly, M.A.; Polansky, M.M.; Anderson, R.A. A polyphenol mixture from cinnamon targets p38 MAP kinase-regulated signaling pathways to produce G2/M arrest. *J. Nutr. Biochem.* **2009**, *20*, 614–620.
108. Kawai, K.; Tsuno, N.H.; Kitayama, J.; Sunami, E.; Takahashi, K.; Nagawa, H. Catechin inhibits adhesion and migration of peripheral blood B cells by blocking CD11b. *Immunopharmacol. Immunotoxicol.* **2011**, *33*, 391–397.
109. Yano, S.; Umeda, D.; Maeda, N.; Fujimura, Y.; Yamada, K.; Tachibana, H. Dietary apigenin suppresses IgE and inflammatory cytokines production in C57BL/6N mice. *J. Agric. Food Chem.* **2006**, *54*, 5203–5207.
110. Chung, S.-Y.; Champagne, E.T. Reducing the allergenic capacity of peanut extracts and liquid peanut butter by phenolic compounds. *Food Chem.* **2009**, *115*, 1345–1349.

111. Wang, C.-C.; Lin, Y.-R.; Liao, M.-H.; Jan, T.-R. Oral supplementation with areca-derived polyphenols attenuates food allergic responses in ovalbumin-sensitized mice. *Bmc Complementary Altern. Med.* **2013**, *13*, 154.
112. Bansode, R.R.; Randolph, P.D.; Plundrich, N.J.; Lila, M.A.; Williams, L.L. Peanut protein-polyphenol aggregate complexation suppresses allergic sensitization to peanut by reducing peanut-specific IgE in C3H/HeJ mice. *Food Chem.* **2019**, *299*, 125025.
113. Peérot, M.; Lupi, R.; Guyot, S.; Delayre-Orthez, C.; Gadonna-Widehem, P.; Theébaudin, J.-Y.; Bodinier, M.; Larreé, C. Polyphenol interactions mitigate the immunogenicity and allergenicity of gliadins. *J. Agric. Food Chem.* **2017**, *65*, 6442–6451.
114. Anderson, K.C.; Teuber, S.S. Ellagic acid and polyphenolics present in walnut kernels inhibit in vitro human peripheral blood mononuclear cell proliferation and alter cytokine production. *Ann. N. Y. Acad. Sci.* **2010**, *1190*, 86–96.
115. Labuckas, D.O.; Maestri, D.M.; Perello, M.; Martínez, M.L.; Lamarque, A.L. Phenolics from walnut (Juglans regia L.) kernels: Antioxidant activity and interactions with proteins. *Food Chem.* **2008**, *107*, 607–612.
116. Graff, J.C.; Jutila, M.A. Differential regulation of CD11b on γδ T cells and monocytes in response to unripe apple polyphenols. *J. Leukoc. Biol.* **2007**, *82*, 603–607.
117. Parkar, S.G.; Stevenson, D.E.; Skinner, M.A. The potential influence of fruit polyphenols on colonic microflora and human gut health. *Int. J. Food Microbiol.* **2008**, *124*, 295–298.
118. Tominaga, T.; Kawaguchi, K.; Kanesaka, M.; Kawauchi, H.; Jirillo, E.; Kumazawa, Y. Suppression of type-I allergic responses by oral administration of grape marc fermented with Lactobacillus plantarum. *Immunopharmacol. Immunotoxicol.* **2010**, *32*, 593–599.
119. Katsarou, A.; Davoy, E.; Xenos, K.; Armenaka, M.; Theoharides, T.C. Effect of an antioxidant (quercetin) on sodium-lauryl-sulfate-induced skin irritation. *Contact Dermat.* **2000**, *42*, 85–89.
120. Neukam, K.; Stahl, W.; Tronnier, H.; Sies, H.; Heinrich, U. Consumption of flavanol-rich cocoa acutely increases microcirculation in human skin. *Eur. J. Nutr.* **2007**, *46*, 53–56.
121. Mehrbani, M.; Choopani, R.; Fekri, A.; Mehrabani, M.; Mosaddegh, M.; Mehrabani, M. The efficacy of whey associated with dodder seed extract on moderate-to-severe atopic dermatitis in adults: A randomized, double-blind, placebo-controlled clinical trial. *J. Ethnopharmacol.* **2015**, *172*, 325–332.
122. Kojima, T.; Akiyama, H.; Sasai, M.; Taniuchi, S.; Goda, Y.; Toyoda, M.; Kobayashi, Y. Anti-allergic effect of apple polyphenol on patients with atopic dermatitis: A pilot study. *Allergol. Int.* **2000**, *49*, 69–73.
123. Singh, A.; Demont, A.; Actis-Goretta, L.; Holvoet, S.; Lévêques, A.; Lepage, M.; Nutten, S.; Mercenier, A. Identification of epicatechin as one of the key bioactive constituents of polyphenol-enriched extracts that demonstrate an anti-allergic effect in a murine model of food allergy. *Br. J. Nutr.* **2014**, *112*, 358–368.
124. Abril-Gil, M.; Massot-Cladera, M.; Pérez-Cano, F.J.; Castellote, C.; Franch, À.; Castell, M. A diet enriched with cocoa prevents IgE synthesis in a rat allergy model. *Pharmacol. Res.* **2012**, *65*, 603–608.
125. Enomoto, T.; Nagasako-Akazome, Y.; Kanda, T.; Ikeda, M.; Dake, Y. Clinical effects of apple polyphenols on persistent allergic rhinitis: A randomized double-blind placebo-controlled parallel arm study. *J. Investig. Allergol. Clin. Immunol.* **2006**, *16*, 283.
126. Belcaro, G.; Luzzi, R.; Cesinaro, P.D.R.; Cesarone, M.R.; Dugall, M.; Feragalli, B.; Errichi, B.M.; Ippolito, E.; Grossi, M.G.; Hosoi, M. Pycnogenol® improvements in asthma management. *Panminerva Med.* **2011**, *53*, 57–64.
127. Kishi, K.; Saito, M.; Saito, T.; Kumemura, M.; Okamatsu, H.; Okita, M.; Takazawa, K. Clinical efficacy of apple polyphenol for treating cedar pollinosis. *Biosci. Biotechnol. Biochem.* **2005**, *69*, 829–832.
128. Spergel, J.M. Epidemiology of atopic dermatitis and atopic march in children. *Immunol. Allergy Clin.* **2010**, *30*, 269–280.
129. Katiyar, S.K.; Elmets, C.A.; Agarwal, R.; Mukhtar, H. Protection against ultraviolet-B radiation-induced local and systemic suppression of contact hypersensitivity and edema responses in C3H/HeN mice by green tea polyphenols. *Photochem. Photobiol.* **1995**, *62*, 855–861.
130. Ichikawa, D.; Matsui, A.; Imai, M.; Sonoda, Y.; Kasahara, T. Effect of various catechins on the IL-12p40 production by murine peritoneal macrophages and a macrophage cell line, J774. 1. *Biol. Pharm. Bull.* **2004**, *27*, 1353–1358.
131. Meydani, M. Potential health benefits of avenanthramides of oats. *Nutr. Rev.* **2009**, *67*, 731–735.
132. Guo, W.; Wise, M.L.; Collins, F.W.; Meydani, M. Avenanthramides, polyphenols from oats, inhibit IL-1β-induced NF-κB activation in endothelial cells. *Free Radic. Biol. Med.* **2008**, *44*, 415–429.
133. Papaliodis, D.; Boucher, W.; Kempuraj, D.; Theoharides, T.C. The flavonoid luteolin inhibits niacin-induced flush. *Br. J. Pharmacol.* **2008**, *153*, 1382–1387.
134. Djukanovic, R.; Roche, W.; Wilson, J.; Beasley, C.; Twentyman, O.; Howarth, P.; Holgate, S. Mucosal Inflammation In Asthma1. 2. *Am. Rev. Respir. Dis.* **1990**, *142*, 434–457.
135. Bisset, L.R.; Schmid-Grendelmeier, P. Chemokines and their receptors in the pathogenesis of allergic asthma: Progress and perspective. *Curr. Opin. Pulm. Med.* **2005**, *11*, 35–42.
136. Lee, M.; Kim, S.; Kwon, O.-K.; Oh, S.-R.; Lee, H.-K.; Ahn, K. Anti-inflammatory and anti-asthmatic effects of resveratrol, a polyphenolic stilbene, in a mouse model of allergic asthma. *Int. Immunopharmacol.* **2009**, *9*, 418–424.
137. Park, H.-j.; Lee, C.-M.; Jung, I.D.; Lee, J.S.; Jeong, Y.-i.; Chang, J.H.; Chun, S.-H.; Kim, M.-J.; Choi, I.-W.; Ahn, S.-C. Quercetin regulates Th1/Th2 balance in a murine model of asthma. *Int. Immunopharmacol.* **2009**, *9*, 261–267.
138. Lim, J.-Y.; Lee, J.-H.; Lee, B.-R.; Kim, M.; Lee, Y.-M.; Kim, D.-K.; Choi, J.K. Extract of Boehmeria nivea Suppresses Mast Cell-Mediated Allergic Inflammation by Inhibiting Mitogen-Activated Protein Kinase and Nuclear Factor-κB. *Molecules* **2020**, *25*, 4178.

139. Lin, C.-H.; Shen, M.-L.; Zhou, N.; Lee, C.-C.; Kao, S.-T.; Wu, D.C. Protective Effects of the Polyphenol Sesamin on Allergen-Induced TH 2 Responses and Airway Inflammation in Mice. *PLoS ONE* **2014**, *9*, e96091.
140. Khan, H.; Sureda, A.; Belwal, T.; Çetinkaya, S.; Süntar, İ.; Tejada, S.; Devkota, H.P.; Ullah, H.; Aschner, M. Polyphenols in the treatment of autoimmune diseases. *Autoimmun. Rev.* **2019**, *18*, 647–657.
141. Sudres, M.; Verdier, J.; Truffault, F.; Le Panse, R.; Berrih-Aknin, S. Pathophysiological mechanisms of autoimmunity. *Ann. N. Y. Acad. Sci.* **2018**, *1413*, 59–68.
142. Thomas, N.J.; Jones, S.E.; Weedon, M.N.; Shields, B.M.; Oram, R.A.; Hattersley, A.T. Frequency and phenotype of type 1 diabetes in the first six decades of life: A cross-sectional, genetically stratified survival analysis from UK Biobank. *Lancet Diabetes Endocrinol.* **2018**, *6*, 122–129.
143. Apaya, M.K.; Kuo, T.-F.; Yang, M.-T.; Yang, G.; Hsiao, C.-L.; Chang, S.-B.; Lin, Y.; Yang, W.-C. Phytochemicals as modulators of β-cells and immunity for the therapy of type 1 diabetes: Recent discoveries in pharmacological mechanisms and clinical potential. *Pharmacol. Res.* **2020**, *156*, 104754.
144. Stojanović, I.; Šavikin, K.; Đedović, N.; Živković, J.; Saksida, T.; Momčilović, M.; Koprivica, I.; Vujičić, M.; Stanisavljević, S.; Miljković, Đ. Pomegranate peel extract ameliorates autoimmunity in animal models of multiple sclerosis and type 1 diabetes. *J. Funct. Foods* **2017**, *35*, 522–530.
145. Ravikumar, N.; Kavitha, C.N. Immunomodulatory effect of Quercetin on dysregulated Th1/Th2 cytokine balance in mice with both type 1 diabetes and allergic asthma. *J. Appl. Pharm. Sci.* **2020**, *10*, 80–87.
146. Jeong, G.-S.; Lee, D.-S.; Song, M.-Y.; Park, B.-H.; Kang, D.-G.; Lee, H.-S.; Kwon, K.-B.; Kim, Y.-C. Butein from Rhus verniciflua protects pancreatic β cells against cytokine-induced toxicity mediated by inhibition of nitric oxide formation. *Biol. Pharm. Bull.* **2011**, *34*, 97–102.
147. Bae, U.-J.; Jang, H.-Y.; Lim, J.M.; Hua, L.; Ryu, J.-H.; Park, B.-H. Polyphenols isolated from Broussonetia kazinoki prevent cytokine-induced β-cell damage and the development of type 1 diabetes. *Exp. Mol. Med.* **2015**, *47*, e160.
148. Glossop, J.R.; Dawes, P.T.; Mattey, D.L. Association between cigarette smoking and release of tumour necrosis factor α and its soluble receptors by peripheral blood mononuclear cells in patients with rheumatoid arthritis. *Rheumatology* **2006**, *45*, 1223–1229.
149. Mateen, S.; Moin, S.; Zafar, A.; Khan, A.Q. Redox signaling in rheumatoid arthritis and the preventive role of polyphenols. *Clin. Chim. Acta* **2016**, *463*, 4–10.
150. Kloesch, B.; Becker, T.; Dietersdorfer, E.; Kiener, H.; Steiner, G. Anti-inflammatory and apoptotic effects of the polyphenol curcumin on human fibroblast-like synoviocytes. *Int. Immunopharmacol.* **2013**, *15*, 400–405.
151. Mateen, S.; Moin, S.; Khan, A.Q.; Zafar, A.; Fatima, N. Increased reactive oxygen species formation and oxidative stress in rheumatoid arthritis. *PLoS ONE* **2016**, *11*, e0152925.
152. Yang, G.; Chang, C.-C.; Yang, Y.; Yuan, L.; Xu, L.; Ho, C.-T.; Li, S. Resveratrol alleviates rheumatoid arthritis via reducing ROS and inflammation, inhibiting MAPK signaling pathways, and suppressing angiogenesis. *J. Agric. Food Chem.* **2018**, *66*, 12953–12960.
153. Khojah, H.M.; Ahmed, S.; Abdel-Rahman, M.S.; Elhakeim, E.H. Resveratrol as an effective adjuvant therapy in the management of rheumatoid arthritis: A clinical study. *Clin. Rheumatol.* **2018**, *37*, 2035–2042.
154. Morinobu, A.; Biao, W.; Tanaka, S.; Horiuchi, M.; Jun, L.; Tsuji, G.; Sakai, Y.; Kurosaka, M.; Kumagai, S. (−)-Epigallocatechin-3-gallate suppresses osteoclast differentiation and ameliorates experimental arthritis in mice. *Arthritis Rheum. Off. J. Am. Coll. Rheumatol.* **2008**, *58*, 2012–2018.
155. Park, M.-K.; Park, J.-S.; Cho, M.-L.; Oh, H.-J.; Heo, Y.-J.; Woo, Y.-J.; Heo, Y.-M.; Park, M.-J.; Park, H.-S.; Park, S.-H. Grape seed proanthocyanidin extract (GSPE) differentially regulates Foxp3+ regulatory and IL-17+ pathogenic T cell in autoimmune arthritis. *Immunol. Lett.* **2011**, *135*, 50–58.
156. Gonçalves, G.A.; Soares, A.A.; Correa, R.C.G.; Barros, L.; Haminiuk, C.W.I.; Peralta, R.M.; Ferreira, I.C.F.R.; Bracht, A. Merlot grape pomace hydroalcoholic extract improves the oxidative and inflammatory states of rats with adjuvant-induced arthritis. *J. Funct. Foods* **2017**, *33*, 408–418.
157. Stamer, D.K.; Nizami, S.A.; Lee, F.Y.; Soung, D.Y. Whole grape alleviates inflammatory arthritis through inhibition of tumor necrosis factor. *J. Funct. Foods* **2017**, *35*, 458–465.
158. Rosillo, M.Á.; Alcaraz, M.J.; Sánchez-Hidalgo, M.; Fernández-Bolaños, J.G.; Alarcón-de-la-Lastra, C.; Ferrándiz, M.L. Anti-inflammatory and joint protective effects of extra-virgin olive-oil polyphenol extract in experimental arthritis. *J. Nutr. Biochem.* **2014**, *25*, 1275–1281.
159. Javadi, F.; Ahmadzadeh, A.; Eghtesadi, S.; Aryaeian, N.; Zabihiyeganeh, M.; Rahimi Foroushani, A.; Jazayeri, S. The effect of quercetin on inflammatory factors and clinical symptoms in women with rheumatoid arthritis: A double-blind, randomized controlled trial. *J. Am. Coll. Nutr.* **2017**, *36*, 9–15.
160. Riccio, P. The molecular basis of nutritional intervention in multiple sclerosis: A narrative review. *Complementary Ther. Med.* **2011**, *19*, 228–237.
161. Nair, M.P.; Mahajan, S.; Reynolds, J.L.; Aalinkeel, R.; Nair, H.; Schwartz, S.A.; Kandaswami, C. The flavonoid quercetin inhibits proinflammatory cytokine (tumor necrosis factor alpha) gene expression in normal peripheral blood mononuclear cells via modulation of the NF-κβ system. *Clin. Vaccine Immunol.* **2006**, *13*, 319–328.
162. Verbeek, R.; Plomp, A.C.; van Tol, E.A.F.; van Noort, J.M. The flavones luteolin and apigenin inhibit in vitro antigen-specific proliferation and interferon-gamma production by murine and human autoimmune T cells. *Biochem. Pharmacol.* **2004**, *68*, 621–629.

163. Sternberg, Z.; Chadha, K.; Lieberman, A.; Hojnacki, D.; Drake, A.; Zamboni, P.; Rocco, P.; Grazioli, E.; Weinstock-Guttman, B.; Munschauer, F. Quercetin and interferon-β modulate immune response (s) in peripheral blood mononuclear cells isolated from multiple sclerosis patients. *J. Neuroimmunol.* **2008**, *205*, 142–147.
164. Hendriks, J.J.A.; de Vries, H.E.; van der Pol, S.M.A.; van den Berg, T.K.; van Tol, E.A.F.; Dijkstra, C.D. Flavonoids inhibit myelin phagocytosis by macrophages; a structure–activity relationship study. *Biochem. Pharmacol.* **2003**, *65*, 877–885.
165. Fonseca-Kelly, Z.; Nassrallah, M.; Uribe, J.; Khan, R.S.; Dine, K.; Dutt, M.; Shindler, K.S. Resveratrol neuroprotection in a chronic mouse model of multiple sclerosis. *Front. Neurol.* **2012**, *3*, 84.
166. Ghaiad, H.R.; Nooh, M.M.; El-Sawalhi, M.M.; Shaheen, A.A. Resveratrol promotes remyelination in cuprizone model of multiple sclerosis: Biochemical and histological study. *Mol. Neurobiol.* **2017**, *54*, 3219–3229.
167. Siahpoosh, A.; Majdinasab, N.; Derakhshannezhad, N.; Khalili, H.R.; Malayeri, A. Effect of grape seed on quality of life in multiple sclerosis patients. *J. Contemp. Med Sci.* **2018**, *4*. Available online: http://www.jocms.org/index.php/jcms/article/view/453/243 (accessed on 10 December 2020).

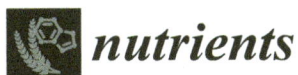

Article

ROS Modulating Effects of Lingonberry (*Vaccinium vitis-idaea* L.) Polyphenols on Obese Adipocyte Hypertrophy and Vascular Endothelial Dysfunction

Katarzyna Kowalska [1], Radosław Dembczyński [1], Agata Gołąbek [1], Mariola Olkowicz [2] and Anna Olejnik [1,*]

[1] Department of Biotechnology and Food Microbiology, Poznan University of Life Sciences, 48 Wojska Polskiego St., 60-627 Poznan, Poland; katarzyna.kowalska@up.poznan.pl (K.K.); radoslaw.dembczynski@up.poznan.pl (R.D.); agata.golabek@up.poznan.pl (A.G.)
[2] Jagiellonian Centre for Experimental Therapeutics, Jagiellonian University, 14 Bobrzynskiego St., 30-348 Krakow, Poland; mariola.olkowicz@jcet.eu
* Correspondence: anna.olejnik@up.poznan.pl

Abstract: Oxidative stress and dysregulated adipocytokine secretion accompanying hypertrophied adipose tissue induce chronic inflammation, which leads to vascular endothelial dysfunction. The present study investigated the ability of anthocyanin (ACN) and non-anthocyanin polyphenol (PP) fractions from lingonberry fruit to mitigate adipose tissue hypertrophy and endothelial dysfunction using 3T3-L1 adipocytes and human umbilical vein endothelial cells (HUVECs). This study showed that the PP fraction decreased intracellular ROS generation in hypertrophied adipocytes by enhancing antioxidant enzyme expression (*SOD2*) and inhibiting oxidant enzyme expression (*NOX4*, *iNOS*). Moreover, PP and ACN fractions reduced triglyceride content in adipocytes accompanied by downregulation of the expression of lipogenic genes such as *aP2*, *FAS*, and *DAGT1*. Treatment with both fractions modulated the mRNA expression and protein secretion of key adipokines in hypertrophied adipocytes. Expression and secretion of leptin and adiponectin were, respectively, down- and upregulated. Furthermore, PP and ACN fractions alleviated the inflammatory response in TNF-α-induced HUVECs by inhibiting the expression of pro-inflammatory genes (*IL-6*, *IL-1β*) and adhesion molecules (*VCAM-1*, *ICAM-1*, *SELE*). The obtained results suggest that consuming polyphenol-rich lingonberry fruit may help prevent and treat obesity and endothelial dysfunction due to their antioxidant and anti-inflammatory actions.

Keywords: polyphenols; anthocyanins; lingonberry; antioxidant potential; anti-obesity; anti-inflammatory; 3T3-L1 adipocytes; hypertrophy; adipokines; endothelial dysfunction

Citation: Kowalska, K.; Dembczyński, R.; Gołąbek, A.; Olkowicz, M.; Olejnik, A. ROS Modulating Effects of Lingonberry (*Vaccinium vitis-idaea* L.) Polyphenols on Obese Adipocyte Hypertrophy and Vascular Endothelial Dysfunction. *Nutrients* **2021**, *13*, 885. https://doi.org/10.3390/nu13030885

Academic Editors: Emad Al-Dujaili and Elena González-Burgos

Received: 27 January 2021
Accepted: 5 March 2021
Published: 9 March 2021

Publisher's Note: MDPI stays neutral with regard to jurisdictional claims in published maps and institutional affiliations.

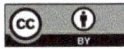

Copyright: © 2021 by the authors. Licensee MDPI, Basel, Switzerland. This article is an open access article distributed under the terms and conditions of the Creative Commons Attribution (CC BY) license (https://creativecommons.org/licenses/by/4.0/).

1. Introduction

Obesity is an independent risk factor for cardiovascular disease and one of the leading causes of the increased risk of dyslipidemia, insulin resistance, hypertension, and atherosclerosis both in adults and children [1]. In obesity, white adipose tissue (WAT) by excessive fat accumulation in hypertrophied adipocytes becomes dysfunctional, which leads to chronic inflammation, oxidative stress, and dysregulated adipokine secretion that contributes to type 2 diabetes mellitus and is also independently associated with coronary endothelial dysfunction [2,3]. Hypertrophic adipocytes are the essential factor linking positive energy balance, diabetes, and cardiometabolic diseases [2]. WAT acts as an endocrine organ and via secreted adipokines and cytokines mediates cross-talk between visceral or subcutaneous WAT and cardiovascular tissues. Adipokines such as leptin, adiponectin and resistin, cytokines, TNF-α, IL-1β, IL-6, IL-8, and MCP-1, and reactive oxygen and nitrogen species (ROS and RNS) affect endothelial dysfunction development through direct and indirect mechanisms [4]. In addition, perivascular adipose tissue (PVAT), mainly from obese individuals, promotes local inflammation and endothelial function impairment.

PVAT contributes to vascular homeostasis by producing vasoactive compounds such as adipokines, ROS, and nitric oxide (•NO). By secreting a wide range of bioactive molecules, PVAT influences vascular smooth muscle cell contraction, proliferation, and migration [4].

The endothelial cells that line the vasculature's inner wall regulate homeostatic functions, and their dysfunction is an early predictor of atherosclerosis and cardiovascular diseases [5]. Oxidative stress contributes to endothelial cell activation, priming it for adhesion, infiltration, and immune cell activation, leading to a low-grade inflammatory phenotype in the vasculature [5,6]. ROS can alter endothelium-dependent vascular relaxation via enhanced degradation of NO [6]. Endothelial dysfunction can be reversed, which might delay or even prevent the progression of atherosclerosis and improve arterial function and reduce the incidence of cardiovascular events [5]. Recent clinical studies have demonstrated that non-pharmacological and pharmacological therapies targeting obesity and insulin resistance ameliorate endothelial function and reduce low-grade inflammation [7]. These findings have shown the association of obesity, insulin resistance, and endothelial dysfunction; therefore, reducing pathological adipocyte function in obesity should be the goal in cardiovascular disease prevention. Therapeutic and nutritional strategies that decrease oxidative stress and inflammation in hypertrophied adipose tissue may become a key target to prevent cardiovascular disease [7].

Berries are rich sources of polyphenols, such as flavonols, phenolic acids, and anthocyanins, and epidemiological studies have reported an association between an increase in berry fruit intake with a decrease in obesity and cardiovascular disease [8]. Berry fruits are known as natural antioxidants, and due to their high antioxidant potential, they are increasingly often referred to as natural functional foods [9]. Lingonberries are classed as "superfruits", being particularly rich in antioxidants such as vitamins C, A, and E (tocopherol) and polyphenols [10]. In vitro and in vivo studies have indicated various health beneficial effects of lingonberries such as anti-inflammatory [11], antioxidant [11], and antiproliferative activities [8,9]. Moreover, lingonberries have been shown to prevent diet-induced obesity and low-grade inflammation in diabetic animals [12]. Our previous study showed the anti-inflammatory potential of aqueous extract of freeze-drying lingonberry fruit [11]. The extract regulated pro-inflammatory (IL-6, MCP-1, and IL-1β) and anti-inflammatory (IL-10) gene expression in inflamed TNF-α-induced 3T3-L1 adipocytes and suppressed the inflammatory response in activated RAW 264.7 macrophages by downregulating expression of proinflammatory mediators (TNF-α, IL-1β, IL-6, MCP-1, iNOS, COX-2). In addition, significant antioxidant effects were observed in inflamed adipocytes treated with the lingonberry fruit extract. The intracellular ROS accumulation decreased as a result of enhanced expression of antioxidant defense enzymes (SOD, catalase, GPx) and inhibited pro-oxidant enzyme (NADPH oxidase 4) [11].

The present study investigated the lingonberry fruit anthocyanin (ACN) fraction and non-anthocyanin polyphenol (PP) fraction ability to prevent and treat hypertrophic obesity and endothelial dysfunction imitated in the in vitro models. The effect of ACN and PP fractions on the molecular pathways in oxidative stress, inflammation, and dysregulated adipokine secretion was analyzed in obese hypertrophied 3T3-L1 adipocytes. Protective potential against endothelial dysfunction was evaluated using TNF-α-induced human umbilical vein endothelial cells (HUVECs).

2. Materials and Methods

2.1. Preparation of Anthocyanin and Non-Anthocyanin Polyphenol Fractions

The frozen lingonberry (*Vaccinium vitis-idaea* L.) fruit obtained from the DANEX company (PHU "DANEX", Wieleń, Poland) were homogenized to fruit pulp, which was subsequently frozen at $-80\ °C$ and subjected to freeze-drying according to the procedure described previously [11]. The fruit powder was suspended in a water solution of 0.75% (v/v) acetic acid. The proportion of solids (g) and the extractant (mL) was 1:10. After mixing in a vortex mixer for 30 s, the suspension was placed in a sonic bath (5 min, 20 °C). Again, the extraction mixture was stirred in a vortex mixer for 30 s and left to stand at 20 °C.

After 10 min, the sample was centrifuged at 3600× g (10 min, 20 °C), and the obtained supernatant was collected. The fresh extractant was poured into the remaining solids to start the second extraction stage. The procedure of the second stage was the same as the first one. The extracts of both stages were combined and centrifuged at 12,000× g to remove tiny fruit residues.

In the next step of fraction preparation, removal of sugars and organic acids from the extract was performed. The separation was carried out with AKTA Explorer 100 Air (GE Healthcare, Chicago, IL, USA) chromatography system equipped with an XK 26/20 glass column (GE Healthcare, Chicago, IL, USA). The column was filled with 40 mL of Amberlite XAD-7 HP macroporous adsorbent resin (DuPont, Wilmington, DE, USA). Before injection to the column, the solution (50 mL of the extract obtained in the extraction stage) was filtered using a 0.45-µm pore size syringe filter (Millex-HV Durapore® PVDF) membrane with glass fiber prefilter (Merck Millipore, Burlington, MA, USA). Three eluents were applied: A—5% (v/v) formic acid, B—methanol, C—0.1% (v/v) formic acid. The solutions of formic acid were prepared by mixing an appropriate amount of formic acid with deionized water. The eluent flow rate was adjusted at 5 mL/min. During separation, the following chromatographic program was employed: Column equilibration: 95% A, 5% B, 3 CV (column volume); sample injection-50 mL of the extract; washing unbound substances-1: 100% C, 6 CV; washing unbound substances-2: 100% A, 1 CV; elution: 20% A, 80% B, 5 CV; column wash: 100% B, 2.5 CV.

The whole effluent of the elution stage which showed the absorbance (monitored at λ = 280, 320, and 520 nm) was evaporated to dryness at 30 °C using a rotary evaporator (Laborota 4003 HB control, Heidolph, Germany). The solids were dissolved in a water solution of 0.75% (v/v) acetic acid. The solution was transferred to glass vials and frozen at −85 °C, and then placed in a freeze dryer Beta 1-16 (Martin Christ, Germany). Freeze-drying was carried out for 48 h. The actual drying took place under the pressure of 10 Pa for 40 h (20 h at a shelf temperature of −15 °C and 20 h at 15 °C). The final drying was performed at a temperature of 22 °C for 8 h without pressure control. Solid preparations were stored in hermetically sealed vials under the nitrogen atmosphere at −85 °C.

The vial solid content was dissolved in the water solution of 5% (v/v) formic acid and filtered using a 0.45-µm pore size filter (Merck Millipore). The separation of anthocyanins from the other polyphenol compounds in the samples was performed using an ÄKTA Explorer 100 Air chromatograph, equipped with a UV/VIS detector and an Agilent Zorbax SB C18 column (250 × 21.2 mm). The separation was carried out at 20 °C. The flow rate of the liquid phase was 21 mL/min. Two eluents were applied: A-5% (v/v) formic acid in water and B-methanol. After the column equilibration (95% A, 5% B, 3 CV) and sample injection in the volume of 2 mL, the separation was performed in a complex gradient. The gradient program was as follows: 5% B-0.5 CV; 20% B-2 CV; 20% B-1.2 CV; 30% B-3.5 CV; 30% B-1.2 CV; 45% B-3.5 CV; 45% B-1.2 CV; 100% B-2.5 CV; 100% B-2.5 CV. The effluent with absorbance at λ = 520 nm was collected and denoted as an anthocyanin (ACN) fraction. The outflow showing absorbance at λ = 320 nm was also gathered and denoted as the non-anthocyanin polyphenol fraction (PP). Both fractions were evaporated, dissolved in a water solution of acetic acid, freeze-dried, and stored as described above. All chemicals used to prepare the ACN and PP fractions were purchased from Sigma–Aldrich (Merck Group, Poznań, Poland).

2.2. Polyphenol Identification and Quantification in ACN and PP Fractions

Polyphenol composition of ACN and PP fractions was analyzed by the HPLC-DAD-ESI-MS method on an Agilent 1200 series HPLC system (Agilent Technologies, Inc., Santa Clara, CA, USA) equipped with a G1315D photodiode array detector and coupled online with an Agilent 6224 time-of-flight MS system. Chromatographic separations were carried out on a 150 × 2.1 mm, 3-µm C18 column (Advanced Chromatography Technologies, Aberdeen, Scotland). A previously published study details the separation conditions (mobile phase, gradient elution program, flow rate, sample injection volume) [11].

The HPLC chromatograms were recorded at 280, 325, 355, and 520 nm, recommended to detect flavan-3-ols, hydroxycinnamic acid derivatives, flavonols, and anthocyanins, respectively.

Polyphenol compounds in ACN and PP fractions were quantified as equivalents of cyanidin-3-O-glucoside (anthocyanins), catechin ((epi)catechin and procyanidins), 4-hydroxybenzoic acid (hydroxybenzoic acid derivatives), ferulic acid (ferulic acid derivative), chlorogenic acid (3-O-caffeoylquinic acid), p-coumaric acid (coumaric acid derivative), trihydroxybenzoic acid-gallic acid (benzoic acid and arbutin derivatives), and quercetin (quercetin glycosides). All samples were injected in triplicate from independently prepared solutions of ACN and PP fractions.

After passing through the DAD detector, column eluate was directed to the MS system fitted with an electrospray ionization (ESI) source operated in positive ion and negative ion mode. A previously published article presents ESI-MS parameters employed for identifying phenolic compounds in ACN and PP fractions [11]. Instrument control, data collection, and analysis were achieved with MassHunter B.04.00 software (Agilent Technologies, Inc., Santa Clara, CA, USA). Sigma–Aldrich supplied phenolic standards and other reagents for HPLC/DAD/MS analysis.

2.3. 3T3-L1 Adipocyte Culture and Treatment

Mouse preadipocyte 3T3-L1 cells were obtained from the American Type Culture Collection (ATCC, CL-173). The cells were cultured at 37 °C under a 5% CO_2 atmosphere in Dulbecco's modified eagle's medium (DMEM) (Sigma–Aldrich, Poznań, Poland) with 10% (v/v) fetal bovine serum (FBS) (Gibco, Thermo Fisher Scientific Polska, Warsaw, Poland) supplementation. 3T3-L1 preadipocytes were subjected to the differentiation process following the protocol described previously [11]. Preadipocytes were seeded at a density of 2.5×10^4 cells/cm^2 into 12-well plates and cultured until they reached confluence. Then they were stimulated for 2 days by a differentiation mixture which contained 0.25 μM of dexamethasone (Sigma–Aldrich, Poznań, Poland), 0.5 mM 3-isobutyl-1-methylxanthine (Sigma–Aldrich, Poznań, Poland) and 1 μM of insulin (Sigma–Aldrich, Poznań, Poland) in DMEM with 10% FBS. The medium was replaced with DMEM supplemented with 10% FBS and 1 μM insulin. After 2 days, the culture medium was replaced with DMEM with 10% FBS addition and refreshed at 2-day intervals until analysis on day 12. 3T3-L1 adipocytes were treated for 24 h with ACN and PP fractions at concentrations of 5, 10, and 20 μg/mL.

2.4. HUVEC Culture and Treatment

Human umbilical vein endothelial cells (HUVECs) were obtained from ATCC (CRL-1730). HUVECs were cultivated in F-12K medium (ATCC) supplemented with 10% FBS (Gibco), endothelial cell growth supplement from bovine neural tissue (30 μg/mL) (Sigma–Aldrich, Poznań, Poland), and heparin (100 μg/mL) (Sigma–Aldrich, Poznań, Poland). HUVECs were seeded at a density of 6×10^3 cells/cm^2 onto 24-well plates coated with rat tail collagen solution (Sigma–Aldrich, Poznań, Poland). Then 24-h cultures of HUVECs were exposed for 3 h to ACN and PP fractions at the concentrations of 0.1, 1, and 10 μg/mL and subsequently treated with TNF-α (10 ng/mL) (Sigma–Aldrich, Poznań, Poland) for an additional 3 h to induce inflammation.

2.5. Cell Viability Assay

The viability of hypertrophied 3T3-L1 adipocytes and TNF-α-induced HUVECs, non-treated and treated with ACN and PP fractions, were analyzed applying the MTT (3-(4,5-dimethylthiazol-2-yl)-2,5-diphenyltetrazolium bromide) assay (Sigma–Aldrich, Poznań, Poland) following the procedure described previously [13]. Low concentrations of ACN and PP fractions applied for cell treatment did not affect the color of medium and absorbance reading in the MTT test.

2.6. Determination of Intracellular ROS Production

ROS generation in 3T3-L1 adipocytes was measured using the nitro blue tetrazolium (NBT) assay based on the procedure described previously [14]. After 90-min incubation in 0.2% NBT (Sigma–Aldrich, Poznań, Poland) solution, cells were washed with phosphate-buffered saline and fixed with methanol. After extraction of the formazan using KOH and DMSO, absorbance was read at 620 nm (Tecan Infinite M200, Tecan Group Ltd., Männedorf, Switzerland).

2.7. Measurement of Intracellular Lipid Content

The effect of PP and ACN fractions on lipid content in hypertrophied adipocytes was determined by the Oil Red O (Sigma–Aldrich, Poznań, Poland) staining method described previously [13] and by total triglycerides (TG) measurement using the Adipogenesis Assay Kit (Sigma–Aldrich, Poznań, Poland) in accordance with the manufacturer's instruction. Intracellular TG content was determined by an enzyme assay. A colorimetric product corresponding to the TG present was measured at 570 nm. TG concentration was calculated based on the curve plotted for the TG standard.

2.8. RNA Extraction and Real-Time PCR Analysis

3T3-L1 adipocytes and HUVECs were treated with TRI-Reagent (Sigma–Aldrich, Poznań, Poland) for total RNA isolation. First-strand cDNA synthesis was performed with 1 µg of total RNA using a Transcriptor First Strand cDNA Synthesis Kit (Roche Diagnostics, Poland) based on the manufacturer's instruction. Gene expression quantification was conducted using a real-time PCR system (SmartCycler DX real-time PCR System Cepheid, Sunnyvale, CA, USA). PCR mixture in a final volume of 25 µL included a cDNA sample (1 µL), specific forward and reverse primers (5 µM/1 µL), and SYBR® Select Master Mix (12.5 µL) (Life Technologies, Carlsbad, CA, USA). Primer sequences are shown in Table S1. The PCR cycling conditions included an initial denaturation at 94 °C for 10 min, followed by 40 PCR cycles: 40 s at 95 °C, 30 s at 59 °C, and 30 s at 72 °C. The relative gene expression was calculated using the $2^{-\Delta\Delta CT}$ method. Transcript levels were normalized to β-actin for 3T3-L1 adipocytes and GAPDH for HUVECs. Relative mRNA expression was expressed as fold change compared with control (untreated) cells. All reactions were performed in triplicate.

2.9. Determination of Adipokine Production

Leptin and adiponectin concentrations were measured with ELISA kits (Sigma–Aldrich, Poznań, Poland) following the manufacturer's protocols. Quantitation was performed using the calibration of standards. Each standard and sample was assayed in triplicate. Inter-assay and intra-assay coefficients of variability were calculated respectively at 12.5% and 9.3% for leptin and 11.2% and 7.9% for adiponectin.

2.10. Statistical Analysis

Statistical analysis was performed using the STATISTICA version 13.3 software (Statsoft, Inc., Tulsa, OK, USA). One-way analysis of variance (ANOVA) and Tukey's post hoc test were applied to estimate the differences between multiple groups' mean values. Levene's test verified the equality of variances assumption. Statistical significance was set at $p < 0.05$.

3. Results and Discussion

3.1. Polyphenol Composition in the Lingonberry ACN and PP Fractions

The study focused on two polyphenolic preparations separated from lingonberry fruit: the anthocyanin ACN fraction and non-anthocyanin PP fraction. The polyphenol profiles in ACN and PP fractions determined based on HPLC-DAD-ESI-MS analysis are presented in Table 1. ACN fraction consisted of three main anthocyanin compounds, contained in lingonberry fruit extract [11], which are cyanidin-based derivatives, including 3-O-galactoside (82.5%), 3-O-arabinoside (13.0%), and 3-O-glucoside (4.5%) (Table 1A).

Table 1. Compounds identified in anthocyanin (ACN) fraction (**A**) and non-anthocyanin polyphenol (PP) fraction (**B**) obtained from lingonberry fruit.

(A)					
Compound	RT (min)	Precursor Ion (m/z)	Ionization Mode	Product Ion (m/z)	Contribution (%)
Cyanidin-3-O-galactoside	16.25	449.1126	(+)	287.0611	82.5
Cyanidin-3-O-glucoside	17.17	449.1124	(+)	287.0589	4.5
Cyanidin-3-O-arabinoside	18.24	419.1021	(+)	287.0607	13
(B)					
Compound	RT (min)	Precursor Ion (m/z)	Ionization Mode	Product Ion (m/z)	Contribution (%)
Flavan-3-ols					40.4
B-type procyanidin dimer	8.46	577.134	(−)	407.0763	6.3
(+)/(−)-Catechin	10.49	289.1139	(−)	245.1203	8.3
(+)/(−)-Epicatechin	12.42	289.114	(−)	245.121	4.2
B-type procyanidin dimer	13.16	577.1338	(−)	407.0762	1.6
B-type procyanidin dimer	13.74	577.1349	(−)	407.0769	3.1
A-type procyanidin dimer	19.36	575.1195	(−)	449.0887	6.2
A-type procyanidin trimer	22.31	863.1829	(−)	575.1217	10.7
Hydroxycinnamic acid derivatives					22.8
3-O-Caffeoylquinic acid	12.42	353.134	(−)	191.0907	8.1
Ferulic acid–hexoside	13.71	355.1037	(−)	193.05	2.9
Ferulic acid–hexoside	14.14	355.1041	(−)	193.0503	2.6
2'-O-Caffeoylarbutin	19.36	433.1137	(−)	179.0337	5
Ferulic acid–hexoside	21.7	355.1031	(−)	193.0509	2.5
Coumaroyl-hexose–hydroxyphenol	22.25	417.1065	(−)	163.0396	1.8
Flavonols					31
Quercetin-3-O-galactoside	23.46	463.0874	(−)	301.0334	7.8
Quercetin-3-O-glucoside	24.17	463.0882	(−)	301.0354	1.3
Quercetin-3-O-xyloside	24.85	433.0777	(−)	301.0336	1.9
Quercetin-3-O-arabinofuranoside	27.05	433.0776	(−)	301.0327	6.3
Quercetin-3-O-rhamnoside	27.87	447.0935	(−)	301.0349	8.1
Quercetin	34.37	301.0356	(−)	151.0031	5.6
Anthocyanins					5.8
Cyanidin-3-O-galactoside	16.28	449.1126	(+)	287.0611	2.6
Cyanidin-pentoside	21.33	419.1033	(+)	287.0618	2
Cyanidin 3-O-(6''-acetyl)-glucoside	23.82	491.1507	(+)	287.0621	1.2

The purity of ACN preparation was evaluated at 97.3%; among the non-anthocyanin constituents, 1-O-Benzoyl-β-glucose was identified by HPLC-ESI-MS analysis in positive ion mode (precursor ion at m/z 307.079, product ion at m/z 185.0432). The PP fraction contained polyphenolic compounds belonging to three predominant groups: Flavan-3-ols, hydroxycinnamic acid derivatives, and flavonols, which accounted for 40.4%, 22.8%, and 31.0%, respectively. In addition, the anthocyanin compounds' residue (5.8%) was detected in the PP fraction with cyanidin-3-O-galactoside as dominant anthocyanin, cyanidin-pentoside, and cyanidin 3-O-(6''-acetyl)-glucoside (Table 1B), trace amounts of which have been identified previously in the original lingonberry fruit extract [11]. In the PP fraction, the following polyphenols were quantified in a significant amount (>5%): A- and B-type procyanidins, catechin, 3-O-caffeoylquinic acid, ferulic acid–hexoside, quercetin and its derivatives (3-*O*-galactoside, 3-*O*-arabinofuranoside, 3-*O*-rhamnoside). Table 1B shows mass spectral data of all polyphenolic compounds tentatively identified in the PP fraction of lingonberry fruit.

3.2. The Effect of PP and ACN Fractions on ROS Generation in Hypertrophied 3T3-L1 Adipocytes

An animal study has shown that obesity is characterized by increased vascular oxidative stress and endothelial dysfunction [15]. Enzymatic sources contributing to increased ROS production in pathophysiological states such as obesity are xanthine oxidase, NADH/NADPH oxidase, and inducible nitric oxide synthase (iNOS) [16]. Oxidative stress contributes to endothelium dysfunction via inactivation of nitric oxide (NO) by superoxide and other ROS; thus, diet intervention rich in antioxidants which prevent their production might ultimately correct endothelial dysfunction [16]. Therefore, the potential of ACN and PP fractions derived from lingonberry fruit to mitigate oxidative stress in hypertrophied adipocytes was evaluated. The results obtained in the NBT assay indicate that the PP fraction decreased ROS accumulation in adipocytes in a dose-dependent manner (Figure 1A). The PP fraction at concentrations of 5, 10, and 20 µg/mL reduced the ROS production by 10.5%, 12.1%, and 15%, respectively ($p < 0.01$). In contrast, the ACN fraction did not significantly influence intracellular ROS production (Figure 1B). Moreover, it should be noted that both PP and ACN fraction did not affect adipocyte viability (Figure 2A), indicating that the PP inhibitory effect on intracellular ROS generation was not due to cytotoxicity. NADPH oxidase 4 (NOX4) from NOX family NADPH oxidases is considered the primary ROS synthesis source in adipose tissue [16]. The NOX-enhanced ROS generation in hypertrophied adipocytes decreased the production of the insulin-sensitizing, antiatherogenic and anti-inflammatory factors. It decreased the mRNA expression of antioxidant defense enzymes, including superoxide dismutase (SOD), catalase, and glutathione peroxidase (GPx) [17]. Furthermore, iNOS, an inducible pro-inflammatory enzyme, is overexpressed in obese adipose tissue, and disruption of the iNOS gene protected obese mice from insulin resistance development [18]. The oxidant imbalance in obese patients causes endothelial dysfunction and leads to increased blood pressure and coronary artery disease [19]. Our previous study has shown that lingonberry fruit extract reduces ROS generation in inflamed adipocytes by increasing the expression of antioxidant enzymes (SOD2, catalase, GPx) and decreasing a pro-oxidant enzyme (NOX4) [11]. In the current study, the antioxidant effect of lingonberry-derived ACN and PP fractions was evaluated in hypertrophied 3T3-L1 adipocytes. Real-time PCR analysis showed that the PP fraction at the highest dose of 20 µg/mL significantly downregulated *NOX4* (↓40%, $p < 0.01$) and *iNOS* (↓37%, $p < 0.05$), and upregulated *SOD2* (↑82%, $p < 0.001$) mRNA expression (Figure 1C). The ACN fraction at a dose of 20 µg/mL inhibited *NOX4* by 33% ($p < 0.01$), *iNOS* by 37% ($p < 0.01$), and enhanced the expression of *SOD2* by 23% ($p > 0.05$) (Figure 1D). The obtained results indicate that the lingonberry fruit antioxidant potential is probably associated with upregulation of *SOD2* expression and downregulation of *iNOS* expression by the PP fraction and ACN fraction. In addition, the compounds from both PP and ACN fractions were found to inhibit *NOX4* expression.

Yen et al. (2011) investigated the effect of 21 polyphenolic compounds on oxidative stress in 3T3-L1 adipocytes induced by TNF-α. They found that that *p*-coumaric acid, quercetin, and resveratrol enhance antioxidant defense enzymes, including SOD2, GPx, glutathione, and glutathione S-transferase [20]. Cyanidin-3-glucoside, an anthocyanin derivative commonly found in different berries, reduced the intracellular ROS production in adipocytes induced by H_2O_2 or TNF-α [21].

Polyphenol-rich plant extracts significantly reduced ROS generation induced in 3T3-L1 cells by H_2O_2, and this effect was associated with an increase in SOD2 gene expression [22]. Animals fed a diet inducing oxidative stress and supplemented with lingonberry extract (23 mg/kg of body weight) had a decreased total oxidant status by 25%, and increased levels of antioxidant enzymes: SOD, catalase, and glutathione reductase in red blood cells and liver [23].

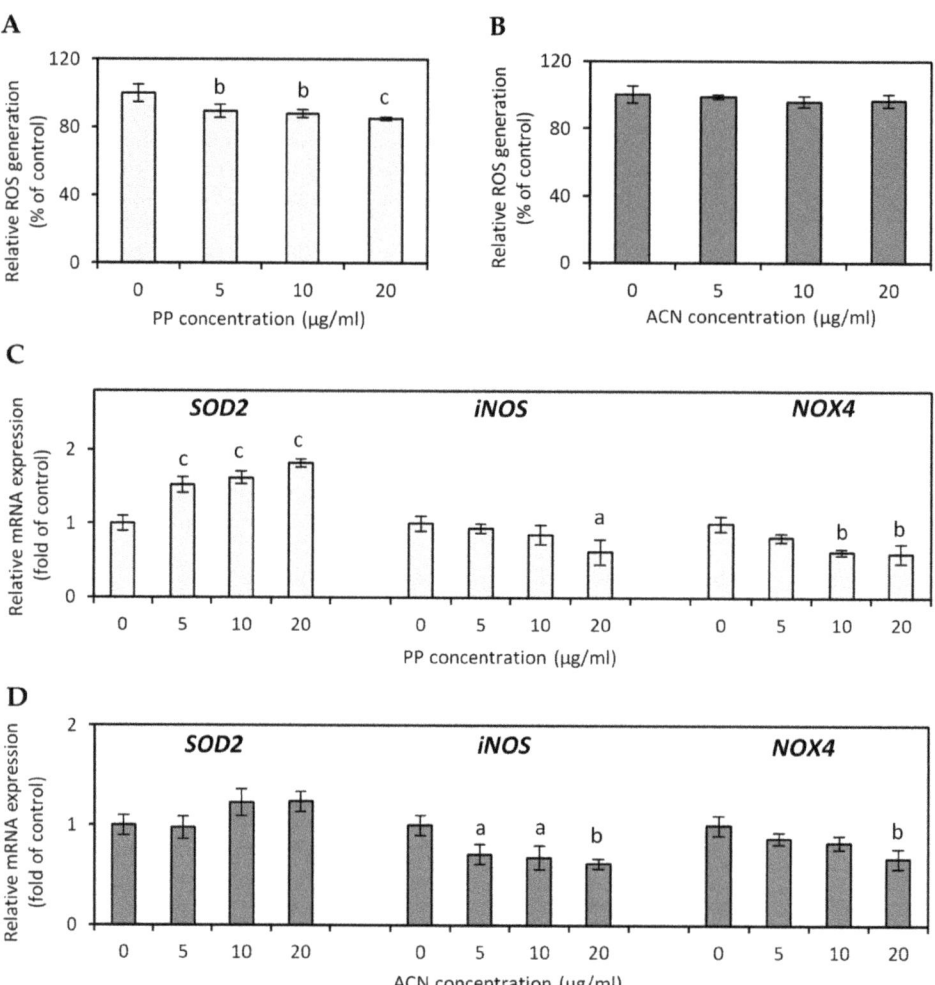

Figure 1. Effect of anthocyanin (ACN) and non-anthocyanin polyphenol (PP) fraction on the intracellular ROS production (**A**,**B**) and antioxidant and pro-oxidant enzymes mRNA expression (**C**,**D**) in hypertrophied 3T3-L1 adipocytes. Data are the mean values ± SD (n = 3). [a] $p < 0.05$, [b] $p < 0.01$, [c] $p < 0.001$.

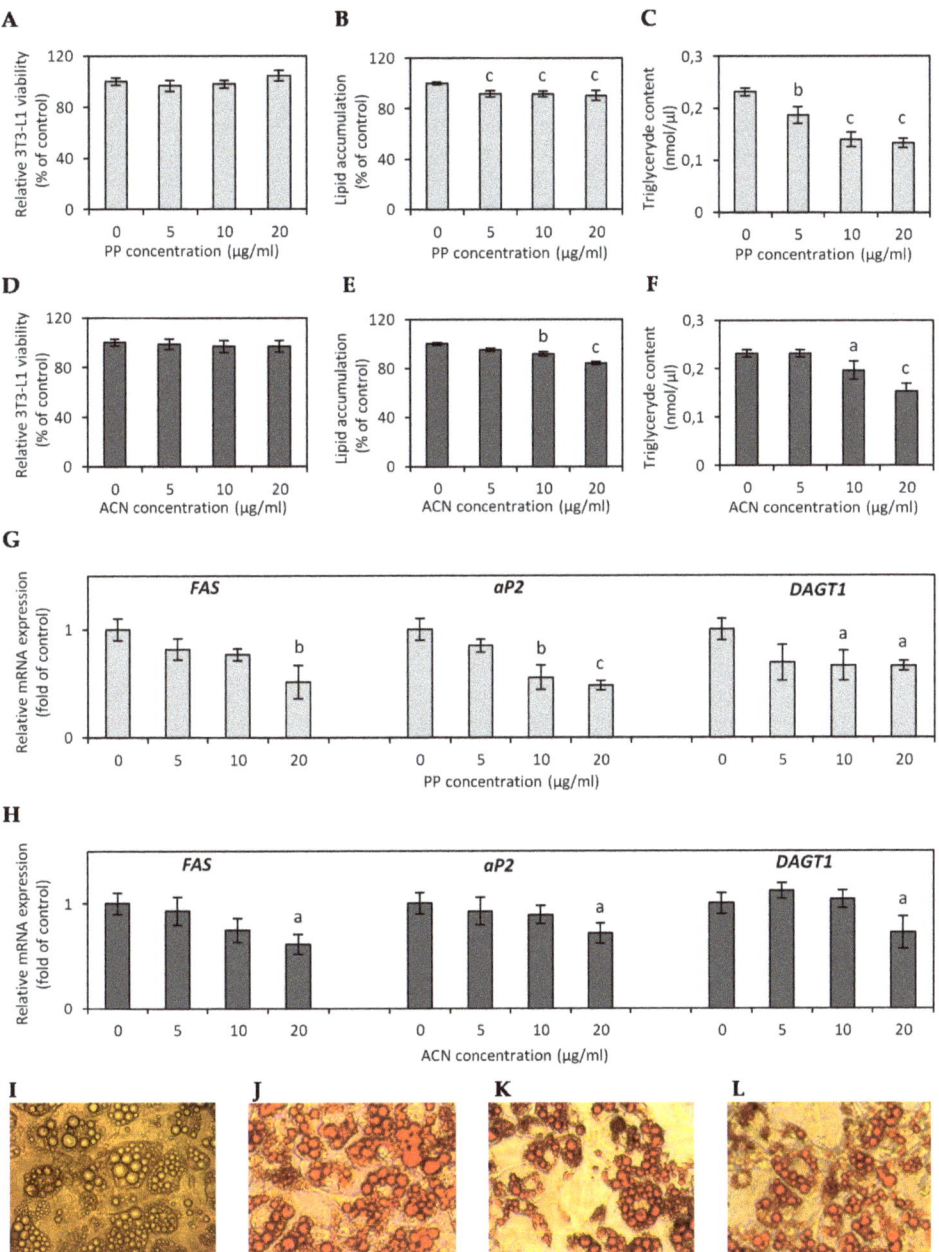

Figure 2. Effect of non-anthocyanin polyphenol (PP) fraction and anthocyanin (ACN) fraction on cell viability (**A,D**), lipid accumulation (**B,E**), triglyceride content (**C,F**), and lipogenic gene expression (**G,H**) in hypertrophied 3T3-L1 adipocytes. Data are the mean values ± SD ($n = 3$).[a] $p < 0.05$, [b] $p < 0.01$, [c] $p < 0.001$. The photos present hypertrophied 3T3-L1 adipocytes on day 12 after differentiation (**I**), Oil Red-stained hypertrophied 3T3-L1 adipocytes non-treated (**J**), and treated with PP fraction (**K**) and ACN fraction (**L**) at the concentrations of 20 µg/mL. The cells were photographed at a magnification of 100×.

3.3. Effect of ACN and PP Fractions on Lipid Accumulation in Hypertrophied 3T3-L1 Adipocytes

In this study, hypertrophic 3T3-L1 adipocytes, formed following the prolonged cultivation of differentiated mature adipocytes in high glucose conditions with medium replacement in 2-day intervals, displayed a morphological pattern typical for adipocyte hypertrophy with disturbance of the lipid handling processes. The 3T3-L1 adipocytes reached the critical cell size and became lipid-overloaded, largely occupied by fat droplets, as shown in Figure 2I. The effect of ACN and PP fractions on lipid content in the hypertrophied 3T3-L1 adipocytes was determined by Oil Red O staining and measurement of the total TG concentration on the cellular level. Semi-quantitative Oil Red O staining revealed that the PP fraction at concentrations of 5, 10, and 20 µg/mL reduced lipid accumulation by 4.9%, 8.4%, and 16% ($p < 0.001$) compared to untreated cells (Figure 2B,J,K), while the ACN fraction at the same concentrations reduced lipid content by 8.4%, 8.6% ($p < 0.01$), and 9.8% ($p < 0.001$), respectively (Figure 2E,J,L). Quantitative analysis of TG content in the cells have shown that 24-h treatment of hypertrophied adipocytes with the PP fraction decreased the TG content by 19.4% ($p < 0.01$), 49.6%, and 42.4% ($p < 0.001$) at a concentration of 5, 10, and 20 µg/mL, respectively (Figure 2C). The effect of the ACN fraction on TG content was less profound, and only the highest dose of ACN fraction 20 µg/mL decreased lipid accumulation by 9.8% ($p < 0.001$), and TG content by 33.9% ($p < 0.001$) (Figure 3F).

The effect of both fractions on lipid accumulation was confirmed by real-time PCR analysis of the expression of genes *FAS (fatty acid synthase)*, *DGAT1 (diacylglycerol acyltransferase 1)*, and *aP2 (fatty acid-binding protein)* involved in fatty acid (FA) and TG synthesis. Animal models with genetic modifications have shown that adipogenic and lipogenic genes, including *FAS*, *DGAT1*, and *aP2*, play a fundamental role in FA and TG synthesis and lipid storage, and a high-fat (HF) diet significantly increased the relative expression of these genes in adipose tissue [24]. DGAT1 is highly expressed in adipose tissue and catalyzes the final reaction of TG synthesis. DGAT1-deficient animals are resistant to obesity and more sensitive to insulin and leptin; therefore, inhibition of DGAT1 may be a potential strategy for decreasing TG synthesis for treating obesity [25]. Fatty acid-binding protein 4 (FABP4), also named adipocyte FABP or aP2, is mostly expressed in fat cells and plays significant roles in developing insulin resistance and atherosclerosis concerning metabolically driven low-grade and chronic inflammation [26]. Circulating aP2 levels are associated with several aspects of metabolic syndrome and endothelial dysfunction; thus, inhibition of the aP2 function could be a novel therapeutic strategy for several diseases, including obesity and cardiovascular disease [27]. FAS is also highly expressed in adipose tissue, and enhanced FAS expression correlates to visceral fat accumulation, impaired insulin sensitivity, and intensified pro-inflammatory cytokine production [28].

In our study, real-time PCR analysis showed that the PP and ACN fraction treatment dose-dependently inhibited *DAGT1*, *aP2*, and *FAS* mRNA expression (Figure 2G,H), but the PP effect was more significant. The PP fraction decreased expression of *DAGT1* in the range of 31–34% ($p < 0.05$). The effect of the PP fraction with statistical significance on *aP2* and *FAS* expression was observed only at concentrations of 10 and 20 µg/mL with 44.7% ($p < 0.01$) and 51.9% ($p < 0.001$) decreases in *aP2* expression and with 23.3% and 48.6% ($p < 0.01$) decreases in *FAS* expression (Figure 2G). The ACN fraction only at the highest dose of 20 µg/mL downregulated *FAS*, *aP2*, and *DAGT1* expression by approximately 28% ($p < 0.05$) (Figure 2H).

In vivo study has shown that DGAT1-deficient mice ($Dgat1^{-/-}$) had less adipose mass and smaller adipocytes. Despite reduced tissue TG levels, the diacylglycerol and fatty acyl CoA, substrates of the DGAT reaction, were not significantly elevated in skeletal muscle and liver. Moreover, the serum TG level was normal in $Dgat1^{-/-}$ mice [25]. DGAT1 deficiency also altered the endocrine function of WAT. Adiponectin mRNA expression in WAT was increased 2-fold in $Dgat1^{-/-}$ mice fed an HF diet [29]. The aP2-deficient mouse model revealed a slight increase in plasma FA. An elevated FA was found to link with the development of obesity and insulin resistance, but paradoxically, mice lacking aP2 were more sensitive to insulin [30].

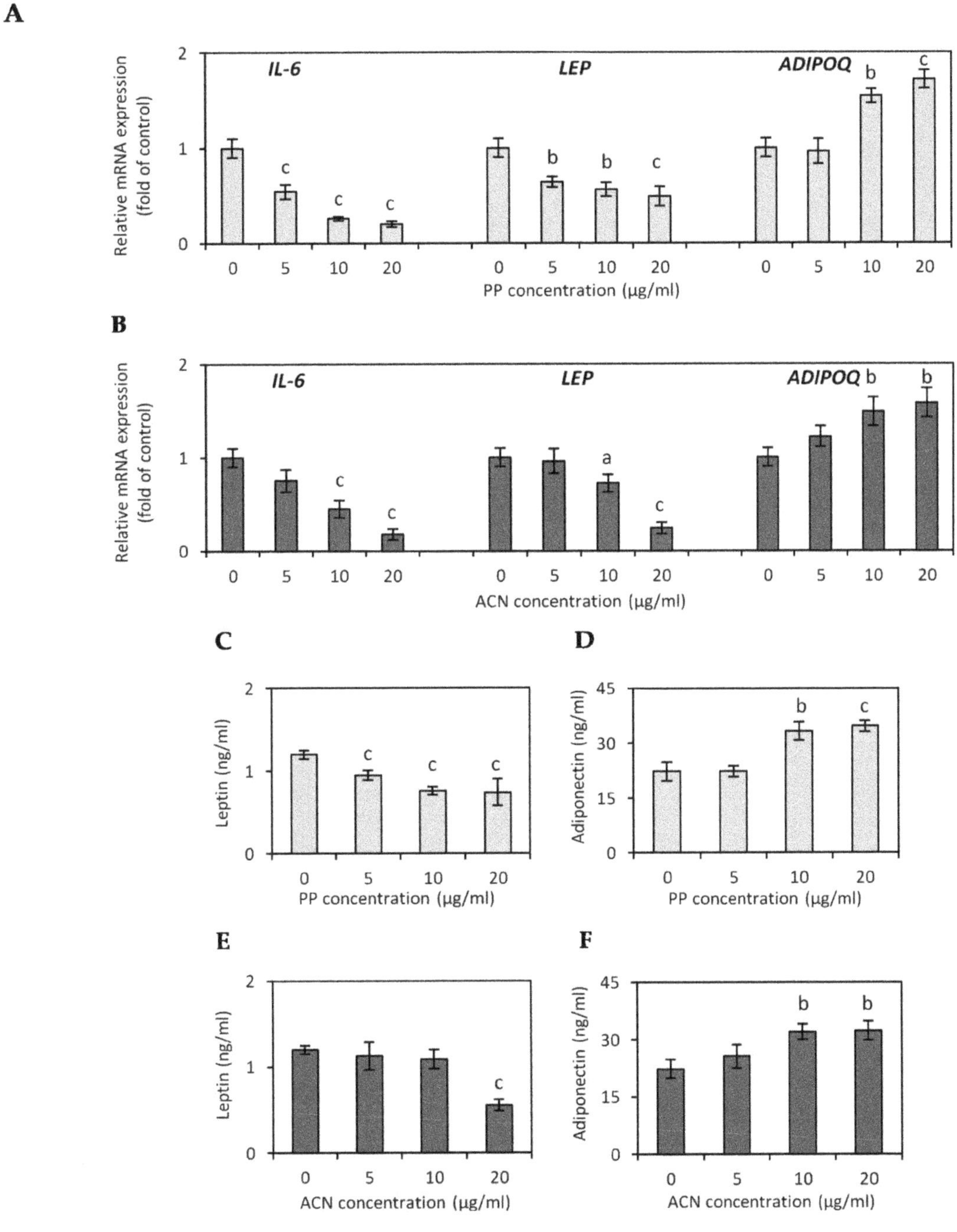

Figure 3. Effect of non-anthocyanin polyphenol (PP) and anthocyanin (ACN) fractions on adiponectin (ADIPOQ), leptin (LEP), and interleukin-6 (IL-6) gene expression (**A**,**B**), and adiponectin (**D**,**F**) and leptin (**C**,**E**) protein secretion by hypertrophied 3T3-L1 adipocytes. Data are the mean values ± SD (n = 3). [a] $p < 0.05$, [b] $p < 0.01$, [c] $p < 0.001$.

Many natural products from plants have been identified as potent DGAT inhibitors [31]. Rose petals, rich in polyphenols and free gallic acid had high antioxidant activity and the ability to inhibit TG synthesis. An extract of rose petals showed selective DGAT inhibition without suppressing other microsomal enzymes [32]. Anthocyanin-rich extracts effectively decreased body weight gain and accumulation of lipids by decreasing the mRNA level and inhibiting FA and TG synthesis enzymes and lipogenic activity [33]. Heyman et al. (2014) have found that lingonberries prevented adiposity, hepatic lipid accumulation, and dyslipidemia in mice fed an HF diet [34]. Qin et al. (2011) have found that consumption of the chokeberry extract, rich in polyphenols, reduces weight gain and epididymal fat accumulation; at the molecular level, it inhibits *aP2*, *FAS*, and *LPL* mRNA expression [35].

3.4. Effect of ACN and PP Fractions on Adipokine and Inflammatory Cytokine Expression in Hypertrophied 3T3-L1 Adipocytes

Adiponectin is the most abundant peptide secreted by adipocytes. Adiponectin production, which has a beneficial effect on insulin sensitivity and cardiovascular function, is significantly reduced in obese adipose tissue. Numerous epidemiological studies have shown that adiponectin deficiency is an independent risk factor for endothelial dysfunction [36]. Adiponectin exerts protective effects by inhibiting TNF-α, resistin, and adhesion molecules (VCAM-1, ICAM-1, and E-selectin) in endothelium and increasing endothelial NO production [37]. The most available therapy for cardiovascular diseases is lifestyle modifications by calorie restriction and dietary interventions that increase plasma levels of adiponectin. There is also a growing interest in the pharmaceutical industry to search for natural compounds that can increase adiponectin production [36].

In our study, adiponectin mRNA expression in hypertrophied adipocytes after PP treatment was upregulated, with a significant enhancement by 57.0% ($p < 0.01$) and 72.7% ($p < 0.001$) at the concentrations of 10 and 20 µg/mL (Figure 3A). The ACN fraction at concentrations of 10 and 20 µg/mL increased adiponectin expression by 50.5% and 59.6%, respectively ($p < 0.01$) (Figure 3B). Contrary to adiponectin, the serum level of leptin is elevated in obesity due to increased leptin release from large hypertrophic adipocytes compared with small fat cells [38]. Evidence from clinical trials and animal experiments suggests that hyperleptinemia is involved in the pathogenesis of obesity-related cardiovascular disease and endothelial dysfunction due to ROS-mediated NO inactivation [39]. In vitro studies have shown that leptin increases ROS production in endothelial cells [40]. In this research, a significant reduction in leptin expression was found after treatment of adipocytes with ACN and PP fractions (Figure 3A,B). Reduction of leptin expression by 27.3% and 75.8% was obtained in hypertrophied adipocytes treated with the ACN fraction at the concentrations of 10 ($p < 0.05$) and 20 µg/mL ($p < 0.001$) (Figure 3B). The PP fraction decreased leptin mRNA expression by 35.0%, 43.4%, and 50.5% at a concentration of 5, 10 ($p < 0.01$), and 20 µg/mL ($p < 0.001$), respectively (Figure 3A). A similar effect of PP and ACN fractions was observed on leptin (Figure 3C,E) and adiponectin (Figure 3D,F) secretion. Treatment of hypertrophied adipocytes with the PP fraction increased the secretion of adiponectin by 49.3% and 55.2% at a concentration of 10 ($p < 0.01$) and 20 µg/mL ($p < 0.001$), respectively (Figure 3D). All tested concentrations of PP fraction (5, 10, and 20 µg/mL) decreased leptin secretion ($\downarrow$20.8%, $\downarrow$36.7%, and $\downarrow$38.1%; $p < 0.001$) (Figure 3C). Only at a concentration of 20 µg/mL did the ACN fraction significantly decrease leptin secretion ($\downarrow$53.9%, $p < 0.001$) (Figure 4E). At doses of 10 and 20 µg/mL, the ACN fraction increased adiponectin production by 43.3% and 44.8% ($p < 0.01$), respectively (Figure 3F).

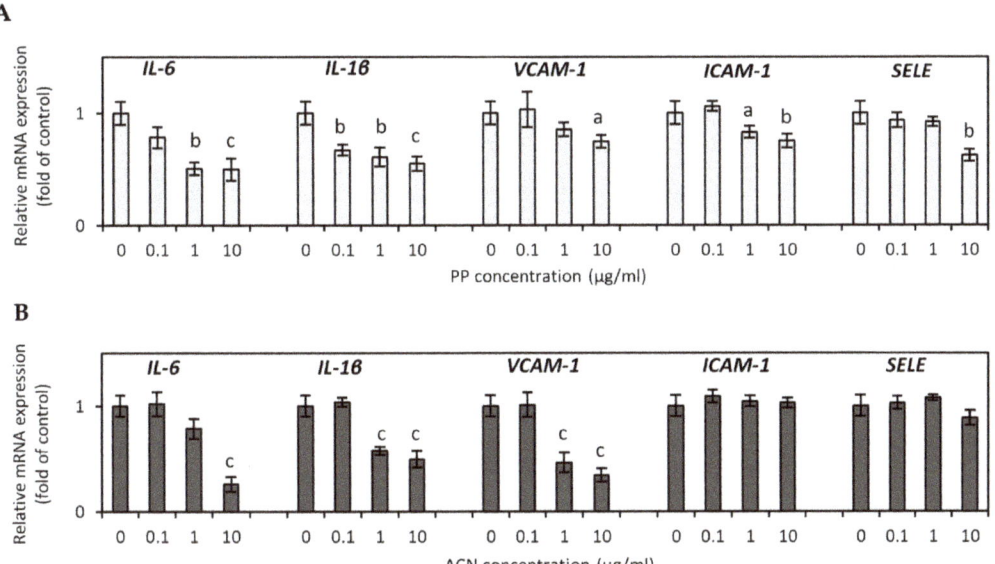

Figure 4. Effect of non-anthocyanin polyphenol (PP) fraction (**A**) and anthocyanin (ACN) fraction (**B**) on inflammatory-related gene expression in HUVECs. Data are the mean values ± SD (n = 3). ^{a} $p < 0.05$, ^{b} $p < 0.01$, ^{c} $p < 0.001$.

Moreover, adipocytokines such as IL-1 and IL-6 are closely linked to endothelial dysfunction and subclinical inflammation [41]. Yudkin et al. (2002) have shown, in healthy subjects, relationships between levels of a hepatic acute-phase C-reactive protein (CRP) and levels of IL-6 released from obese adipose tissue, indicating adipose tissue as a major source for circulating IL-6 [41]. The study with 368 participants showed that persistently high levels of IL-6 were associated with a higher body mass index and an increased number of cardiovascular diseases compared to persistently lower levels of IL-6 [42]. Therefore, we investigated the effect of ACN and PP fractions on the expression of IL-6 in hypertrophied adipocytes after 24-h treatment. Compared to the control adipocytes, the PP fraction downregulated the expression of IL-6 by 45.5%, 73.7%, and 79.8% at a dose of 5, 10, and 20 µg/mL ($p < 0.001$) (Figure 3A). The ACN fraction suppressed IL-6 mRNA expression by 54.5% and 82.0% at a concentration of 10 and 20 µg/mL ($p < 0.001$), compared to untreated adipocytes (Figure 3B).

Our previous study showed that lingonberry fruit extract suppressed pro-inflammatory cytokines IL-6, IL-1β, and leptin expression, and significantly enhanced the expression of anti-inflammatory cytokines IL-10 and adiponectin in TNF-α-induced 3T3-L1 cells [11]. In mice fed the HF diet and supplemented with chokeberry juice concentrate, a higher plasma adiponectin level was observed [43]. Qin et al. (2012) have found that chokeberry extract elevated plasma adiponectin and inhibited plasma TNF-α and IL-6 levels in rats fed a high-fructose diet [35]. C57BL/6J mice fed the HF diet had elevated serum levels of TG, cholesterol, and leptin. Purified ACNs provided along with the HF diet led to decreasing serum TG, cholesterol, and leptin to the low-fat diet levels [44]. Tsuda et al. (2004) also found that adiponectin gene expression was upregulated in the WAT of ACN-fed mice [45].

Twenty healthy volunteers supplemented for 4 weeks with 200 mL/day of ACN-rich Queen Garnet plum juice for 4 weeks had a significantly reduced body weight and BMI with an average decrease of 0.6 kg in body weight and 0.2 units in BMI. Furthermore, consumption of ACN-rich plum juice significantly increased adiponectin blood levels (average increase of 3.8 µg/mL) and decreased leptin blood levels (average decrease of 1.3 ng/mL) [46]. A study conducted by Vugic et al. (2020) showed that the regular intake of ACNs reduced obesity-associated inflammation in obese subjects. The supplementation with purified ACNs for 28 days significantly reduced the plasma IL-6 level [47]. Several in vitro and in vivo studies confirmed that ACN-rich food consumption prevents obesity-related consequences such as diabetes, inflammation and oxidative stress. ACN supplementation favorably alters genes involved in glucose, FA and lipid metabolism, immune and inflammatory system, antioxidant defense, and the antiangiogenic system [48].

3.5. The Effects of PP and ACN Fractions on TNF-α-Induced Endothelial Dysfunction

The endothelium plays a vital role in vascular homeostasis and response to various stimuli, synthesizing and releasing many vasoactive substances, growth modulators, and other elements that mediate/influence these functions. The loss of balance between pro-atherogenic and antiatherogenic factors production leads to endothelial dysfunction [49]. The plasma levels of markers of endothelial activation, such as vascular cell adhesion molecule (VCAM), intercellular adhesion molecule (ICAM), endothelin 1 (ET-1), E-selectin (SELE), and markers of low-grade inflammation such as CRP, IL-1β, and IL-6 indicate the endothelial dysfunction [7]. Obesity has been confirmed to activate endothelial cell functions. It has been shown that endothelial cells of obese mice express higher levels of ICAM-1 [50].

Our study examined the ability of ACN and PP fractions to decrease endothelial dysfunction in HUVECs induced by TNF-α. Accumulating evidence from clinical trials and basic research proves a crucial role of TNF-α in vascular dysfunction and vascular disease [51]. TNF-α is a proinflammatory cytokine with multiple immune response functions, playing a pivotal role in low-grade systemic inflammation. TNF-α-mediated signaling pathways initiate and stimulate atherosclerosis, thrombosis, vasculitis, vascular oxidative stress, and endothelial cell apoptosis, contributing to vascular impairment [51]. A close relationship between TNF-α upregulation and lipid metabolism and HF and high-carbohydrate diets has been reported in several studies. Significantly increased plasma levels of TNF-α, IL-6, ICAM-1, and VCAM-1 have been observed in patients with hyperlipidaemia, obesity, metabolic syndrome, and type 2 diabetes [51,52]. In our study, TNF-α significantly stimulated several inflammation-related genes and adhesion molecules such as IL-6, IL-1β, VCAM-1, ICAM-1, and SELE in HUVECs. Compared to control cells, PP and ACN fractions decreased TNF-α-induced increase in IL-6, IL-1β, VACM-1, and ICAM-1 expression in a dose-dependent manner (Figure 4A,B). After incubation of HUVECs with a PP fraction at a concentration of 10 µg/mL, *IL-6* and *IL-1β* mRNA expression decreased by 49.6% and 45.0% ($p < 0.001$), respectively. The mRNA expression of *VCAM-1*, *ICAM-1*, and *SELE* decreased by 25.5% ($p < 0.05$), 25.0% ($p < 0.01$), and 38.0% ($p < 0.01$) (Figure 4A). The ACN fraction at a dose of 10 µg/mL suppressed *IL-6*, *IL-1β*, and *VCAM-1* mRNA expression by 74.0%, 50.0%, and 65.6%, respectively ($p < 0.001$). The ACN fraction did not affect *ICAM-1* and *SELE* expression (Figure 4B). In TNF-α-induced HUVECs, the upregulated VCAM-1, ICAM-1, and E-selectin were meaningfully reduced by pretreatment with quercetin [53]. ACNs and hydroxycinnamic acids present in blueberry and cranberry fruits reduced TNF-α-induced upregulation of various inflammatory mediators (IL-8, MCP-1, and ICAM-1) in HUVECs [54]. A clinical study with 27 subjects with metabolic syndrome has shown that consumption of freeze-dried strawberry for 8 weeks decreased circulating levels of VCAM-1 by 18%, while no effects were noted in ICAM-1 [55]. Ruel et al. (2008) reported a significant decrease in adhesion molecules (ICAM-1 and VCAM-1) in healthy volunteers after a 12-week supplementation with low-calorie cranberry juice [56]. Mechanisms that link obesity and endothelial dysfunctions are multidirectional and complex. Several clinical studies have shown that reducing WAT hypertrophy leads to decreased plasma levels of various adipocytokines, attenuates the pro-inflammatory state, and improves endothelial functions [57].

In summary, the results have shown that PP and ACN fractions obtained from lingonberry fruit ameliorate adipocyte hypertrophy by acting directly on the molecular and cellular pathways. Both fractions decreased intracellular ROS generation by enhancing the expression of antioxidant defense enzyme SOD2 and inhibiting oxidant enzymes such as NOX4 and iNOS. Moreover, PP and ACN fractions downregulated the expression of *FAS*, *DGAT1*, and *aP2*, which resulted in reduced TG content in adipocytes. Both fractions downregulated the expression of pro-inflammatory mediators (IL-6 and leptin), and upregulated adiponectin expression. To our knowledge, the present study is the first to show the protective effect of PP and ACN fractions from lingonberry fruit on endothelial functions by significantly decreasing the expression of several inflammation-related genes and adhesion molecules such as *IL-6*, *IL-1β*, *VCAM-1*, *ICAM-1* and *SELE* in TNF-α-induced HUVECs. These results suggest that consuming polyphenol-rich lingonberry fruit may help prevent and treat obesity and endothelial dysfunction due to their antioxidant and anti-inflammatory actions. Thus, lingonberries could be a dietary recommendation for preventing and managing obesity and cardiovascular complications, although further in vivo studies in animal models, followed by clinical trials, are needed.

Supplementary Materials: The following are available online at https://www.mdpi.com/2072-6643/13/3/885/s1, Table S1: The primers sequence used for real-time PCR.

Author Contributions: Conceptualization, K.K. and A.O.; methodology, K.K., R.D., and A.O.; validation, K.K. and A.G.; formal analysis, A.O.; investigation, K.K., R.D., A.G., and M.O.; writing—original draft preparation, K.K.; writing—review and editing, A.O.; visualization, K.K.; project administration, A.O.; funding acquisition, A.O. All authors have read and agreed to the published version of the manuscript.

Funding: This research was funded by the NATIONAL SCIENCE CENTRE, POLAND, grant number 2015/19/B/NZ9/01054.

Conflicts of Interest: The authors declare no conflict of interest. The funders had no role in the design of the study; in the collection, analyses, or interpretation of data; in the writing of the manuscript; or in the decision to publish the results.

References

1. Barroso, T.A.; Marins, L.B.; Alves, R.; Gonçalves, A.C.S.; Barroso, S.G.; Rocha, G.D.S. Association of central obesity with the incidence of cardiovascular diseases and risk factors. *Int. J. Cardiovasc. Sci.* **2017**, *30*, 416–424. [CrossRef]
2. Lafontan, M. Adipose tissue and adipocyte dysregulation. *Diabetes Metab.* **2013**, *40*, 16–28. [CrossRef] [PubMed]
3. Al Suwaidi, J.; Higano, S.T.; Holmes, D.R., Jr.; Lennon, R.; Lerman, A. Obesity is independently associated with coronary endothelial dysfunction in patients with normal or mildly diseased coronary arteries. *J. Am. Coll. Cardiol.* **2001**, *37*, 1523–1528. [CrossRef]
4. Brown, N.K.; Zhou, Z.; Zhang, J.; Zeng, R.; Wu, J.; Eitzman, D.T.; Chen, Y.E.; Chang, L. Perivascular adipose tissue in vascular function and disease: A review of current research and animal models. *Arterioscler. Thromb. Vasc. Biol.* **2014**, *34*, 1621–1630. [CrossRef] [PubMed]
5. Daiber, A.; Steven, S.; Weber, A.; Shuvaev, V.V.; Muzykantov, V.R.; Laher, I.; Li, H.; Lamas, S.; Munzel, T. Targeting vascular (endothelial) dysfunction. *Br. J. Pharmacol.* **2017**, *174*, 1591–1619. [CrossRef] [PubMed]
6. Heitzer, T.; Schlinzig, T.; Krohn, K.; Meinertz, T.; Munzel, T. Endothelial dysfunction, oxidative stress, and risk of cardiovascular events in patients with coronary artery disease. *Circulation* **2001**, *104*, 2673–2678. [CrossRef]
7. Caballero, A.E. Endothelial dysfunction in obesity and insulin resistance: A road to diabetes and heart disease. *Obes. Res.* **2003**, *11*, 1278–1289. [CrossRef]
8. Kowalska, K.; Olejnik, A. Current evidence on the health-beneficial effects of berry fruits in the prevention and treatment of metabolic syndrome. *Curr. Opin. Clin. Nutr. Metab. Care* **2016**, *19*, 446–452. [CrossRef]
9. Szajdek, A.; Borowska, E.J. Bioactive compounds and health-promoting properties of berry fruits: A review. *Plant Foods Hum. Nutr.* **2008**, *63*, 147–156. [CrossRef]
10. Szakiel, A.; Pączkowski, C.; Koivuniemi, H.; Huttunen, S. Comparison of the triterpenoid content of berries and leaves of lingonberry *Vaccinium vitis-idaea* from Finland and Poland. *J. Agric. Food Chem.* **2012**, *60*, 4994–5002. [CrossRef]
11. Kowalska, K.; Olejnik, A.; Zielińska-Wasielica, J.; Olkowicz, M. Inhibitory effects of lingonberry (*Vaccinium vitis-idaea* L.) fruit extract on obesity-induced inflammation in 3T3-L1 adipocytes and RAW 264.7 macrophages. *J. Funct. Foods* **2019**, *54*, 371–380. [CrossRef]
12. Eid, H.M.; Ouchfoun, M.; Brault, A.; Vallerand, D.; Musallam, L.; Arnason, J.T.; Haddad, P.S. Lingonberry (*Vaccinium vitis-idaea* L.) exhibits antidiabetic activities in a mouse model of diet-induced obesity. *Evid. Based Complement. Alternat. Med.* **2014**, *2014*, 645812. [CrossRef] [PubMed]

13. Kowalska, K.; Olejnik, A.; Rychlik, J.; Grajek, W. Cranberries (Oxycoccus quadripetalus) inhibit adipogenesis and lipogenesis in 3T3-L1 cells. *Food Chem.* **2014**, *148*, 246–252. [CrossRef] [PubMed]
14. Choi, H.S.; Kim, J.W.; Cha, Y.N.; Kim, C. A quantitative nitroblue tetrazolium assay for determining intracellular superoxide anion production in phagocytic cells. *J. Immunoass. Immunochem.* **2006**, *27*, 31–44. [CrossRef] [PubMed]
15. Galili, O.; Versari, D.; Sattler, K.J.; Olson, M.L.; Mannheim, D.; McConnell, J.P.; Chade, A.R.; Lerman, L.O.; Lerman, A. Early experimental obesity is associated with coronary endothelial dysfunction and oxidative stress. *Am. J. Physiol. Heart Circ. Physiol.* **2007**, *292*, H904–H911. [CrossRef]
16. Cai, H.; Harrison, D.G. Endothelial dysfunction in cardiovascular diseases. The role of oxidant stress. *Circ. Res.* **2000**, *87*, 840–844. [CrossRef] [PubMed]
17. Furukawa, S.; Fujita, T.; Shimabukuro, M.; Iwaki, M.; Yamada, Y.; Nakajima, Y.; Nakayama, O.; Makishima, M.; Matsuda, M.; Shimomura, I. Increased oxidative stress in obesity and its impact on metabolic syndrome. *J. Clin. Investig.* **2004**, *114*, 1752–1761. [CrossRef]
18. Perreault, M.; Marette, A. Targeted disruption of inducible nitric oxide synthase protects against obesity-linked insulin resistance in muscle. *Nat. Med.* **2001**, *7*, 1138–1143. [CrossRef]
19. Hopps, E.; Noto, D.; Caimi, G.; Averna, M.R. A novel component of the metabolic syndrome: The oxidative stress. *Nutr. Metab. Cardiovasc. Dis.* **2010**, *20*, 72–77. [CrossRef] [PubMed]
20. Yen, G.C.; Chen, Y.C.; Chang, W.T.; Hsu, C.L. Effects of polyphenolic compounds on tumor necrosis factor-α (TNF-α)-induced changes of adipokines and oxidative stress in 3T3-L1 adipocytes. *J. Agric. Food Chem.* **2011**, *59*, 546–551. [CrossRef] [PubMed]
21. Guo, H.; Ling, W.; Wang, Q.; Liu, C.; Hu, Y.; Xia, M. Cyanidin 3-glucoside protects 3T3-L1 adipocytes against H_2O_2- or TNF-alpha-induced insulin resistance by inhibiting c-Jun NH2-terminal kinase activation. *Biochem. Pharmacol.* **2008**, *75*, 1393–1401. [CrossRef]
22. Marimoutou, M.; Le Sage, F.; Smadja, J.; Lefebvre d'Hellencourt, C.; Gonthier, M.P.; Robert-Da Silva, C. Antioxidant polyphenol-rich extracts from the medicinal plants Antirhea borbonica, Doratoxylon apetalum and Gouania mauritiana protect 3T3-L1 preadipocytes against H_2O_2, TNFα and LPS inflammatory mediators by regulating the expression of superoxide dismutase and NF-κB genes. *J. Inflamm.* **2015**, *12*, 10. [CrossRef]
23. Mane, C.; Loonis, M.; Juhel, C.; Dufour, C.; Malien-Aubert, C. Food grade lingonberry extract: Polyphenolic composition and in vivo protective effect against oxidative stress. *J. Agric. Food Chem.* **2011**, *59*, 3330–3339. [CrossRef]
24. Yang, X.F.; Qiu, Y.Q.; Wang, L.; Gao, K.G.; Jiang, Z.Y. A high-fat diet increases body fat mass and up-regulates expression of genes related to adipogenesis and inflammation in a genetically lean pig. *J. Zhejiang Univ. Sci. B* **2018**, *19*, 884–894. [CrossRef]
25. Chen, H.C.; Farese, R.V., Jr. Inhibition of triglyceride synthesis as a treatment strategy for obesity: Lessons from DGAT1-deficient mice. *Arterioscler. Thromb. Vasc. Biol.* **2005**, *25*, 482–486. [CrossRef]
26. Hotamisligil, G.S. Inflammation, metaflammation and immunometabolic disorders. *Nature* **2017**, *542*, 177–185. [CrossRef] [PubMed]
27. Furuhashi, M. Fatty Acid-Binding Protein 4 in Cardiovascular and Metabolic Diseases. *J. Atheroscler. Thromb.* **2019**, *26*, 216–232. [CrossRef] [PubMed]
28. Berndt, J.; Kovacs, P.; Ruschke, K.; Klöting, N.; Fasshauer, M.; Schön, M.R.; Körner, A.; Stumvoll, M.; Blüher, M. Fatty acid synthase gene expression in human adipose tissue: Association with obesity and type 2 diabetes. *Diabetologia* **2007**, *50*, 1472–1480. [CrossRef] [PubMed]
29. Chen, H.C.; Jensen, R.; Myers, H.M.; Eckel, R.H.; Farese, R.V., Jr. Obesity resistance and enhanced glucose metabolism in mice transplanted with white adipose tissue lacking acyl CoA:diacylglycerol acyltransferase 1. *J. Clin. Investig.* **2003**, *111*, 1715–1722. [CrossRef] [PubMed]
30. Makowski, L.; Hotamisligil, G.S. Fatty acid binding proteins—The evolutionary crossroads of inflammatory and metabolic responses. *J. Nutr.* **2004**, *134*, 2464S–2468S. [CrossRef]
31. Naik, R.; Obiang-Obounou, B.W.; Kim, M.; Choi, Y.; Lee, H.S.; Lee, K. Therapeutic strategies for metabolic diseases: Small-molecule diacylglycerol acyltransferase (DGAT) inhibitors. *Chem. Med. Chem.* **2014**, *9*, 2410–2424. [CrossRef]
32. Kondo, H.; Hashizume, K.; Shibuya, Y.; Hase, T.; Murase, T. Identification of diacylglycerol acyltransferase inhibitors from Rosa centifolia petals. *Lipids* **2011**, *46*, 691–700. [CrossRef]
33. Belwal, T.; Nabavi, S.F.; Nabavi, S.M.; Habtemariam, S. Dietary Anthocyanins and Insulin Resistance: When Food Becomes a Medicine. *Nutrients* **2017**, *9*, 1111. [CrossRef]
34. Heyman, L.; Axling, U.; Blanco, N.; Sterner, O.; Holm, C.; Berger, K. Evaluation of beneficial metabolic effects of berries in high-fat fed C57BL/6J mice. *J. Nutr. Metab.* **2014**, 403041. [CrossRef] [PubMed]
35. Qin, B.; Anderson, R.A. An extract of chokeberry attenuates weight gain and modulates insulin, adipogenic and inflammatory signalling pathways in epididymal adipose tissue of rats fed a fructose-rich diet. *Br. J. Nutr.* **2012**, *108*, 581–587. [CrossRef] [PubMed]
36. Zhu, W.; Cheng, K.K.; Vanhoutte, P.M.; Lam, K.S.; Xu, A. Vascular effects of adiponectin: Molecular mechanisms and potential therapeutic intervention. *Clin. Sci.* **2008**, *114*, 361–374. [CrossRef] [PubMed]
37. Li, C.J.; Sun, H.W.; Zhu, F.L.; Chen, L.; Rong, Y.Y.; Zhang, Y.; Zhang, M. Local adiponectin treatment reduces atherosclerotic plaque size in rabbits. *J. Endocrinol.* **2007**, *193*, 137–145. [CrossRef] [PubMed]

38. Lonnqvist, F.; Nordfors, L.; Jansson, M.; Thorne, A.; Schalling, M.; Arner, P. Leptin secretion from adipose tissue in women: Relationship to plasma levels and gene expression. *J. Clin. Investig.* **1997**, *99*, 2398–2404. [CrossRef]
39. Beltowski, J.; Wójcicka, G.; Marciniak, A.; Jamroz, A. Oxidative stress, nitric oxide production, and renal sodium handling in leptin-induced hypertension. *Life Sci.* **2004**, *74*, 2987–3000. [CrossRef]
40. Bouloumie, A.; Marumo, T.; Lafontan, M.; Busse, R. Leptin induces oxidative stress in human endothelial cells. *FASEB J.* **1999**, *13*, 1231–1238. [CrossRef]
41. Yudkin, J.S.; Kumari, M.; Humphries, S.E.; Mohamed-Ali, V. Inflammation, obesity, stress and coronary heart disease: Is interleukin-6 the link? *Atherosclerosis* **2000**, *148*, 209–214. [CrossRef]
42. McDermott, M.M.; Liu, K.; Ferrucci, L.; Tian, L.; Guralnik, J.M.; Tao, H.; Ridker, P.M.; Criqui, M.H. Relation of interleukin-6 and vascular cellular adhesion molecule-1 levels to functional decline in patients with lower extremity peripheral arterial disease. *Am. J. Cardiol.* **2011**, *107*, 1392–1398. [CrossRef]
43. Baum, J.I.; Howard, L.R.; Prior, R.L.; Lee, S.O. Effect of Aronia melanocarpa (Black Chokeberry) supplementation on the development of obesity in mice fed a high-fat diet. *J. Berry Res.* **2016**, *6*, 203–212. [CrossRef]
44. Prior, R.L.; Wu, X.; Gu, L.; Hager, T.; Hager, A.; Wilkes, S.; Howard, L. Purified berry anthocyanins but not whole berries normalize lipid parameters in mice fed an obesogenic high fat diet. *Mol. Nutr. Food Res.* **2009**, *53*, 1406–1418. [CrossRef]
45. Tsuda, T.; Ueno, Y.; Aoki, H.; Koda, T.; Horio, F.; Takahashi, N.; Kawada, T.; Osawa, T. Anthocyanin enhances adipocytokine secretion and adipocyte-specific gene expression in isolated rat adipocytes. *Biochem. Biophys. Res. Commun.* **2004**, *316*, 149–157. [CrossRef]
46. Tucakovic, L.; Colson, N.; Santhakumar, A.B.; Kundur, A.R.; Shuttleworth, M.; Singh, I. The effects of anthocyanins on body weight and expression of adipocyte's hormones: Leptin and adiponectin. *J. Funct. Foods* **2018**, *45*, 173–180. [CrossRef]
47. Vugic, L.; Colson, N.; Nikbakht, E.; Gaiz, A.; Holland, O.J.; Kundur, A.R.; Singh, I. Anthocyanin supplementation inhibits secretion of pro-inflammatory cytokines in overweight and obese individuals. *J. Funct. Foods* **2020**, *64*, 103596. [CrossRef]
48. Sivamaruthi, B.S.; Kesika, P.; Chaiyasut, C. The Influence of Supplementation of Anthocyanins on Obesity-Associated Comorbidities: A Concise Review. *Foods* **2020**, *9*, 687. [CrossRef] [PubMed]
49. Quyyumi, A.A. Endothelial function in health and disease: New insights into the genesis of cardiovascular disease. *Am. J. Med.* **1998**, *105*, 32S–39S. [CrossRef]
50. Fernández-Alfonso, M.S.; Somoza, B.; Tsvetkov, D.; Kuczmanski, A.; Dashwood, M.; Gil-Ortega, M. Role of Perivascular Adipose Tissue in Health and Disease. *Compr. Physiol.* **2017**, *8*, 23–59. [CrossRef]
51. Zhang, H.; Park, Y.; Wu, J.; Chen, X.; Lee, S.; Yang, J.; Dellsperger, K.C.; Zhang, C. Role of TNF-alpha in vascular dysfunction. *Clin. Sci.* **2009**, *116*, 219–230. [CrossRef]
52. Esposito, K.; Ciotola, M.; Sasso, F.C.; Cozzolino, D.; Saccomanno, F.; Assaloni, R.; Ceriello, A.; Giugliano, D. Effect of a single high-fat meal on endothelial function in patients with the metabolic syndrome: Role of tumor necrosis factor-α. *Nutr. Metab. Cardiovasc. Dis.* **2007**, *17*, 274–279. [CrossRef]
53. Chen, T.; Zhang, X.; Zhu, G.; Liu, H.; Chen, J.; Wang, Y.; He, X. Quercetin inhibits TNF-α induced HUVECs apoptosis and inflammation via downregulating NF-kB and AP-1 signaling pathway in vitro. *Medicine* **2020**, *99*, e22241. [CrossRef]
54. Youdim, K.A.; McDonald, J.; Kalt, W.; Joseph, J.A. Potential role of dietary flavonoids in reducing microvascular endothelium vulnerability to oxidative and inflammatory insults. *J. Nutr. Biochem.* **2002**, *13*, 282–288. [CrossRef]
55. Basu, A.; Fu, D.X.; Wilkinson, M.; Simmons, B.; Wu, M.; Betts, N.M.; Du, M.; Lyons, T.J. Strawberries decrease atherosclerotic markers in subjects with metabolic syndrome. *Nutr. Res.* **2010**, *30*, 462–469. [CrossRef] [PubMed]
56. Ruel, G.; Pomerleau, S.; Couture, P.; Lemieux, S.; Lamarche, B.; Couillard, C. Low-calorie cranberry juice supplementation reduces plasma oxidized LDL and cell adhesion molecule concentrations in men. *Br. J. Nutr.* **2008**, *99*, 352–359. [CrossRef] [PubMed]
57. Ziccardi, P.; Nappo, F.; Giugliano, G.; Esposito, K.; Marfella, R.; Cioffi, M.; D'Andrea, F.; Molinari, A.M.; Giugliano, D. Reduction of inflammatory cytokine concentrations and improvement of endothelial functions in obese women after weight loss over one year. *Circulation* **2002**, *105*, 804–809. [CrossRef] [PubMed]

Review

Redox and Anti-Inflammatory Properties from Hop Components in Beer-Related to Neuroprotection

Gustavo Ignacio Vazquez-Cervantes [1], Daniela Ramírez Ortega [1], Tonali Blanco Ayala [1], Verónica Pérez de la Cruz [1], Dinora Fabiola González Esquivel [1], Aleli Salazar [2] and Benjamín Pineda [2,*]

[1] Laboratory of Neurobiochemistry and Behavior, National Institute of Neurology and Neurosurgery, 14269 Mexico City, Mexico; guigvace@gmail.com (G.I.V.-C.); drmz_ortega@hotmail.com (D.R.O.); tonaliblaya@gmail.com (T.B.A.); veped@yahoo.com.mx (V.P.d.l.C.); dinora.gonzlez@gmail.com (D.F.G.E.)
[2] Laboratory of Neuroimmunology, National Institute of Neurology and Neurosurgery, 14269 Mexico City, Mexico; ajsalazar27@gmail.com
* Correspondence: benpio76@hotmail.com; Tel.: +52-55-5606-3822 (ext. 2003)

Abstract: Beer is a fermented beverage widely consumed worldwide with high nutritional and biological value due to its bioactive components. It has been described that both alcoholic and non-alcoholic beer have several nutrients derived from their ingredients including vitamins, minerals, proteins, carbohydrates, and antioxidants that make beer a potential functional supplement. Some of these compounds possess redox, anti-inflammatory and anticarcinogenic properties making the benefits of moderate beer consumption an attractive way to improve human health. Specifically, the hop cones used for beer brewing provide essential oils, bitter acids and flavonoids that are potent antioxidants and immune response modulators. This review focuses on the redox and anti-inflammatory properties of hop derivatives and summarizes the current knowledge of their neuroprotective effects.

Keywords: hop; antioxidant; xanthohumol; prenylflavonoids; beer

1. Generalities

Beer is an alcoholic natural beverage, not distilled, from barley extract. The traditional ingredients for brewing beer are barley (malt), hops (*Humulus lupulus* L.), yeast, and water. The brewing steps and brewing conditions are essential to generate specific beer characteristics and quality. In general, the first step of brewing is the malting process which consists of germinating the barley grains in water; subsequently, the flavor and color of the beer are given by roasting the grains. Afterward, a sweet mixture is obtained by grinding the cereal at the appropriate temperature. After boiling, the female inflorescences of the hop plant (*Humulus lupulus* L., Cannabaceae) are added, giving a colloidal strength to beer. It should be noted that beer bitterness is attributable to the hop plant. The final step of brewing is fermentation, which begins just after yeast addition. The most used yeast strains are *Saccharomyces cerevisiae* (stout, ale and porter beers) and *Saccharomyces uvarum* (lager beers); however, non-conventional yeast strains have also been used [1,2]. According to the fermentation parameters used during brewing, beers are classified into two major classes: top and bottom-fermented beers. In top-fermented beers (ale-type beers), yeast growth occurs in the upper part of the container and the fermentation temperature ranges between 16 °C and 24 °C; while in the bottom-fermented beers (lagers), yeast growth occurs in the base of the container and the fermentation temperature ranges between 8 °C and 15 °C [3].

The moderate consumption of beer has been related to beneficial human health effects; however, harmful effects have been described by the consumption of beverages with high alcohol content. Low-moderate intake of alcohol is considered up to one drink per day for women and up to two in men (considering that typically a can of beer has 330 mL containing about 4% *w/v* alcohol). Drinking beer contributes to the intake of carbohydrates and it can be an important risk factor for obesity and overweight; nevertheless, an inconsistency between beer consumption and obesity has been observed due to the contribution of other risk factors such as individual diet, physical activity, or the consumption of other alcoholic beverages [2,4,5]. On the other hand, it has been described that the regular and moderate consumption of beer confers cardiovascular protection similar to that of wine; and also reduces mortality both in healthy adults and in cardiovascular patients [6]. However, alcohol abuse is harmful to several human organs and a major social and health problem associated with addictions, accidents, violence, and crime [7–10]. Additionally, moderate beer consumption has been associated with lipid profile improvement in blood plasma; reduction in leukocyte adhesion molecules and inflammatory markers improving the prognosis of cardiovascular diseases such as atherosclerosis and thrombotic ailments. Other studies regarding beer consumption showed better beneficial effects in vascular endothelial function and pressure wave reflections compared to other kinds of alcoholic beverages [2,6,11,12]. Clinical studies have suggested that the moderate consumption of beer is beneficial for human health, mainly due to the phenolic compounds with antioxidant and anti-inflammatory properties.

Beer is a beverage rich in phenolic compounds derived from hop (30%) and malt (70–80%) [13]. It has been described that its phenolic acid content ranges from 3 to 12 mg/L and its total polyphenol content ranges from 74 to 256 mg/L in 34 different lager beers brewed in various geographic locations [14]. Specifically, the resin secreted by lupulin glands contains bitter acids, essential oils, and prenylated flavonoids (Figure 1) that have received particular attention because of their high antioxidant, anti-inflammatory and anticarcinogenic effects, among others. Recently, a study focused on the biosynthesis and regulation of these compounds demonstrated an increased expression of transcription factors and structural genes in lupulin glands after leaf development, which correlated with increased levels of bitter acids and prenylflavonoids in these glands [15]. Derived compounds from hop are used as a source of bitterness, herbal aroma and natural preservative.

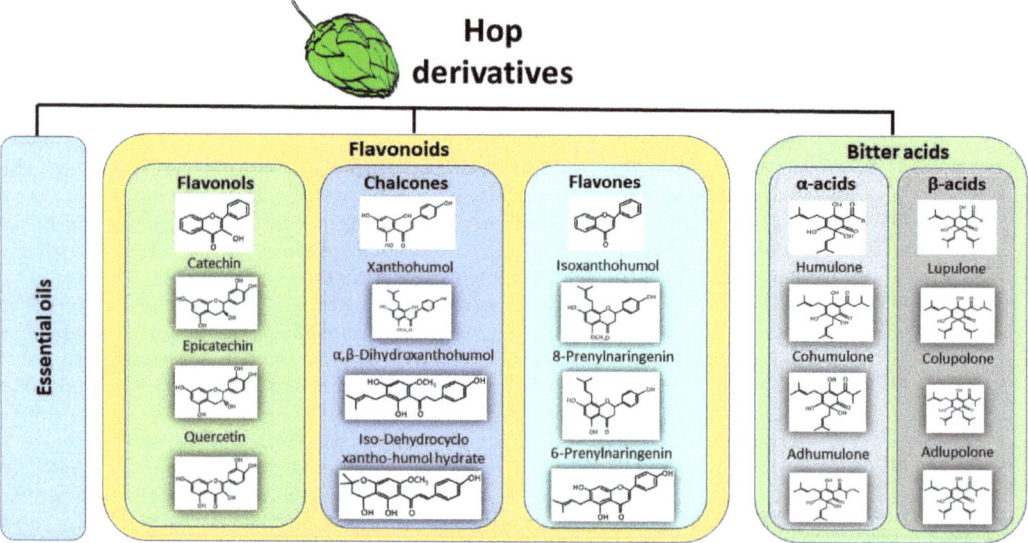

Figure 1. The main derived compounds from hop cones. Hop cones are the main source of bioactive compounds during the brewing process. Hops contribute essential oils, phenolic compounds such as flavonoids which can be further classified into flavonols, chalcones, and flavones. Hop cones contain α-acids and β-acids also known as bitter acids.

Essential oils represent 0.5–3.0% from hop dry weight and can be classified into hydrocarbons (50–80% of total oil) such as limonene, myrcene, and pinene; oxygenated compounds (30% of total oil), such as linalool, caryophyllene, geraniol, and farnesol; and sulfur-containing compounds (around 1% of total oil) [16]. The bitter acids found in hops are α-acids (humulone, cohumulone, and adhumulone) and β-acids (lupulone, colupulone, and adlupulone) that differ from each other because the β-acids contain an extra isoprenyl group [17]. After thermal isomerization during the brewing process, α-acids are transformed into iso-α-acids (which occurs favorably at temperatures around 100–130 °C and pH of 8–9) which are considered the primary drivers of hop-derived beer bitterness, meanwhile, β-acids are oxidized during the brewing process [16,18,19]. Additionally, hops are a source of polyphenols; however, brewing malt is the major source of these compounds [20]. The main hop polyphenols are flavonoids, catechins, phenolic acids, prenylated-chalcones and proanthocyanidins. Prenylated flavonoids combine a flavonoid skeleton with a lipophilic prenyl side-chain, increasing the lipophilicity of flavonoids [21]. Xanthohumol is the principal prenylated chalcone in the lupulin glands (0.1–1% in dry weight), but it is a minor prenylflavonoid in beer since it contains a free 2′-hydroxy group which, after thermal isomerization during the brewing process, produces its corresponding flavanone isoxanthohumol (ranging from 0.04 to 3.44 mg/L), which is the most abundant flavonoid in beer [22–24]. A pharmacokinetic study performed in healthy subjects (24 males of 31 ± 2 years old and 24 females 35 ± 2 years old) showed that after a single oral dose of 20, 60 or 180 mg of xanthohumol, the maximum xanthohumol concentrations were 33, 48 and 120 mg/L, respectively, with isoxanthohumol being the main circulating metabolite [25]. Beer is the principal dietary source of xanthohumol and related prenylflavonoids [23], their health benefits as well as the mechanism by which these hop derivatives act are the subject of several investigations.

The next section describes the current knowledge on redox, anti-inflammatory and immunomodulatory effects of hop components in experimental models, mainly focused in xanthohumol and its derivative isoxanthohumol, which represents the major prenylflavonoid in beer. Subsequently, a comprehensive compilation of human beer consumption effects as well as hop components on redox, anti-inflammatory and immunomodulatory markers are summarized. Some novel information of selected beer hop components on neuroprotection is also provided.

2. Redox Properties from Hop Derivatives on Beer

Free radicals and reactive oxygen species (ROS) are highly reactive compounds that easily oxidize other molecules by taking up electrons [26]. ROS are normally produced during cell metabolism mainly in the mitochondrial electron transport chain, which has been described as an important role of ROS in the regulation of metabolism, cell cycle and survival, among others [26,27]. However, when excessive ROS are produced, the oxidation of biomolecules such as lipids, proteins, and nucleic acids occurs, leading to cellular stress and oxidative damage. The role of oxidative stress in the progression of several diseases and aging has been widely reported, which is the reason why much investigation is focused on the search for compounds that attenuate the oxidation processes [26–29].

The benefits of hop derivatives contained in beer are associated with their ability to modulate the redox environment since they can scavenge a wide range of reactive oxygen species, but it has also been described that hop components can modulate the expression and activity of antioxidant enzymes and the glutathione (GSH) levels, thus protecting against toxic stimulus.

Several studies have evaluated the antioxidant capacity of beer varieties, finding that their redox activity depends on their polyphenolic amount. The polyphenolic content varies depending on the type of beer from 366 gallic acid equivalents (GAEs) mg/L in alcohol-free beers to 875 GAE mg/L in bock beers [30]. In general, beers are able to scavenge free radicals in ferric antioxidant power (FRAP) and 2,2-azino-bis (3-ethylbenzothiazoline-6-6sulphonic acid) (ABTS) assays, among others, as well as to prevent DNA oxidation [30–34]. In recent years, many research groups have studied the redox properties of beers characterizing the fractions obtained during brewing or testing individual components.

In 2009, Gerhauserin [35] analyzed the scavenging capacity of 51 phenolic beer compounds. The redox activity of polyphenols is determined in part by the OH groups found in the aromatic nucleus, mainly in the C4′ and C3′ positions. General radical scavenging potential was determined by the reaction with 1,1-diphenyl-2-picrylhydrazyl (DPPH), the group of proanthocyanidins and flavonols that had a better scavenging potential considering their half maximal scavenging concentration (SC_{50} 7.6–16 µM and 10.4–23.7 µM, respectively). When the phenolic compounds were exposed to a system able to chemically generate superoxide, the best scavenging profile was shown by protoanthocyanidins, catechins, flavonols and flavones. However, when the superoxide was produced by an enzymatic reaction, the catechins and proanthocyanidins were identified as the most potent scavengers of the beer phenolic compounds tested. Furthermore, xanthohumol, saponaretin and 4-ketopinoresinol were the only compounds that showed the inhibition of superoxide production, stimulated with phorbolmyristate acetate (PMA) in HL60 human promyelocytic leukemia cells with an IC_{50} of 5.5 µM, 4.7 µM and 7.1 µM, respectively. Proanthocyanidins, catechins, flavonols, xanthohumol, and isoxanthohumol showed a better peroxyl radical scavenging potential than Trolox (vitamin E analogous with high antioxidant capacity) at 1 µM. The hydroxyl radical scavenging profile was also evaluated in phenolic beer compounds, most of them were able to scavenge this radical. However, xanthohumol was the best compound to scavenge hydroxyl radical followed by caffeic acid, myricetin and cinnamic acid when compared to Trolox [35].

Hop bitter acids, humulone and lupulone have a radical scavenging activity with an IC_{50} around $2–3 \times 10^{-5}$ M and lipid peroxidation inhibitory activity (7.9×10^{-6} and 3.9×10^{-5}, respectively), these effects were similar to those obtained with α-tocopherol and ascorbic acid. It has been suggested that the 5-hydroxyl group of bitter acids is the active site for radical scavenging activity since those analogs lacking this group do not have this activity [36].

One of the most studied and the most abundant prenylated chalcones (open C-ring flavonoids) from hops is the xanthohumol [22]. Xanthohumol is 9-fold and 3-fold more effective than Trolox in scavenging peroxyl and hydroxyl radicals, respectively. However, isoxanthohumol was more potent than xanthohumol for peroxyl radical scavenging and showed the same effect as Trolox for scavenging hydroxyl radicals. According to these data, xanthohumol (1.5 and 3 µM) reduced the electron spin resonance signal intensity of hydroxyl radical formation in a cell-free system (H_2O_2/NaOH/DMSO) [37]. Xanthohumol inhibited the production of superoxide in the xanthine/xanthine oxidase system with an IC_{50} 27.7 ± 4.9 µM, while xanthohumol showed an IC_{50} of 2.6 ± 0.4 µM for superoxide scavenging in TPA-stimulated HL-60 cells [38]. Both xanthohumol and isoxanthohumol reduced nitric oxide (NO) production (IC_{50} 12.9 ± 1.2 µM and 21.9 ± 2.6 µM, respectively) induced by lipopolysaccharide (LPS) in RAW 264.7 mouse macrophages [38]. An additional study showed that xanthohumol inhibited the production of NO with an IC_{50} 8.3 µM in RAW 264.7 macrophages exposed to LPS and IFN-γ [39]. According to these data, it was reported that the ethyl acetate soluble fraction of *Humulus lupulus* L. that contains chalcones including xanthohumol inhibits the production of NO by suppressing the expression of iNOS in RAW 264.7 cells exposed to LPS and IFN-γ [40].

Additionally, xanthohumol was able to neutralize around 60% of ABTS free radicals and decrease 30% of the thiobarbituric acid-reactive substances (TBARS) formation induced by free radicals in erythrocyte ghosts [41]. Furthermore, xanthohumol and other prenylated chalcones found in beers were able to inhibit the oxidation of human low-density lipoprotein (LDL), the formation of TBARS, and the oxidation of tryptophan residues in LDL induced by Cu^{2+} [42]. An additional study found that xanthohumol decreased lipid peroxidation in rat liver microsomes induced by Fe^{2+}-ascorbate or *tert*-butyl hydroperoxide (TBH). The protective effect of xanthohumol (0.1 and 0.5 µM) was observed in PC12 cells from H_2O_2-induced and 6-hydroxydopamine-induced cellular damage due to a reduction in both ROS production and caspase-3 activity [41]. It was also shown that 5 µM and 10 µM of this chalcone decreased lactate dehydrogenase activity (by around 25 and 50%, respectively) in the primary cultures of rat hepatocytes treated with TBH; this anti-cytotoxic effect showed by xanthohumol was related to its antioxidant activity [43].

The protective effects shown by xanthohumol can be in part related to the activation of nuclear factor erythroid-2-related factor 2 (Nrf2) and the expression of the Nrf2-driven antioxidant/detoxifying genes. Under normal conditions, Nrf2 is bonded to the Kelch-like ECH-associated protein 1 (Keap1) in the cytoplasm, and Nrf2 is ubiquitinated for its proteasomal degradation; however, under oxidative stress conditions, the Nrf2-Keap1 complex is dissociated and Nrf2 is translocated to the nucleus where it binds to the antioxidant-responsive element (ARE), thus promoting the transcription of antioxidant-protective genes such as heme oxygenase-1 (HO-1), NAD(P)H: quinone oxidoreductase 1 (NQO1), thioredoxin (Trx1), thioredoxin reductase 1 (TrxR1), glutamate cysteine ligase (GCL). It has been shown that xanthohumol increases the content of nuclear Nrf2 and decreases its cytosolic localization, indicating its nuclear translocation and promoting the antioxidant response. Moreover, it was demonstrated that xanthohumol (0.5 µM) increased the mRNA expression of HO-1, NQO1, Trx1, TrxR1, GCL after 6 and 12 h, with HO-1 and TrxR1 mRNAs being the most highly transcribed (by around 2.8- and 2.3-fold). In line with the upregulation of phase II enzymatic expression, the protein and activity of these enzymes as well as GSH levels were also increased by xanthohumol [41]. Likewise, it has been suggested that the anti-inflammatory effect shown by xanthohumol could be related to its Nrf2-ARE signaling modulation [44].

The antioxidant cellular modulation by hop components contributes to the beneficial effects of beer intake. There is in vivo evidence that beer intake (0.5 mL/day) reduces lipid peroxidation and TNFα over-expression induced by the oral administration of aluminum in mice. These effects were related to the restoration of the antioxidant enzymatic expression of catalase and superoxide dismutase [45]. Another study demonstrated that treatment with beer fractions derived from the brewing process reduced oxidative stress as well as the senescence induced by H_2O_2 in dental-derived stem cells and human intestinal epithelial lines (Caco-2 cells) [13]. Moreover, the consumption of beer with or without alcohol restored the enzymatic activity of complex I and IV and prevented the oxidation of coenzymes Q_9 and Q_{10} in the heart and liver mitochondria from rats treated with adriamycin [46]. In addition to redox modulation, the immunomodulatory and anti-inflammatory effects of the hop components were extensively studied and are described in the following section.

3. Anti-Inflammatory and Immunomodulatory Effects of Beer Compounds

Crosstalk between the oxidative and pro-inflammatory signals has been described, making these two important factors in the progression of age-related disorders. Inflammation is the response elicited by the immune system to counteract noxious agents, which is a complex process that requires the precise balance of intracellular and extracellular signals, first elicited by the innate immune system cell populations including neutrophils, macrophages, dendritic cells and natural killer cells, later reinforced by the components of the adaptive immune response, T and B lymphocytes [47]. The synchronic orchestration of both innate and adaptive immune responses leads to the beginning and control of inflammation, and the reestablishment of the organism homeostasis. However, dysregulated inflammation is associated with the development of age-related disorders such as cancer, neurodegenerative diseases, and chronic inflammation disorders [48].

Thus, in addition to the search for natural compounds with antioxidant properties, finding anti-inflammatory or immunomodulatory characteristics in the same molecules would be ideal. In light of this, both the anti-inflammatory role of isolated beer compounds as well as the effect of moderate beer consumption on the immune system have been investigated. It was reported that beer consumption in healthy rats, considering a daily ethanol consumption of 1.16 g/kg, has no impact on the relative abundance of the different lymphocytic populations [49]. Additionally, the positive effects of beer consumption have been demonstrated, since this prevented the formation of atherosclerotic plaques in addition to the decrease in the expression of the endothelial adhesion molecules: intercellular adhesion molecules (ICAMs) and vascular cell adhesion molecules (VCAMs), together with a decreased expression of the nuclear factor κB (NF-κB, an important transcription factor that drives the production of pro-inflammatory signals), indicating an anti-inflammatory effect in atherosclerotic rats [50]. Moreover, beer consumption promoted anti-tumor immune responses and increased the number of T lymphocytes on tumor-bearing rats [51].

As mentioned above, the female cones of hop are a major source of beer polyphenols and bioactive compounds. Thus, the effect as immunomodulators of the whole hop extracts in the immune system has been studied (Figure 2). In vitro treatments using hop extracts on LPS-stimulated macrophages and peripheral blood mononuclear cells (PBMCs) decreased the levels of the proinflammatory cytokines interleukin (IL)-1β, IL-6, tumor necrosis factor (TNF)-α and the monocyte chemo-attractant protein (MCP)-1; in addition, they decreased the production of nitric oxide (NO), a diffusible ROS involved in vasodilation and immune infiltration [52–54]. The anti-inflammatory activity of hop extracts is attributed to the inhibition of the NF-κB activation. Hop extracts also decreased the activity of the enzyme cyclo-oxygenase 2 (COX-2) leading to the reduction in the inflammatory mediator prostaglandin E2 (PGE2) in a mouse model of zymosan-induced arthritis [55]. Likewise, these anti-inflammatory effects of hop extracts (1–10 µg/mL) have been described in epithelial cells stimulated with viral double-stranded RNA where they decreased the production of TNF-α and the thymic stromal lymphopoietin (TSLP), a cytokine involved in allergic reactions, thus suggesting a role of hop extracts on the modulation of allergic responses [56]. More refined hop extracts contain only the α-acids, β-acids and iso-acids, also known as bitter acids. The bitter acids (1–50 mg/kg) prevented brain inflammation and depressive behavior in mice exposed to LPS-induced brain intoxication [57]. Moreover, these molecules also decreased the production of TNF-α and IL-1β in TNF-α-stimulated fibroblasts and activated the hepatic stellate cells, suggesting a role of bitter acids in the prevention of fibrosis [58,59].

Iso-α-acids have been widely studied in the modulation of the innate immune system within the brain and its implications in neurodegenerative disorders. Iso-α-acids promoted the phagocytic activity of microglial cells in vitro together with a shift from a pro-inflammatory towards an anti-inflammatory phenotype, as evidenced by reduced levels of NO, TNF-α, IL-1β, IL-6, IL-12 and MCP-1, while the number of the anti-inflammatory microglial marker CD206 was increased [60–63]. In addition to its role in preventing neuroinflammation, iso-α-acids prevented the hepatic damage observed in non-alcoholic steatohepatitis induced by a Western diet, reducing hepatic fibrosis, inflammation and oxidative damage [64]. In the case of β-acids, it has been observed to have an inhibitory effect on the activation of NF-κB, thus inhibiting tumor generation in mice exposed to 12-O-tetrahydrophorbol 13-acetate [65]; however, the role of separated β-acids in immune activation remains poorly explored.

To specifically identify which beer compounds are responsible for these effects, several studies have focused on studying them individually (Table 1).

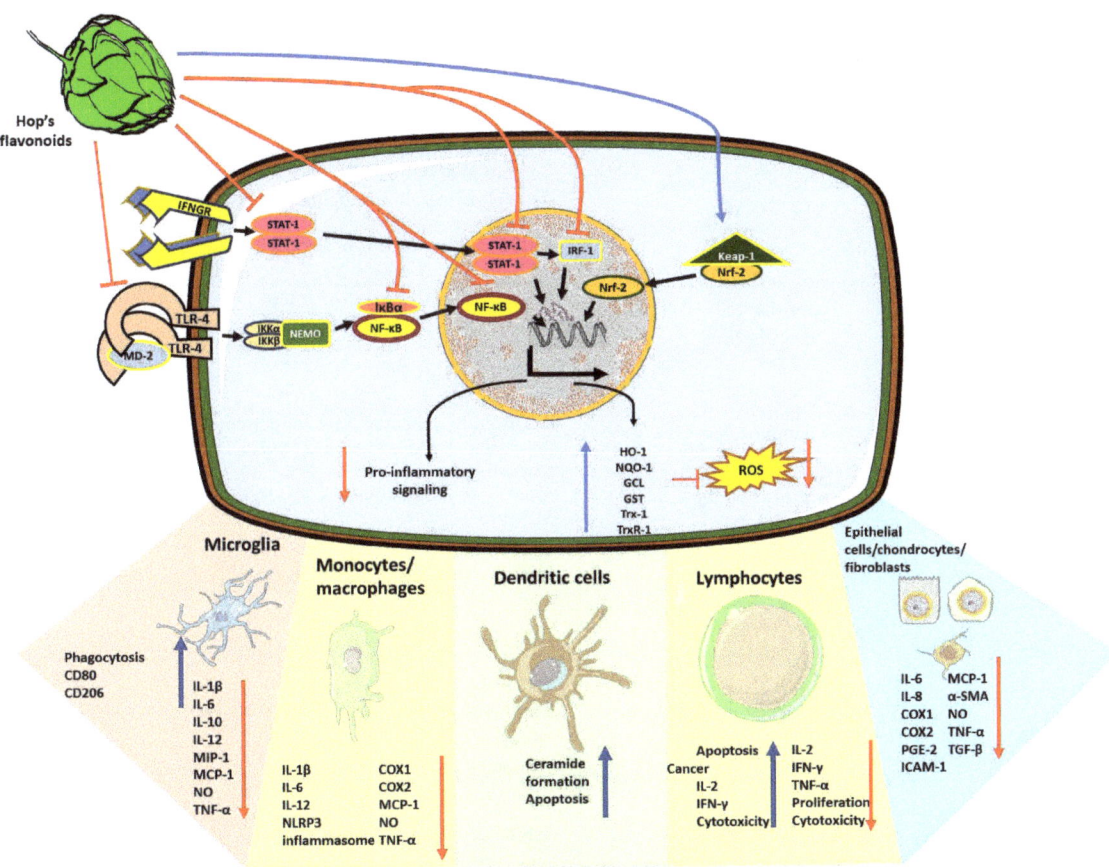

Figure 2. Cellular mechanisms of the anti-inflammatory, immunomodulatory and antioxidant effects exerted by hop compounds. Polyphenols extracted from *H. lupulus* such as xanthohumol, isoxanthohumol and bitter acids can interfere with intracellular immune signaling pathways at different levels. Due to the inhibition of TLR4 activation through preventing the association of TLR4 dimers with the co-stimulatory molecule MD2, NF-κB nuclear translocation was prevented. Hop compounds inhibit NF-κB signaling pathway due to both, the inhibition of TLR4 activation through preventing the association of TLR4 dimers with the co-stimulatory molecule MD2, and in a TLR-independent fashion. Hop compounds can inhibit other pro-inflammatory signaling pathways driven by STAT-1 and IRF-1. Thus, reducing the expression of the subset of pro-inflammatory mediators such as IL-1β, IL-6, IL-8, IL-10, IL-12, TNF-α, inflammasome subunits, nitric oxide, cyclooxygenases, and prostaglandin production, adhesion molecules such as ICAM-1, MCP-1, and MIP-1. Simultaneously, hop compounds promote microglial phagocytic activity together with the switching to M2 phenotype. In different cell types, hop compounds also prevent fibrotic processes by reducing the expression of α-SMA or TGF-β. However, hop compounds also promote the pro-inflammatory and cytotoxic responses from lymphocytes to elicit anti-tumor responses. Finally, in many cases, the anti-inflammatory effects of hop compounds are accompanied by the activation of the antioxidant response regulator, Nrf-2, and the increase in the production of HO-1, NQO-1, GST, GCL, Trx-1 and TrxR-1.

Table 1. Effects of beer compounds on immunomodulation.

Beer Compound	In Vitro/In Vivo/Clinical Study	Effect	References
		In vitro	
Xanthohumol or Isoxanthohumol	Monocytes/macrophages (0.5–20 μM).	- Decreased expression of TLR-4. - Interference with TLR-4/MD-2 association. - Inhibition of NF-κB signaling. - Decreased expression of inflammasome subunits. - Decreased production of IL-1β, IL-6, IL-12, MCP-1, TNF-α, and NO.	[44,66–70]
	Dendritic cells (2–50 μM).	- Increased formation of ceramide. - Activation of caspase-8-mediated apoptosis.	[71]
	T lymphocytes (1.25–40 μM).	- Antiproliferative. - Increased apoptosis. - Reduced lymphocyte cytotoxic activity. - Inhibition of JAK/STAT and NF-κB signaling. - Decreased production of IL-2, TNF-α and IFN-γ.	[72,73]
	Mice primary chondrocytes. (10–50 μM).	- Inhibition of NF-κB signaling. - Reduced production of TNF-α, IL-8, PGE-2 and NO.	[74]
	IEC-6 intestinal epithelium (25 μM).	- Inhibition of NF-κB signaling.	[75]
	Primary hepatocytes and hepatic stellate cells (5–10 μM).	- Inhibition of NF-κB signaling. - Decreased production of IL-8 and MCP-1.	[75,76]
	HUVEC cells (0.001–10 μM).	-Inhibited capillary-like structure formation.	[77]
		In vivo	
	Mice, dextran sodium sulfate-induced colitis (0.1–10 mg/kg orally).	- Inhibition of NF-κB signaling. - Decreased levels of IL-1β, TNF-α and COX2.	[75]
	Liver inflammation, non-alcoholic steatohepatitis, CCl$_4$-induced liver injury, ischemia/reperfusion-induced liver injury (0.5% w/w food).	- Inhibition of NF-κB signaling. - Decreased levels of IL-1α, IL-6, MCP-1, TNF-α and ICAM-1. - Decreased levels of TGF-β, α-SMA and collagen.	[76,78,79]
	Oxalazone-induced inflammation (0.1–5% topically).	- Reduction in ear thickness.	[69]
	LPS-induced lung injury (10–50 mg/kg intraperitoneally).	- Reduced neutrophil count and MPO activity. - Decreased expression of inflammasome subunits. - Reduced levels of IL-1β, IL-6, TNF-α and NO.	[67]
	Skin wound healing (10 mg/L beverage or 50 μM topically).	- Decreased levels of IL-1β, NO and VEGF. - Decreased angiogenesis.	[77,80]
	High-fat diet-induced inflammation (0.01%).	- Reduced levels of circulating IL-1β and TNF-α.	[81]

Table 1. Cont.

Beer Compound	In Vitro/In Vivo/Clinical Study	Effect	References
	Mice, breast cancer (25–50 mg/kg gavage).	- Increased levels of IL-2 and IFN-γ. - Lymphocyte polarization towards TH1 phenotype. - Increased anti-tumor lymphocyte activity. - Reduced tumor volume.	[82]
8-prenylnaringenin	In vitro		
	RAW 264.7 macrophages (1–30 µM).	- Inhibition of NF-κB activation. - Decreased expression of TNF-α, iNOS, COX1 and COX2.	[83]
	HUVEC cells (0.001–10 µM).	- Decreased expression of COX2. - Decreased PGI-2 production. - Promoted capillary-like structure formation.	[77,83]
	Spleenic adherent cells (5 µg/mL).	- Decreased production of IL-12.	[69]
	In vivo		
	Rat skin wound healing (50 µM topically)	- Increased level of IL-1β. - Increased angiogenesis.	[77]
Hop iso-α-acids	In vitro		
	Primary hepatocytes and hepatic stellate cells (10–20 µg/mL).	- Decreased production of IL-8, ICAM-1, TGF-β and α-SMA. - Increased proliferation.	[64]
	BV-2 microglial cells (1–100 µM).	- Decreased production of NO on LPS-stimulated cells.	[60]
	Mice primary microglia culture. (0.1–40 µM).	- Increased amyloid-β phagocytosis. - Decreased production of TNF-α IL-1β, IL-6, IL-10, IL-12, MIP-1 and MCP-1.	[61,63]
	In vivo		
	Western diet-induced non-alcoholic liver disease mice. (0.5% w/w in food)	- Decreased levels of IL-1α and TNF-α. - Reduced expression of adhesion molecules. - Decreased levels of TGF-β, MMP-1 and α-SMA. - Decreased lymphocyte infiltration into the liver.	[64]
	Rat intracerebral hemorrhage. (10 mg/kg intraperitoneally).	- Microglial polarization towards M2 phenotype. - Decreased NF-κB expression. - Reduced levels of IL-1β and TNF-α.	[84]
	5xFAD mice (Alzheimer's experimental model) (0.4–20 mg/kg orally).	- Microglial polarization towards M2 phenotype. - Increased phagocytic activity. - Decreased soluble amyloid-β. - Prevention of amyloid-β deposition. - Decreased production of IL-1β, IL-12 and MIP-1α. - Amelioration of cognitive impairment.	[61,63]
	rTg4510 mice (tauopathy experimental model) (0.5% w/w in food).	- Reduced levels of IL-1β, IL-12, TNF-α and MIP-1. - Decreased levels of phosphorylated tau.	[62]

Table 1. Cont.

Beer Compound	In Vitro/In Vivo/Clinical Study	Effect	References
	Aged mice. (0.5% w/w in food).	- Microglial polarization towards M2 phenotype. - Reduced levels of TNF-α and IL-1β. - Reduced level of amyloid-β and glutamate. - Increased level of dopamine. - Improved age-related cognitive impairment.	[85]
Hop β-acids	In vivo		
	TPA-induced skin inflammation in mice (5–50 µg/mL topically).	- Inhibition of NF-KB signaling. - Decreased pro-inflammatory markers iNOS, COX1 and COX2. - Decreased infiltrated lymphocytes in the skin. - Prevention of tumor formation.	[65]
Hop bitter acids mix	In vitro		
	Hepatic stellate cells (10 µg/mL).	- Decreased activation of NF-κB signaling. - Reduced production of MCP-1 and RANTES. - Decreased α-SMA expression.	[58]
	L929sA fibroblasts (0–200 µM).	- Reduced NF-κB activation. - Reduced IL-6 production.	[59]
	In vivo		
	Vagotomized and LPS-intoxicated mice (1–50 mg/kg).	- Reduced blood levels of IL-1β. - Prevention of dendritic spine loss. - Improved depression-like behavior.	[57]
Hop extract	In vitro		
	RAW 264.7 macrophages (0.1–100 µg/mL).	- Decreased production of IL-1β, IL-6, TNF-α, MCP-1 and NO.	[52,53]
	THP-1 myeloid cells (0.1–2%).	- Decreased production of IL-10 and TNF-α. - Inhibition of NF-κB activation.	[54]
	PBMCs (3.6–30 µg/mL).	- Decreased COX-2 activity and PGE-2 production.	[55]
	Human nasal epithelial cells (0.1–50 µg/mL).	- Decreased TSLP and TNF-α production.	[56]
Beer	In vivo		
	42 mL beer/kg body weight.	- Decreased expression of ICAM, VCAM, NF-κB. - Prevention of atherosclerotic plaque formation.	[50]
	Drinkable beer ad libitum.	- Increased number of anti-tumor reactive lymphocytes. - No difference in tumor growth.	[51]
	Clinical study on healthy subjects Short term (30 min–4 h after single ingestion).		
	Alcoholic beer (355–700 mL).	- Prevented radiation-induced lymphocyte DNA damage (ex vivo). - Reduced lymphocyte cytotoxic activity.	[86,87]

Table 1. Cont.

Beer Compound	In Vitro/In Vivo/Clinical Study	Effect	References
	\multicolumn{2}{l}{Long term. (21–45 days of beer consumption).}	
Alcoholic beer (330 mL/day women, 660 mL/day men).		- No changes in cell adhesion molecules. - Increased number of circulating lymphocytes (women). - Increased serum levels of IgM, IgA and IgG. - Increased monocyte oxidative burst capacity (ex vivo). - Increased cytokine production capacity (ex vivo).	[8,88,89]
Non-alcoholic beer (500–1500 mL daily).		- Unchanged levels of complement system molecules. - Decreased the acute rise of IL-6 and leukocyte after endurance aerobic exercise.	[90,91]
	Clinical study on cardiovascular risk subjects. Long term. (14–28 days of beer consumption).		
Alcoholic beer (500–660 mL/day men).		- Increased level of macrophage microRNA: miR-145a-5p. - Decreased levels of lymphocyte adhesion molecules and IL-5. - Increased levels of IL-1 receptor antagonist.	[92,93]
Non-alcoholic beer (500–990 mL/day men).		- Decreased level of macrophage microRNAs: miR-320a-3p, miR-92a-5p, miR-20a-5p and miR-17-5p. - Decreased level of monocyte and lymphocyte adhesion molecules. - Decreased level of IL-6r, IL-15 and RANTES.	[92,93]

Immunomodulatory Effect of Xanthohumol

The isolated compounds of hop extracts have been tested in several models. Regarding the immune system and inflammatory process, xanthohumol and its derivative isoxanthohumol have been described as potent anti-inflammatory molecules. In vitro studies demonstrated that both xanthohumol and isoxanthoumol, at concentrations ranging between 0.5 and 20 µM, suppressed the production of pro-inflammatory cytokines such as IL-1β, IL-6, IL-12, MCP-1, and TNF-α, together with a decreased expression of the inducible nitric oxide synthase (iNOS) and reduced levels of NO on macrophages and monocytes stimulated with LPS or interferon-γ (IFN-γ) [44,66–69]. The mechanisms through which xanthohumol exerts its anti-inflammatory effects have been attributed to its intervention at different levels of the macrophage inflammatory signals. Xanthohumol interferes with the Toll-like receptor 4 (TLR-4) signaling by binding directly to its co-receptor, the myeloid differentiation protein 2 (MD-2) and decreases TLR-4 expression [68,70]. Additionally, it blocks the interferon response factor 1 (IRF1)/STAT1 cascade [66] and inhibits the activation of the NF-κB [44,66,67,69], which also leads to reduced levels of the inflammasome components NLRP-3 and caspase-1, and finally to the reduction in IL-1β levels [67]. Conversely, the mechanism of action of isoxanthohumol in the pro-inflammatory signaling cascade only points to the inhibition of the NF-κB cascade but no changes in TLR-4 expression have been described [68,75].

The anti-inflammatory role of xanthohumol has been observed in vitro in different tissue resident cell types that contribute to the innate immune response such as chondrocytes, intestinal epithelial cells, hepatocytes and hepatic stellate cells. In these cells, xanthohumol decreased the production of inflammatory markers NO, IL-6, IL-8, TNF-α, MCP-1, COX-2, and PGE2 [74–76]. In contrast, a deleterious role of xanthohumol has been reported in dendritic cells, another cellular subset of the innate immune response. In this context, xanthohumol, at 50 μM, induced apoptosis triggered by caspase-8 in a mechanism dependent on the activity of the enzyme acid sphingomyelinase that led to an increased ceramide production in vitro [71].

The anti-inflammatory role of xanthohumol in vivo has been tested in models of acute and chronic inflammation in different organs. The topical administration of xanthohumol prevented skin inflammation in oxazolone-induced dermatitis [69] and its intraperitoneal administration showed anti-inflammatory and antioxidant effects as well as the prevention of fibrosis on acute lung injury induced by LPS injection [67].

Supplementation of a standard rodent diet with xanthohumol in different murine experimental models including ischemia/reperfusion, carbon tetrachloride acute liver toxicity and non-alcoholic steatohepatitis was shown to prevent the increase in proinflammatory markers IL-1α, IL-6, MCP-1, TNF-α and ICAM-1; it also decreased the levels of the transforming growth factor β (TGF-β), TIMP1, collagen-1 and α-smooth muscle actin (α-SMA) and contributed to the prevention of liver fibrosis in these models [76,78,79]. The oral administration of xanthohumol decreased the inflammatory markers and the severity of dextran sulfate sodium-induced colitis where TNF-α, IL-1β and COX-2 decline was associated with xanthohumol-induced inhibition of NF-κB signaling [75]. Moreover, xanthohumol-supplemented beverages given to animals decreased the levels of the pro-inflammatory markers IL-1β and NO in addition to the decrease in the vascular endothelial growth factor (VEGF) and the number of new blood vessels in a skin wound healing model, suggesting that xanthohumol also modulates the angiogenic process [80]. These results are in line with previous studies showing that both xanthohumol and isoxanthohumol prevented the assembly of capillary-like structures from endothelial cells by inducing apoptosis on these cells [77]. The anti-inflammatory role of isoxanthohumol has been demonstrated in models of high-fat diet-induced insulin resistance where it decreased levels of the pro-inflammatory cytokines IL-1β and TNF-α and improved the glucose tolerance; these effects were attributed to isoxanthohumol-induced changes in the abundance and diversity of mice microbiota [81].

Despite the described mechanisms of xanthohumol in the function of the innate immune system cells, the role of this chalcone on the modulation of adaptive immune response remains poorly understood. In vitro studies evidenced that xanthohumol exerts an antiproliferative role on concanavalin-A or IL-12-activated T lymphocytes, an effect which was accompanied by cell cycle arrest but also with the increase in apoptotic cells [72,73] and it has been attributed to the inhibition of STAT and NF-κB signaling as occurred in cells of the innate immune response [72,73]. Moreover, xanthohumol suppressed the cytotoxic activity and the production of IL-2, TNF-α and IFN-γ on T lymphocytes suggesting the inhibition of pro-inflammatory T cell responses (TH1) in vitro [72]. However, xanthohumol showed opposite effects on the stimulation of TH1 lymphocytes in vivo on a breast cancer mouse model, where xanthohumol induced the reduction in tumor mass, the increase in cytotoxic lymphocytes together with an increase in IFN-γ and IL-2. Additionally, it produced a reduction in the lymphocyte-produced anti-inflammatory cytokines IL-4 and IL-10, favoring an anti-tumor TH1 phenotype instead of an anti-inflammatory TH2 phenotype on T lymphocytes [82]. This contradictory evidence suggests that the role of xanthohumol is beyond its anti-inflammatory properties, as further research using different models of immune activation would reveal a more complex role of xanthohumol in the modulation of the immune response.

The role of 8-prenylnaringenin on the inflammatory process has also been studied, demonstrating that this compound can reduce the expression of pro-inflammatory markers such as IL-12, TNF-α and NO together with a decrease in the production of ROS and PGE2 [69,83]. Furthermore, contrary to xanthohumol and isoxanthohumol,

8-prenylnaringenin modulates the angiogenic processes by inhibiting the cell death of vascular endothelial cells and promoting the formation of capillary structures in wound healing models [77].

4. Effect of Human Beer Consumption on Redox Environment and Immunomodulation

The role of moderate beer consumption has been studied in the immunological and redox markers of healthy subjects and people with cardiovascular risk. The favorable beer consumption effects can be related to the mechanisms previously described in experimental models. In a randomized feeding trial comparing moderate beer intake (660 mL/day, containing 30 g of ethanol and 1209 mg of polyphenols) with non-alcoholic beer (900 mL/day containing 1243 mg of total polyphenols), reduced serum concentration of inflammatory biomarkers and also beneficial effects on the cardiovascular system with better results than distilled beverages such as gin (100 mL/day, containing 30 g of ethanol) were observed, probably because of the polyphenolic content of beer [93]. Another study showed that non-alcoholic beer intake for 45 days followed by hop supplementation (400 mg/days) decreases lipid peroxidation and carbonyl groups while it increases the GSH and α-tocopherol content in the blood. Interestingly, the inflammatory parameters IL-6 and complement C3 fraction decreased just after hop supplementation [94].

Comparisons between social and problem alcohol drinkers demonstrated that problem drinkers present lower levels of both serum IL-6 and IL-1 receptor agonist, (pro-inflammatory and anti-inflammatory markers, respectively) suggesting that these subjects have a blunted immune response compared to social drinkers, these differences were related to anxiety and motivation behavior in the studied subjects [95]. In the short term, 30 min after consumption, beer decreased the cytotoxic activity of peripheral lymphocytes stimulated with IL-2 or phytohemagglutinin of healthy subjects [86]; this would seem like a detrimental role of beer consumption on the immune response immediately after ingestion, nevertheless, blood lymphocytes were more resistant to radiation-induced damage from 30 min to 4.5 h after beer ingestion [87]; this could be beneficial in the case of cancer patients receiving radiotherapy. Moderate (330 mL for women, 660 mL for men) beer consumption in healthy subjects did not affect the serum levels of the adhesion molecules ICAM-1 and E-selectin [88] nor the levels of cytokines or complement proteins involved in the serum immune response [90]. Moreover, as part of a study to determine the effect of moderate beer consumption on immunocompetence in healthy adults, sixty subjects (29 women and 31 men) between 25 and 50 years consumed, after a month of abstinence, one or two cans of beer as part of a regular diet during a month. An increased number of peripheral leukocytes, neutrophils, basophils, and CD3+ lymphocytes was observed in women while in men it was only a trend [8,89]. There were no differences in CD4+, CD8+, CD19+, TNF-α, and IL-6. Nevertheless, an increase in IgG, IgA, and IgM values was observed both in men and women [8]; ex vivo blood analysis from the same subjects demonstrated that after the beer consumption period, E. coli-stimulated macrophages showed elevated levels of oxidative burst, but no changes in phagocytic activity [89], as well as an improved capacity of PBMCs for the production of IL-2, IL-4, IL-6, IL-10, TNF-α and IFN-γ in both sexes [8]. In this study, the IFN-γ/IL-10 ratio decreased in both women and men, considering that a high IFN-γ/IL-10 ratio has been associated with depressive disorders, moderate beer consumption could have anti-depressive effects without affecting the proinflammatory cytokine production (no changes on TNF- α and IL-6). In addition to this, it has been shown that moderate non-alcoholic beer consumption prevented the acute inflammation caused by aerobic endurance exercise, in this case, alcoholic and non-alcoholic beer prevented the increase in serum IL-6 and the number of circulating leukocytes given after finishing a marathon [91].

In the case of subjects with cardiovascular risk, moderate beer consumption increased the level of macrophage-produced microRNAs that have been related to a decreased expression of inflammatory cytokines [92]; accordingly, moderate beer consumption also decreased the blood levels of inflammatory markers IL-5, IL-15, the receptor of IL-6, and the chemokine regulated upon activation, normal T cell expressed and secreted (RANTES) in cardiovascular risk individuals [93]—however, no changes in IL-6 or TNF-α were reported [9].

Studies focused on moderate beer consumption and the effect of the natural compounds found in beers have shown important roles in the modulation of immune responses, beyond anti-inflammatory effects, beer components seem to play a more complex part in the different immune populations, also depending on the type of immune challenge that is presented. Further research is needed to clarify these complex behaviors and incidentally reinforce the benefits of moderate beer consumption.

5. Hop Derivatives and Neuroprotection

The prevalence of age-related neurodegenerative diseases is exponentially increased due to a longer life expectancy; currently, there are no effective therapies available to ameliorate their progressive disabling characteristics. The processes that contribute to neurodegeneration include excitotoxicity, the dysfunction of cellular organelles such as mitochondria, and lysosomes favoring an oxidative environment and losing the redox homeostasis which together with an immune imbalance lead to inflammatory signaling and altered responses of glia in the brain. These events converge and contribute to misfolded proteins, protein aggregation, cellular communication damage, and altered—which subsequently induce brain cellular loss. These cellular and molecular processes can be reflected in the cognitive impairment and motor deterioration characteristic of aging and neurodegenerative disorders [96–99]. Recently, it has been reported that the moderate drinking of beer shows some positive effects by improving cognitive impairments related to several of these neurological and pathological conditions. These effects have been related to the antioxidative and anti-inflammatory properties of the chemical compounds that can be found in the hops, described above. Specifically, these components have shown effects in neurotransmission, redox modulation, and neurogenesis, providing neuroprotection in different experimental models (Figure 3).

One of the earliest indications showing that hop components could act on the central nervous system was the fact that hop cones have been widely used in folk medicine as a tranquilizer, sedative, and anxiolytic, presumably by an effect on γ-aminobutyric acid (GABA)$_A$ receptors. This idea was supported by evidence showing that extracts from *H. lupulus* decreased the locomotor activity, increased sleeping time, and overall potentiate the sedative effects induced by pentobarbital or ketamine [100–102] through the inhibitory action of GABAergic neurotransmission. In this line, the effect of beer components on GABA$_A$ receptors has been studied in *Xenopus oocytes* injected with cRNAs of α_1 and β_1 subunits of bovine GABA$_A$ receptors to induce their expression. The beer components myrcenol, linalool, geraniol and, 1-octen-3-ol induced a stronger potentiation (2- to 4-fold taking as reference the response elicited by GABA) on the GABA$_A$ receptor activation; while hop oils showed a small potentiation (20–50% compared with the GABA response). In the absence of a preliminary GABA stimulus, these compounds did not induce a response on the GABA$_A$ receptors, therefore, they did not act as agonists but as enhancers. Among all the compounds examined, myrcenol showed the greatest potentiation on the GABA$_A$ receptor using this *Xenopus oocytes* expression system; for this reason, the effect of myrcenol was also tested in vivo where, accordingly, it potentiated the GABA$_A$ response extending the sleeping time induced by pentobarbital [103]. On the other hand, contrasting effects were attributed to the hop β-acids since they reduced the GABA-evoked currents in a concentration-dependent manner in cerebellar granule cells [104].

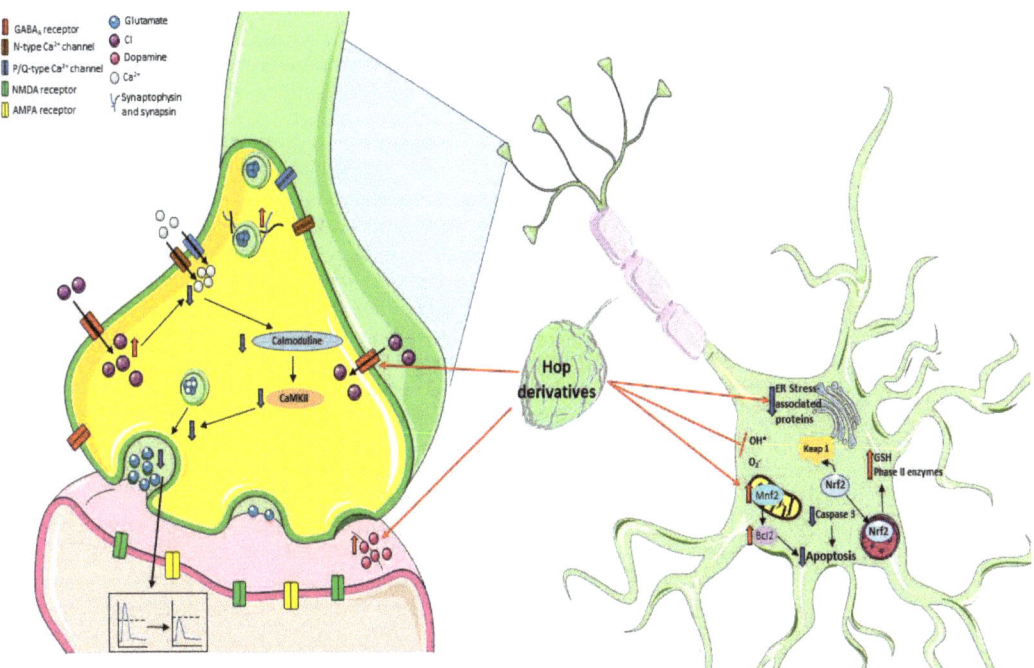

Figure 3. Mechanisms of neuroprotection by prenylflavonoids. It has been described that prenyl flavonoids such as xanthohumol can modulate the $GABA_A$ receptors, thus increasing intracellular Cl^- concentrations and reducing Ca^{2+} influx, leading to a decrease in glutamate release, and preventing an exacerbated excitotoxic neuronal damage. Additionally, hop metabolites can modulate the redox environment through Nrf2 signaling, regulating the expression of mitochondrial proteins, or preventing oxidative damage by directly scavenging ROS.

Recently, it was described that xanthohumol, isoxanthohumol and 8-prenylnaringenin can displace 3-ethynylbicycloorthobenzoate, a noncompetitive blocker of $GABA_A$ receptor, and bind to $GABA_A$ receptors with an IC_{50} of 29.7 ± 0.8 µM, 11.6 ± 0.7 µM and 7.3 ± 0.4 µM, respectively. This effect showed a positive allosteric modulation of the GABA-induced responses where the highest potency was observed for 8-prenylnaringenin with a relatively higher subtype selectivity for those $GABA_A$ receptors containing δ-subunits [105]. The effect of 8-prenylnaringenin suggests that it can directly activate $GABA_A$ receptors considering that this hop derivative can displace almost 50% of radioligand binding ([^{3}H]Ro 15-4513, an inverse agonist of $GABA_A$) [105]. Furthermore, xanthohumol was able to decrease glutamate release from rat hippocampal synaptosomes and reduce miniature excitatory postsynaptic currents in hippocampal slices. This effect was attributed to a presynaptic mechanism, which involved the modulation of $GABA_A$ receptors [106].

Considering that xanthohumol inhibits glutamate release, Wang and coworkers studied the effect of this chalcone in a rat model of excitotoxicity induced by an intraperitoneal injection of kainic acid (KA). In this case, xanthohumol administration (10 and 50 mg/kg) effectively reduced glutamate levels, seizure score and neuronal death after KA administration [107]. Furthermore, the mitochondrial alterations (swelling, disruption, and decreased size) induced by KA and observed in the hippocampal CA3 region were prevented by xanthohumol pretreatment; in fact, this compound restored the downregulated mitofusin-2 and consequently prevented the increase in the apoptotic protease activating factor 1 (Apaf-1) and the levels of cleaved caspase-3. In sum, xanthohumol prevents the excitotoxic damage induced by kainic acid inhibiting glutamate release, preserving the mitochondrial functionality, and hence preventing the mitochondrial-dependent apoptotic process [107].

Other studies have investigated the effect of xanthohumol on cognitive performance, senescence, and neuronal differentiation models. In this context, this chalcone has been shown to reduce brain proinflammatory, TNF-α and IL-1β, and proapoptotic (BAD, BAX and AIF) markers in senescence-accelerated prone mice (SAMP8) and to increase the protein expression of neural trophic factor (BDNF), synapsin and synaptophysin [108]. This evidence suggests a positive effect of xanthohumol on cognitive performance in aging or other neurodegenerative diseases. Particularly, it has been observed that a xanthohumol diet (30 mg/kg body weight/day for 8 weeks) improves cognitive flexibility in young mice [109]. Moreover, its derivative isoxanthohumol and the flavanones 8-prenylnaringenin and 6-prenylnaringenin promote neuronal differentiation in fetal progenitor cells [110,111]. Future studies that integrate new tools related to neurogenesis are the next step to decipher the mechanistic role of xanthohumol and isoxanthohumol in this issue.

There are other mechanisms studied through which xanthohumol exerts its neuroprotective effects (Figure 3). The systemic administration of xanthohumol (0.2 and 0.4 mg/kg) reduced (40 and 60%, respectively) the infarct area in cerebral ischemic rats, improving their neurobehavioral deficits. This protective xanthohumol effect was associated with a decrease in inflammatory and apoptotic proteins' expression such as TNF-α, caspase-3, hypoxia-inducible factor (HIF)-1α, and inducible nitric oxide synthase protein (iNOS) [37].

Xanthohumol activates the Nrf2-ARE signaling pathway in PC12 cells, leading to the upregulation of phase II enzymes expression, therefore preventing the neurotoxicity induced by hydrogen peroxide and 6-hydroxydopamine. The Nrf2-signaling pathway activation as a mechanism by which xanthohumol exerts neuroprotection was confirmed in PC12 cells transfected with shRNAs silencing the rat Nrf2 gene (shNrf2s)—as a result, the cytoprotective effect of this chalcone was lost [41]. Additionally, xanthohumol showed anti-inflammatory activity in a murine microglial cell line (BV2 cells) exposed to LPS. Briefly, the pretreatment with xanthohumol (5 µg/mL) decreased the overproduction of NO, as well as the increased expression of iNOS, COX-2, TNFα, IL-1β, and NF-κB, in LPS-stimulated BV2 cells. The inhibitory effect of this chalcone was related to the fact that xanthohumol pretreatment increased the Nrf2 activation and, in consequence, the NQO1 and HO-1 mRNA and the protein levels as well as the GSH levels increased [44]. Moreover, xanthohumol and quercetin prevented the neuronal morphological alterations, thus contributing to the preservation of cell viability while preventing astrogliosis, attributable to chronic exposure to corticosterone. However, the mechanism by which these polyphenols act is different since xanthohumol involves the Nrf2 pathway while quercetin attenuates the activation of the glucocorticoid receptor (GR) [44].

Additionally, xanthohumol has shown positive effects on neurodegeneration models, for instance, it reduced Aβ accumulation, APP processing and attenuated tau hyperphosphorylation in a cellular model of Alzheimer's disease (AD) (murine neuroblastoma N2a cells expressing the human Swedish mutant amyloid precursor protein). Proteomic analysis comparing the proteins in lysates of N2a/APP cells in the presence or absence of xanthohumol showed 21 differentially expressed proteins involved in endoplasmic reticulum (ER) stress, oxidative stress, proteasome molecular systems, and the neuronal cytoskeleton [112].

In a different mouse model of AD, in a transgenic 5xFAD mouse, it was found that iso-α-acids ameliorated the pro-inflammatory cytokine production, increased microglial phagocytosis of the β-amyloid peptides, prevented tau phosphorylation and tauopathy, and induced the improvement in both memory and cognitive function [61–63]. Similar results have been reported in aged mice fed with iso-α-acids which prevented the age-related cognitive decline by decreasing the levels of pro-inflammatory cytokines and promoted the profile of microglia with an anti-inflammatory phenotype [85]. Moreover, iso-α-acids have shown neuroprotective effects in animal models of brain hematoma through the inhibition of NF-κB signaling, the reduced production of IL-1β and TNF-α, and the promotion of anti-inflammatory microglial activation, which contributed to the improvement in the cognitive functions of these mice [84].

On the other hand, hop bitter acids intake improved spatial and object recognition memory functions and increased hippocampal dopamine levels through vagus nerve activation. The memory improvement induced by hop bitter acids is attenuated when vagotomy is performed, suggesting that iso-α-acids activate the vagus nerve and possibly lead to increased hippocampal dopamine levels and consequently they improve memory function [113]. Moreover, the hop bitter acids diet increased the dopaminergic activity associated with stress resilience in a repeated social defeat stress mouse model [114].

The neuroprotective effect of hop components has also been demonstrated in human studies. In a randomized double-blind placebo-controlled study in healthy adults, it was observed that the consumption of matured hop bitter acids (35 mg/day for 12 weeks) improved mental fatigue, mood state, verbal memory retrieval, and anxiety when compared with the placebo group (45–64 years) [115]. Indeed, hop bitter acids improved cognitive function, attention, and mood state in older people (45–69 years) with subjective cognitive decline [116].

6. Conclusions

Throughout this review, it has been described that beer is one of the most consumed beverages worldwide and its components possess relevant antioxidant and immunomodulatory properties. In particular, hop compounds have demonstrated their effectiveness in improving neurodegenerative processes since they can modulate the cellular redox environment, favoring an antioxidant and anti-inflammatory response, which in turn attenuates the damage of harmful agents or simply prevents physiological alterations due to aging. Based on this evidence, beer consumption and hop compounds represent an excellent research target to prevent or ameliorate cellular processes that lead to neurodegeneration.

Author Contributions: Conceptualization, V.P.d.l.C., T.B.A. and B.P.; investigation, V.P.d.l.C., G.I.V.-C., D.R.O., T.B.A. and A.S.; writing—original draft preparation, G.I.V.-C., D.R.O., D.F.G.E., T.B.A., A.S. and V.P.d.l.C.; writing—review and editing, B.P., T.B.A., D.F.G.E., A.S., G.I.V-C and V.P.d.l.C.; funding acquisition, B.P. All authors have read and agreed to the published version of the manuscript.

Funding: This research was funded by Consejo de Investigación sobre Salud y Cerveza de México, A. C. Fomento a la Investigación 2019, grant number 110-19.

Institutional Review Board Statement: Not applicable.

Informed Consent Statement: Not applicable.

Data Availability Statement: The data presented in this study are available on request from the corresponding author.

Acknowledgments: G.I.V.-C. is a scholarship holder of CONACyT-México (308052) in the Graduate Program in Biological Science, UNAM.

Conflicts of Interest: The authors declare no conflict of interest.

References

1. Almaguer, C.; Schönberger, C.; Gastl, M.; Arendt, E.K.; Becker, T. Humulus Lupulus-A Story that Begs to Be Told. A Review. *J. Inst. Brew.* **2014**, *120*, 289–314. [CrossRef]
2. Osorio-Paz, I.; Brunauer, R.; Alavez, S. Beer and Its Non-Alcoholic Compounds in Health and Disease. *Crit. Rev. Food Sci. Nutr.* **2019**, *60*, 1–14. [CrossRef]
3. Lasanta, C.; Durán-Guerrero, E.; Díaz, A.B.; Castro, R. Influence of Fermentation Temperature and Yeast Type on the Chemical and Sensory Profile of Handcrafted Beers. *J. Sci. Food Agric.* **2021**, *101*, 1174–1181. [CrossRef]
4. Traversy, G.; Chaput, J.-P. Alcohol Consumption and Obesity: An Update. *Curr. Obes. Rep.* **2015**, *4*, 122–130. [CrossRef] [PubMed]
5. Bobak, M.; Skodova, Z.; Marmot, M. Beer and Obesity: A Cross-Sectional Study. *Eur. J. Clin. Nutr.* **2003**, *57*, 1250–1253. [CrossRef]
6. Fernández-Solà, J. Cardiovascular Risks and Benefits of Moderate and Heavy Alcohol Consumption. *Nat. Rev. Cardiol.* **2015**, *12*, 576–587. [CrossRef]

7. de Gaetano, G.; Costanzo, S.; Di Castelnuovo, A.; Badimon, L.; Bejko, D.; Alkerwi, A.; Chiva-Blanch, G.; Estruch, R.; La Vecchia, C.; Panico, S.; et al. Effects of Moderate Beer Consumption on Health and Disease: A Consensus Document. *Nutr. Metab. Cardiovasc. Dis.* **2016**, *26*, 443–467. [CrossRef]
8. Romeo, J.; Wärnberg, J.; Nova, E.; Díaz, L.E.; González-Gross, M.; Marcos, A. Changes in the Immune System after Moderate Beer Consumption. *Ann. Nutr. Metab.* **2007**, *51*, 359–366. [CrossRef]
9. Spaggiari, G.; Cignarelli, A.; Sansone, A.; Baldi, M.; Santi, D. To Beer or Not to Beer: A Meta-Analysis of the Effects of Beer Consumption on Cardiovascular Health. *PLoS ONE* **2020**, *15*, e0233619. [CrossRef]
10. Rundio, A. Understanding Alcoholism. *Nurs. Clin. North Am.* **2013**, *48*, 385–390. [CrossRef] [PubMed]
11. Karatzi, K.; Rontoyanni, V.G.; Protogerou, A.; Georgoulia, A.; Xenos, K.; Chrysou, J.; Sfikakis, P.P.; Sidossis, L.S. Acute Effects of Beer on Endothelial Function and Hemodynamics: A Single-Blind, Crossover Study in Healthy Volunteers. *Nutrition* **2013**, *29*, 1122–1126. [CrossRef]
12. Gorinstein, S.; Zemser, M.; Berliner, M.; Goldstein, R.; Libman, I.; Trakhtenberg, S.; Caspi, A. Moderate Beer Consumption and Positive Biochemical Changes in Patients with Coronary Atherosclerosis. *J. Intern. Med.* **1997**, *242*, 219–224. [CrossRef]
13. Di Domenico, M.; Feola, A.; Ambrosio, P.; Pinto, F.; Galasso, G.; Zarrelli, A.; Di Fabio, G.; Porcelli, M.; Scacco, S.; Inchingolo, F.; et al. Antioxidant Effect of Beer Polyphenols and Their Bioavailability in Dental-Derived Stem Cells (D-dSCs) and Human Intestinal Epithelial Lines (Caco-2) Cells. *Stem Cells Int.* **2020**, *2020*, 1–13. [CrossRef]
14. Oladokun, O.; Tarrega, A.; James, S.; Smart, K.; Hort, J.; Cook, D. The Impact of Hop Bitter Acid and Polyphenol Profiles on the Perceived Bitterness of Beer. *Food Chem.* **2016**, *205*, 212–220. [CrossRef]
15. Mishra, A.K.; Kocábek, T.; Nath, V.S.; Awasthi, P.; Shrestha, A.; Killi, U.K.; Jakse, J.; Patzak, J.; Krofta, K.; Matoušek, J. Dissection of Dynamic Transcriptome Landscape of Leaf, Bract, and Lupulin Gland in Hop (Humulus lupulus L.). *Int. J. Mol. Sci.* **2019**, *21*, 233. [CrossRef]
16. Karabín, M.; Hudcová, T.; Jelínek, L.; Dostálek, P. Biologically Active Compounds from Hops and Prospects for Their Use. *Compr. Rev. Food Sci. Food Saf.* **2016**, *15*, 542–567. [CrossRef]
17. Farag, M.A.; Porzel, A.; Schmidt, J.; Wessjohann, L.A. Metabolite Profiling and Fingerprinting of Commercial Cultivars of Humulus Lupulus L. (hop): A Comparison of MS and NMR Methods in Metabolomics. *Metabolomics* **2012**, *8*, 492–507. [CrossRef]
18. Haseleu, G.; Lagemann, A.; Stephan, A.; Intelmann, D.; Dunkel, A.; Hofmann, T. Quantitative Sensomics Profiling of Hop-Derived Bitter Compounds Throughout a Full-Scale Beer Manufacturing Process. *J. Agric. Food Chem.* **2010**, *58*, 7930–7939. [CrossRef]
19. Malowicki, M.G.; Shellhammer, T.H. Isomerization and Degradation Kinetics of Hop (Humulus lupulus) Acids in a Model Wort-Boiling System. *J. Agric. Food Chem.* **2005**, *53*, 4434–4439. [CrossRef]
20. Aron, P.M.; Shellhammer, T.H. A Discussion of Polyphenols in Beer Physical and Flavour Stability. *J. Inst. Brew.* **2010**, *116*, 369–380. [CrossRef]
21. Yang, X.; Jiang, Y.; Yang, J.; He, J.; Sun, J.; Chen, F.; Zhang, M.; Yang, B. Prenylated Flavonoids, Promising Nutraceuticals with Impressive Biological Activities. *Trends Food Sci. Technol.* **2015**, *44*, 93–104. [CrossRef]
22. Stevens, J.F.; Taylor, A.W.; Deinzer, M.L. Quantitative Analysis of Xanthohumol and Related Prenylflavonoids in Hops and Beer by Liquid Chromatography–Tandem Mass Spectrometry. *J. Chromatogr. A* **1999**, *832*, 97–107. [CrossRef]
23. Stevens, J.F.; Page, E.J. Xanthohumol and Related Prenylflavonoids from Hops and Beer: To Your Good Health! *Phytochemistry* **2004**, *65*, 1317–1330. [CrossRef]
24. Magalhaes, P.J.; Carvalho, D.O.; Cruz, J.M.; Guido, L.F.; Barros, A.A. Fundamentals and Health Benefits of Xan-Thohumol, a Natural Product Derived from Hops and Beer. *Nat. Prod. Commun.* **2009**, *4*, 591–610. [PubMed]
25. Legette, L.; Karnpracha, C.; Reed, R.L.; Choi, J.; Bobe, G.; Christensen, J.M.; Rodriguez-Proteau, R.; Purnell, J.Q.; Stevens, J.F. Human Pharmacokinetics of Xanthohumol, an Antihyperglycemic Flavonoid from Hops. *Mol. Nutr. Food Res.* **2013**, *58*, 248–255. [CrossRef]
26. Lushchak, V.I. Free Radicals, Reactive Oxygen Species, Oxidative Stress and Its Classification. *Chem. Interact.* **2014**, *224*, 164–175. [CrossRef] [PubMed]
27. Di Meo, S.; Venditti, P. Evolution of the Knowledge of Free Radicals and Other Oxidants. *Oxid. Med. Cell. Longev.* **2020**, *2020*, 1–32. [CrossRef] [PubMed]
28. Nissanka, N.; Moraes, C.T. Mitochondrial DNA Damage and Reactive Oxygen Species in Neurodegenerative Disease. *FEBS Lett.* **2018**, *592*, 728–742. [CrossRef] [PubMed]
29. Grimm, A.; Eckert, A. Brain Aging and Neurodegeneration: From a Mitochondrial Point of View. *J. Neurochem.* **2017**, *143*, 418–431. [CrossRef]
30. Piazzon, A.; Forte, M.; Nardini, M. Characterization of phenolics content and antioxidant activity of different beer types. *J. Agric. Food Chem.* **2010**, *58*, 10677–10683. [CrossRef] [PubMed]
31. Andersen, M.L.; Outtrup, H.; Skibsted, L.H. Potential antioxidants in beer assessed by ESR spin trapping. *J. Agric. Food Chem.* **2000**, *48*, 3106–3111. [CrossRef]
32. Spreng, S.; Hofmann, T. Activity-Guided Identification of In Vitro Antioxidants in Beer. *J. Agric. Food Chem.* **2018**, *66*, 720–731. [CrossRef] [PubMed]
33. Rivero, D.; Pérez-Magariño, S.; González-Sanjosé, M.L.; Valls-Belles, V.; Codoñer, A.P.; Muñiz, P. Inhibition of Induced DNA Oxidative Damage by Beers: Correlation with the Content of Polyphenols and Melanoidins. *J. Agric. Food Chem.* **2005**, *53*, 3637–3642. [CrossRef]

34. Ottaviani, I.J.; Carrasquedo, F.; Keen, C.L.; Lazarus, A.S.; Schmitz, H.H.; Fraga, C.G. Influence of Flavan-3-Ols and Procyanidins on UVC-Mediated Formation of 8-oxo-7,8-dihydro-2′-Deoxyguanosine in Isolated DNA. *Arch. Biochem. Biophys.* **2002**, *406*, 203–208. [CrossRef]
35. Gerhäuser, C. Phenolic Beer Compounds to Prevent Cancer. In *Beer in Health and Disease Prevention*; Elsevier BV: Amsterdam, The Netherlands, 2009; pp. 669–684.
36. Tagasgira, M.; Watanabe, M.; Uemitsu, N. Antioxidative Activity of Hop Bitter Acids and Their Analogues. *Biosci. Biotechnol. Biochem.* **1995**, *59*, 740–742. [CrossRef]
37. Yen, T.-L.; Hsu, C.-K.; Lu, W.-J.; Hsieh, C.-Y.; Hsiao, G.; Chou, D.-S.; Wu, G.-J.; Sheu, J.-R. Neuroprotective Effects of Xanthohumol, a Prenylated Flavonoid from Hops (*Humulus lupulus*), in Ischemic Stroke of Rats. *J. Agric. Food Chem.* **2012**, *60*, 1937–1944. [CrossRef] [PubMed]
38. Gerhauser, C.; Alt, A.; Heiss, E.; Gamal-Eldeen, A.; Klimo, K.; Knauft, J.; Neumann, I.; Scherf, H.-R.; Frank, N.; Bartsch, H.; et al. Cancer Chemopreventive Activity of Xanthohumol, a Natural Product Derived from Hop. *Mol. Cancer Ther.* **2002**, *1*, 959–969. [PubMed]
39. Zhao, F.; Watanabe, Y.; Nozawa, H.; Daikonnya, A.; Kondo, K.; Kitanaka, S. Prenylflavonoids and Phloroglucinol Derivatives from Hops (Humulus Lupulus). *J. Nat. Prod.* **2005**, *68*, 43–49. [CrossRef]
40. Zhao, F.; Nozawa, H.; Daikonnya, A.; Kondo, K.; Kitanaka, S. Inhibitors of Nitric Oxide Production from Hops (*Humulus Lupulus* L.). *Biol. Pharm. Bull.* **2003**, *26*, 61–65. [CrossRef]
41. Yao, J.; Zhang, B.; Ge, C.; Peng, S.; Fang, J. Xanthohumol, a Polyphenol Chalcone Present in Hops, Activating Nrf2 Enzymes To Confer Protection against Oxidative Damage in PC12 Cells. *J. Agric. Food Chem.* **2015**, *63*, 1521–1531. [CrossRef]
42. Miranda, C.L.; Stevens, J.F.; Ivanov, V.; McCall, M.; Frei, B.; Deinzer, M.L.; Buhler, D.R. Antioxidant and Prooxidant Actions of Prenylated and Nonprenylated Chalcones and Flavanones In Vitro. *J. Agric. Food Chem.* **2000**, *48*, 3876–3884. [CrossRef]
43. Rodriguez, R.; Miranda, C.; Stevens, J.; Deinzer, M.; Buhler, D. Influence of Prenylated and Non-Prenylated Flavonoids on Liver Microsomal Lipid Peroxidation and Oxidative Injury in Rat Hepatocytes. *Food Chem. Toxicol.* **2001**, *39*, 437–445. [CrossRef]
44. Lee, I.-S.; Lim, J.; Gal, J.; Kang, J.C.; Kim, H.J.; Kang, B.Y.; Choi, H.J. Anti-Inflammatory Activity of Xanthohumol Involves Heme Oxygenase-1 Induction via NRF2-ARE Signaling in Microglial BV2 Cells. *Neurochem. Int.* **2011**, *58*, 153–160. [CrossRef] [PubMed]
45. González-Muñoz, M.; Meseguer, I.; Sánchez-Reus, M.; Schultz, A.; Olivero, R.; Benedi, J.; Sánchez-Muniz, F. Beer Consumption Reduces Cerebral Oxidation Caused by Aluminum Toxicity by Normalizing Gene Expression of Tumor Necrotic Factor Alpha and Several Antioxidant Enzymes. *Food Chem. Toxicol.* **2008**, *46*, 1111–1118. [CrossRef]
46. Valls-Belles, V.; Torres, C.; Muñiz, P.; Codoñer-Franch, P. Effect of Beer Consumption on Levels of Complex I and Complex IV Liver and Heart Mitochondrial Enzymes and Coenzymes Q9 and Q10 in Adriamycin-Treated Rats. *Eur. J. Nutr.* **2009**, *49*, 181–187. [CrossRef] [PubMed]
47. Medzhitov, R. Origin and Physiological Roles of Inflammation. *Nature* **2008**, *454*, 428–435. [CrossRef]
48. López-Otín, C.; Blasco, M.A.; Partridge, L.; Serrano, M.; Kroemer, G. The Hallmarks of Aging. *Cell* **2013**, *153*, 1194–1217. [CrossRef]
49. Diaz, L.E.; Cano, P.; Jimenez-Ortega, V.; Nova, E.; Romeo, J.; Marcos, A.; Esquifino, A.I. Effects of Moderate Consumption of Distilled and Fermented Alcohol on Some Aspects of Neuroimmunomodulation. *Neuroimmunomodulation* **2007**, *14*, 200–205. [CrossRef]
50. Martinez, N.; Urpi-Sarda, M.; Martinez-Gonzalez, M.A.; Andres-Lacueva, C.; Mitjavila, M.T. Dealcoholised Beers Reduce Atherosclerosis and Expression of Adhesion Molecules in apoE-Deficient Mice. *Br. J. Nutr.* **2010**, *105*, 721–730. [CrossRef] [PubMed]
51. Autelitano, D.J.; Howarth, E.A.; Pihl, E. Promoting Effect of Beer and Ethanol on Anti-Tumour Cytotoxicity: Unaffected Growth of a Transplantable Rat Tumour. *Aust. J. Exp. Biol. Med Sci.* **1984**, *62*, 507–514. [CrossRef]
52. Wu, C.-N.; Sun, L.-C.; Chu, Y.-L.; Yu, R.-C.; Hsieh, C.-W.; Hsu, H.-Y.; Hsu, F.-C.; Cheng, K.-C. Bioactive Compounds with Anti-oxidative and Anti-Inflammatory Activities of Hop Extracts. *Food Chem.* **2020**, *330*, 127244. [CrossRef]
53. Lupinacci, E.; Meijerink, J.; Vincken, J.-P.; Gabriele, B.; Gruppen, H.; Witkamp, R.F. Xanthohumol from Hop (Humulus Lupulus L.) Is an Efficient Inhibitor of Monocyte Chemoattractant Protein-1 and Tumor Necrosis Factor-α Release in LPS-Stimulated RAW 264.7 Mouse Macrophages and U937 Human Monocytes. *J. Agric. Food Chem.* **2009**, *57*, 7274–7281. [CrossRef]
54. Schink, A.; Neumann, J.; Leifke, A.L.; Ziegler, K.; Fröhlich-Nowoisky, J.; Cremer, C.; Thines, E.; Weber, B.; Pöschl, U.; Schuppan, D.; et al. Screening of Herbal Extracts for TLR2-and TLR4-Dependent Anti-Inflammatory Effects. *PLoS ONE* **2018**, *13*, e0203907. [CrossRef] [PubMed]
55. Hougee, S.; Faber, J.; Sanders, A.; Berg, W.B.V.D.; Garssen, J.; Smit, H.F.; Hoijer, M.A. Selective Inhibition of COX-2 by a Standardized CO2Extract of Humulus Lupulus in Vitroand Its Activity in a Mouse Model of Zymosan-Induced Arthritis. *Planta Med.* **2006**, *72*, 228–233. [CrossRef] [PubMed]
56. Fuchimoto, J.; Kojima, T.; Kobayashi, N.; Ohkuni, T.; Ogasawara, N.; Masaki, T.; Obata, K.; Nomura, K.; Kondoh, A.; Shigyo, T.; et al. Hop Water Extract Inhibits Double-stranded RNA-induced Thymic Stromal Lymphopoietin Release from Human Nasal Epithelial Cells. *Am. J. Rhinol. Allergy* **2012**, *26*, 433–438. [CrossRef] [PubMed]
57. Fukuda, T.; Ohya, R.; Kobayashi, K.; Ano, Y. Matured Hop Bitter Acids in Beer Improve Lipopolysaccharide-Induced Depression-Like Behavior. *Front. Neurosci.* **2019**, *13*, 41. [CrossRef] [PubMed]

58. Saugspier, M.; Dorn, C.; Thasler, W.E.; Gehrig, M.; Heilmann, J.; Hellerbrand, C. Hop Bitter Acids Exhibit Anti-Fibrogenic Effects on Hepatic Stellate Cells In Vitro. *Exp. Mol. Pathol.* **2012**, *92*, 222–228. [CrossRef] [PubMed]
59. Van Cleemput, M.; Heyerick, A.; Libert, C.; Swerts, K.; Philippé, J.; De Keukeleire, D.; Haegeman, G.; De Bosscher, K. Hop Bitter Acids Efficiently Block Inflammation Independent of GRα, PPARα, or PPARγ. *Mol. Nutr. Food Res.* **2009**, *53*, 1143–1155. [CrossRef] [PubMed]
60. Li, J.; Li, N.; Li, X.; Chen, G.; Wang, C.; Lin, B.; Hou, Y. Characteristic α-Acid Derivatives from Humulus lupulus with Antineuroinflammatory Activities. *J. Nat. Prod.* **2017**, *80*, 3081–3092. [CrossRef] [PubMed]
61. Ano, Y.; Dohata, A.; Taniguchi, Y.; Hoshi, A.; Uchida, K.; Takashima, A.; Nakayama, H. Iso-α-acids, Bitter Components of Beer, Prevent Inflammation and Cognitive Decline Induced in a Mouse Model of Alzheimer's Disease. *J. Biol. Chem.* **2017**, *292*, 3720–3728. [CrossRef]
62. Ano, Y.; Takaichi, Y.; Uchida, K.; Kondo, K.; Nakayama, H.; Takashima, A. Iso-α-Acids, the Bitter Components of Beer, Suppress Microglial Inflammation in rTg4510 Tauopathy. *Molecules* **2018**, *23*, 3133. [CrossRef]
63. Ano, Y.; Yoshikawa, M.; Takaichi, Y.; Michikawa, M.; Uchida, K.; Nakayama, H.; Takashima, A. Iso-α-Acids, Bitter Components in Beer, Suppress Inflammatory Responses and Attenuate Neural Hyperactivation in the Hippocampus. *Front. Pharmacol.* **2019**, *10*, 81. [CrossRef]
64. Mahli, A.; Koch, A.; Fresse, K.; Schiergens, T.; Thasler, W.E.; Schönberger, C.; Bergheim, I.; Bosserhoff, A.; Hellerbrand, C. Iso-alpha Acids from Hops (Humulus Lupulus) Inhibit Hepatic Steatosis, Inflammation, and Fibrosis. *Lab. Investig.* **2018**, *98*, 1614–1626. [CrossRef]
65. Hsu, C.-H.; Ho, Y.-S.; Lai, C.-S.; Hsieh, S.-C.; Chen, L.-H.; Lin, E.; Ho, C.-T.; Pan, M.-H. Hexahydro-β-Acids Potently Inhibit 12-O-Tetradecanoylphorbol 13-Acetate-Induced Skin Inflammation and Tumor Promotion in Mice. *J. Agric. Food Chem.* **2013**, *61*, 11541–11549. [CrossRef]
66. Cho, Y.-C.; Kim, H.J.; Kim, Y.-J.; Lee, K.Y.; Choi, H.J.; Lee, I.-S.; Kang, B.Y. Differential Anti-Inflammatory Pathway by Xanthohumol in IFN-γ and LPS-Activated Macrophages. *Int. Immunopharmacol.* **2008**, *8*, 567–573. [CrossRef]
67. Lv, H.; Liu, Q.; Wen, Z.; Feng, H.; Deng, X.; Ci, X. Xanthohumol Ameliorates Lipopolysaccharide (LPS)-Induced Acute Lung Injury via Induction of AMPK/GSK3β-Nrf2 Signal Axis. *Redox Biol.* **2017**, *12*, 311–324. [CrossRef]
68. Peluso, M.R.; Miranda, C.L.; Hobbs, D.J.; Proteau, R.R.; Stevens, J.F. Xanthohumol and Related Prenylated Flavonoids Inhibit Inflammatory Cytokine Production in LPS-Activated THP-1 Monocytes: Structure-Activity Relationships andIn SilicoBinding to Myeloid Differentiation Protein-2 (MD-2). *Planta Med.* **2010**, *76*, 1536–1543. [CrossRef] [PubMed]
69. Cho, Y.-C.; You, S.-K.; Kim, H.J.; Cho, C.-W.; Lee, I.-S.; Kang, B.Y. Xanthohumol Inhibits IL-12 Production and Reduces Chronic Allergic Contact Dermatitis. *Int. Immunopharmacol.* **2010**, *10*, 556–561. [CrossRef] [PubMed]
70. Liang, G.; Fu, W.; Chen, L.; Wang, Z.; Zhao, C.; Chen, G.; Liu, X.; Cai, Y.; Zhou, J.; Dai, Y.; et al. Determination of the Binding Mode for Anti-Inflammatory Natural Product Xanthohumol with Myeloid Differentiation Protein 2. *Drug Des. Dev. Ther.* **2016**, *ume 10*, 455–463. [CrossRef]
71. Xuan, N.T.; Shumilina, E.; Gulbins, E.; Gu, S.; Götz, F.; Lang, F. Triggering of Dendritic Cell Apoptosis by Xanthohumol. *Mol. Nutr. Food Res.* **2010**, *54*, S214–S224. [CrossRef] [PubMed]
72. Gao, X.; Deeb, D.; Liu, Y.; Gautam, S.; Dulchavsky, S.A.; Gautam, S.C. Immunomodulatory Activity of Xanthohumol: Inhibition of T Cell Proliferation, Cell-Mediated Cytotoxicity and Th1 Cytokine Production through Suppression of NF-κB. *Immunopharmacol. Immunotoxicol.* **2009**, *31*, 477–484. [CrossRef] [PubMed]
73. Liu, Y.; Gao, X.; Deeb, D.; Arbab, A.S.; Dulchavsky, S.A.; Gautam, S.C. Anticancer Agent Xanthohumol Inhibits IL-2 Induced Signaling Pathways Involved in T Cell Proliferation. *J. Exp. Ther. Oncol.* **2012**, *10*, 1–8.
74. Chen, X.; Li, Z.; Hong, H.; Wang, N.; Chen, J.; Lu, S.; Zhang, H.; Zhang, X.; Bei, C. Xanthohumol Suppresses Inflammation in Chondrocytes and Ameliorates Osteoarthritis in Mice. *Biomed. Pharmacother.* **2021**, *137*, 111238. [CrossRef]
75. Cho, J.-M.; Yun, S.-M.; Choi, Y.-H.; Heo, J.; Kim, N.-J.; Kim, S.-H.; Kim, E.-H. Xanthohumol Prevents Dextran Sulfate Sodium-induced Colitis via Inhibition of IKKβ/NF-κB Signaling in Mice. *Oncotarget* **2017**, *9*, 866–880. [CrossRef]
76. Dorn, C.; Kraus, B.; Motyl, M.; Weiss, T.S.; Gehrig, M.; Schölmerich, J.; Heilmann, J.; Hellerbrand, C. Xanthohumol, a Chalcon Derived from Hops, Inhibits Hepatic Inflammation and Fibrosis. *Mol. Nutr. Food Res.* **2010**, *54*, S205–S213. [CrossRef]
77. Negrão, R.; Costa, R.; Duarte, D.; Gomes, T.T.; Mendanha, M.; Moura, L.; Vasques, L.; Azevedo, I.; Soares, R. Angiogenesis and Inflammation Signaling Are Targets of Beer Polyphenols on Vascular Cells. *J. Cell. Biochem.* **2010**, *111*, 1270–1279. [CrossRef]
78. Dorn, C.; Heilmann, J.; Hellerbrand, C. Protective Effect of Xanthohumol on Toxin-Induced Liver Inflammation and Fibrosis. *Int. J. Clin. Exp. Pathol.* **2012**, *5*, 29–36. [CrossRef]
79. Dorn, C.; Massinger, S.; Wuzik, A.; Heilmann, J.; Hellerbrand, C. Xanthohumol Suppresses Inflammatory Response to Warm Ischemia–Reperfusion Induced Liver Injury. *Exp. Mol. Pathol.* **2013**, *94*, 10–16. [CrossRef] [PubMed]
80. Negrão, R.; Costa, R.; Duarte, D.; Gomes, T.T.; Coelho, P.; Guimarães, J.T.; Guardão, L.; Azevedo, I.; Soares, R. Xanthohumol-Supplemented Beer Modulates Angiogenesis and Inflammation in a Skin Wound Healing Model. Involvement of Local Adipocytes. *J. Cell. Biochem.* **2011**, *113*, 100–109. [CrossRef]
81. Yamashita, M.; Fukizawa, S.; Nonaka, Y. Hop-Derived Prenylflavonoid Isoxanthohumol Suppresses Insulin Resistance by Changing the Intestinal Microbiota and Suppressing Chronic Inflammation in High Fat Diet-Fed Mice. *Eur. Rev. Med. Pharmacol. Sci.* **2020**, *24*, 1537–1547. [CrossRef] [PubMed]

82. Zhang, W.; Pan, Y.; Gou, P.; Zhou, C.; Ma, L.; Liu, Q.; Du, Y.; Yang, J.; Wang, Q. Effect of Xanthohumol on Th1/Th2 Balance in a Breast Cancer Mouse Model. *Oncol. Rep.* **2017**, *39*, 280–288. [CrossRef] [PubMed]
83. Paoletti, T.; Fallarini, S.; Gugliesi, F.; Minassi, A.; Appendino, G.; Lombardi, G. Anti-Inflammatory and Vascularprotective Properties of 8-Prenylapigenin. *Eur. J. Pharmacol.* **2009**, *620*, 120–130. [CrossRef] [PubMed]
84. Zhao, J.-L.; Chen, Y.-J.; Yu, J.; Du, Z.-Y.; Yuan, Q.; Sun, Y.-R.; Wu, X.; Li, Z.-Q.; Wu, X.-H.; Hu, J.; et al. ISO-Alpha-Acids Improve the Hematoma Resolution and Prevent Peri-Hematoma Inflammations by Transforming Microglia via PPARgamma-CD36 Axis in ICH Rats. *Int. Immunopharmacol.* **2020**, *83*, 106396. [CrossRef]
85. Ano, Y.; Ohya, R.; Kondo, K.; Nakayama, H. Iso-α-acids, Hop-Derived Bitter Components of Beer, Attenuate Age-Related Inflammation and Cognitive Decline. *Front. Aging Neurosci.* **2019**, *11*, 16. [CrossRef]
86. Bounds, W.; Betzing, K.W.; Stewart, R.M.; Holcombe, R.F. Social Drinking and the Immune Response: Impairment of Lymphokine-Activated Killer Activity. *Am. J. Med Sci.* **1994**, *307*, 391–395. [CrossRef] [PubMed]
87. Monobe, M.; Ando, K. Drinking Beer Reduces Radiation-Induced Chromosome Aberrations in Human Lymphocytes. *J. Radiat. Res.* **2002**, *43*, 237–245. [CrossRef] [PubMed]
88. Imhof, A.; Blagieva, R.; Marx, N.; Koenig, W. Drinking Modulates Monocyte Migration in Healthy Subjects: A Randomised Intervention Study of Water, Ethanol, Red Wine and Beer with or without Alcohol. *Diabetes Vasc. Dis. Res.* **2008**, *5*, 48–53. [CrossRef] [PubMed]
89. Romeo, J.; Wärnberg, J.; Díaz, L.E.; González-Gross, M.; Marcos, A. Effects of Moderate Beer Consumption on First-Line Immunity of Healthy Adults. *J. Physiol. Biochem.* **2007**, *63*, 153–159. [CrossRef] [PubMed]
90. Alvarez, J.R.M.; Bellés, V.V.; López-Jaén, A.B.; Marín, A.V.; Codoñer-Franch, P. Effects of Alcohol-Free Beer on Lipid Profile and Parameters of Oxidative Stress and Inflammation in Elderly Women. *Nutrition* **2009**, *25*, 182–187. [CrossRef]
91. Scherr, J.; Nieman, D.C.; Schuster, T.; Habermann, J.; Rank, M.; Braun, S.; Pressler, A.; Wolfarth, B.; Halle, M. Nonalcoholic Beer Reduces Inflammation and Incidence of Respiratory Tract Illness. *Med. Sci. Sports Exerc.* **2012**, *44*, 18–26. [CrossRef]
92. Daimiel, L.; Micó, V.; Díez-Ricote, L.; Ruiz-Valderrey, P.; Istas, G.; Rodríguez-Mateos, A.; Ordovás, J.M. Alcoholic and Non-Alcoholic Beer Modulate Plasma and Macrophage microRNAs Differently in a Pilot Intervention in Humans with Cardiovascular Risk. *Nutrients* **2020**, *13*, 69. [CrossRef]
93. Chiva-Blanch, G.; Magraner, E.; Condines, X.; Valderas-Martínez, P.; Roth, I.; Arranz, S.; Casas, R.; Navarro, M.; Hervas, A.; Sisó, A.; et al. Effects of Alcohol and Polyphenols from Beer on Atherosclerotic Biomarkers in High Cardiovascular Risk Men: A Randomized Feeding Trial. *Nutr. Metab. Cardiovasc. Dis.* **2015**, *25*, 36–45. [CrossRef] [PubMed]
94. López-Jaén, A.B.; Codoñer-Franch, P.; Martínez-Álvarez, J.R.; Villarino-Marín, A.; Valls-Bellés, V. Effect on Health of Non-Alcohol Beer and Hop Supplementation in a Group of Nuns in a Closed Order. *Proc. Nutr. Soc.* **2010**, *69*, 252. [CrossRef]
95. Milivojevic, V.; Ansell, E.; Simpson, C.; Siedlarz, K.M.; Sinha, R.; Fox, H.C. Peripheral Immune System Adaptations and Motivation for Alcohol in Non-Dependent Problem Drinkers. *Alcohol. Clin. Exp. Res.* **2017**, *41*, 585–595. [CrossRef] [PubMed]
96. Simpson, D.S.A.; Oliver, P.L. ROS Generation in Microglia: Understanding Oxidative Stress and Inflammation in Neurodegenerative Disease. *Antioxidants* **2020**, *9*, 743. [CrossRef]
97. Zádori, D.; Veres, G.; Szalardy, L.; Klivenyi, P.; Vécsei, L. Alzheimer's Disease: Recent Concepts on the Relation of Mitochondrial Disturbances, Excitotoxicity, Neuroinflammation, and Kynurenines. *J. Alzheimer's Dis.* **2018**, *62*, 523–547. [CrossRef]
98. Kovacs, G.G. Concepts and Classification of Neurodegenerative Diseases. *Handb. Clin. Neurol.* **2018**, *145*, 301–307. [CrossRef]
99. Yin, F.; Sancheti, H.; Patil, I.; Cadenas, E. Energy Metabolism and Inflammation in Brain Aging and Alzheimer's Disease. *Free. Radic. Biol. Med.* **2016**, *100*, 108–122. [CrossRef] [PubMed]
100. Lee, K.; Jung, J.; Song, D.; Kräuter, M.; Kim, Y. Effects of Humulus Lupulus Extract on the Central Nervous System in Mice. *Planta Med.* **1993**, *59*, A691. [CrossRef]
101. Schiller, H.; Forster, A.; Vonhoff, C.; Hegger, M.; Biller, A.; Winterhoff, H. Sedating Effects of Humulus Lupulus L. Extracts. *Phytomedicine* **2006**, *13*, 535–541. [CrossRef]
102. Zanoli, P.; Rivasi, M.; Zavatti, M.; Brusiani, F.; Baraldi, M. New Insight in the Neuropharmacological Activity of *Humulus Lupulus* L. *J. Ethnopharmacol.* **2005**, *102*, 102–106. [CrossRef]
103. Aoshima, H.; Takeda, K.; Okita, Y.; Hossain, S.J.; Koda, H.; Kiso, Y. Effects of Beer and Hop on Ionotropic γ-Aminobutyric Acid Receptors. *J. Agric. Food Chem.* **2006**, *54*, 2514–2519. [CrossRef] [PubMed]
104. Zanoli, P.; Zavatti, M.; Rivasi, M.; Brusiani, F.; Losi, G.; Puia, G.; Avallone, R.; Baraldi, M. Evidence that the β-acids Fraction of Hops Reduces Central GABAergic Neurotransmission. *J. Ethnopharmacol.* **2007**, *109*, 87–92. [CrossRef] [PubMed]
105. Benkherouf, A.Y.; Soini, S.L.; Stompor, M.; Uusi-Oukari, M. Positive Allosteric Modulation of Native and Recombinant GABAA Receptors by Hops Prenylflavonoids. *Eur. J. Pharmacol.* **2019**, *852*, 34–41. [CrossRef] [PubMed]
106. Chang, Y.; Lin, T.Y.; Lu, C.W.; Huang, S.K.; Wang, Y.C.; Wang, S.J. Xanthohumol-Induced Presynaptic Reduction of Glutamate Release in the Rat Hippocampus. *Food Funct.* **2016**, *7*, 212–226. [CrossRef]
107. Wang, C.C.; Ho, Y.H.; Hung, C.F.; Kuo, J.R.; Wang, S.J. Xanthohumol, an Active Constituent from Hope, Affords Protection Against Kainic Acid-Induced Excitotoxicity in Rats. *Neurochem. Int.* **2020**, *133*, 104629. [CrossRef]
108. Rancán, L.; Paredes, S.D.; García, I.; Muñoz, P.; García, C.; De Hontanar, G.L.; de la Fuente, M.; Vara, E.; Tresguerres, J.A.F. Protective Effect of Xanthohumol Against Age-Related Brain Damage. *J. Nutr. Biochem.* **2017**, *49*, 133–140. [CrossRef]
109. Zamzow, D.R.; Elias, V.; Legette, L.L.; Choi, J.; Stevens, J.F.; Magnusson, K.R. Xanthohumol Improved Cognitive Flexibility in Young Mice. *Behav. Brain Res.* **2014**, *275*, 1–10. [CrossRef]

110. Oberbauer, E.; Urmann, C.; Steffenhagen, C.; Bieler, L.; Brunner, D.; Furtner, T.; Humpel, C.; Bäumer, B.; Bandtlow, C.; Couillard-Despres, S.; et al. Chroman-Like Cyclic Prenylflavonoids Promote Neuronal Differentiation and Neurite Outgrowth and are Neuroprotective. *J. Nutr. Biochem.* **2013**, *24*, 1953–1962. [CrossRef]
111. Urmann, C.; Oberbauer, E.; Couillard-Despres, S.; Aigner, L.; Riepl, H. Neurodifferentiating Potential of 8-Prenylnaringenin and Related Compounds in Neural Precursor Cells and Correlation with Estrogen-Like Activity. *Planta Med.* **2015**, *81*, 305–311. [CrossRef]
112. Huang, X.; Wang, J.; Chen, X.; Liu, P.; Wang, S.; Song, F.; Zhang, Z.; Zhu, F.; Liu, J.; Song, G.; et al. The Prenylflavonoid Xanthohumol Reduces Alzheimer-Like Changes and Modulates Multiple Pathogenic Molecular Pathways in the Neuro2a/APPswe Cell Model of AD. *Front. Pharmacol.* **2018**, *9*, 199. [CrossRef] [PubMed]
113. Ano, Y.; Hoshi, A.; Ayabe, T.; Ohya, R.; Uchida, S.; Yamada, K.; Kondo, K.; Kitaoka, S.; Furuyashiki, T. Iso-α-acids, the Bitter Components of Beer, Improve Hippocampus-Dependent Memory through Vagus Nerve Activation. *FASEB J.* **2019**, *33*, 4987–4995. [CrossRef]
114. Ano, Y.; Kitaoka, S.; Ohya, R.; Kondo, K.; Furuyashiki, T. Hop Bitter Acids Increase Hippocampal Dopaminergic Activity in a Mouse Model of Social Defeat Stress. *Int. J. Mol. Sci.* **2020**, *21*, 9612. [CrossRef] [PubMed]
115. Fukuda, T.; Obara, K.; Saito, J.; Umeda, S.; Ano, Y. Effects of Hop Bitter Acids, Bitter Components in Beer, on Cognition in Healthy Adults: A Randomized Controlled Trial. *J. Agric. Food Chem.* **2019**, *68*, 206–212. [CrossRef] [PubMed]
116. Fukuda, T.; Ohnuma, T.; Obara, K.; Kondo, S.; Arai, H.; Ano, Y. Supplementation with Matured Hop Bitter Acids Improves Cognitive Performance and Mood State in Healthy Older Adults with Subjective Cognitive Decline. *J. Alzheimer's Dis.* **2020**, *76*, 387–398. [CrossRef]

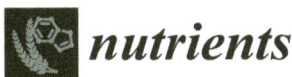 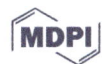

Article

Nutritional Value of *Moringa oleifera* Lam. Leaf Powder Extracts and Their Neuroprotective Effects via Antioxidative and Mitochondrial Regulation

Elena González-Burgos, Isabel Ureña-Vacas, Marta Sánchez and M. Pilar Gómez-Serranillos *

Department of Pharmacology, Pharmacognosy and Botany, Faculty of Pharmacy, Universidad Complutense de Madrid (UCM), 28040 Madrid, Spain; elenagon@ucm.es (E.G.-B.); isabelur@ucm.es (I.U.-V.); martas15@ucm.es (M.S.)
* Correspondence: pserra@ucm.es

Citation: González-Burgos, E.; Ureña-Vacas, I.; Sánchez, M.; Gómez-Serranillos, M.P. Nutritional Value of *Moringa oleifera* Lam. Leaf Powder Extracts and Their Neuroprotective Effects via Antioxidative and Mitochondrial Regulation. *Nutrients* **2021**, *13*, 2203. https://doi.org/10.3390/nu13072203

Academic Editor: Serguei O. Fetissov

Received: 7 June 2021
Accepted: 22 June 2021
Published: 26 June 2021

Publisher's Note: MDPI stays neutral with regard to jurisdictional claims in published maps and institutional affiliations.

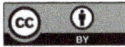

Copyright: © 2021 by the authors. Licensee MDPI, Basel, Switzerland. This article is an open access article distributed under the terms and conditions of the Creative Commons Attribution (CC BY) license (https://creativecommons.org/licenses/by/4.0/).

Abstract: Age-related neurodegenerative disorders are an increasing public health problem. Oxidative stress is one of the major causes. Medicinal plant-based functional foods can be effective for these diseases. The aim of this work is to investigate the neuroprotective role of methanol extracts of *Moringa oleifera* leaf powder on antioxidant/oxidant imbalance and mitochondrial regulation in a H_2O_2-induced oxidative stress model in human neuroblastoma cells. On nutritional analysis, results showed that moringa contained 28.50% carbohydrates, 25.02% proteins, 10.42% fat, 11.83% dietary fiber, 1.108 mg β-carotene, 326.4 µg/100 g vitamin B1 and 15.2 mg/100 g vitamin C. In-vitro assays revealed that moringa methanol extracts had more phenolic content and higher antioxidant activity than acetone extracts. Moreover, pretreatments with methanol extracts showed a protective effect against H_2O_2-induced oxidative damage through increasing cell viability and reducing free radicals. Furthermore, the extract decreased lipid peroxidation and enhanced glutathione levels and antioxidant enzyme activity. Finally, moringa also prevented mitochondrial dysfunction by regulating calcium levels and increasing mitochondrial membrane potential. The most active concentration was 25 µg/mL. In summary, the nutritional and functional properties of *Moringa oleifera* as a neuroprotective agent could be beneficial to protect against oxidative stress and provide necessary nutrients for a healthy diet.

Keywords: *Moringa oleifera*; neurodegenerative disorders; neuroprotection; oxidative stress; nutrients

1. Introduction

Age-related neurodegenerative diseases such as Alzheimer's and Parkinson's disease are heterogeneous clinical diseases with a multi-causal origin. Neurodegenerative diseases affect millions of people, causing disability and great economic impact. Conventional treatments are symptomatic, and there are currently no drugs that cure any of these neurodegenerative diseases. In this context, medicinal plants are an inexhaustible source of molecules with pharmacological properties. The World Health Organization (WHO) and European Medicines Agency (EMA) reported several herbal products for the management of neurodegenerative diseases, such as folium *Ginkgo* [1,2]. Currently, research is aimed at finding new herbal products with protective and therapeutic properties against neurodegenerative disease.

Oxidative stress is one of the major causes implicated in the pathogenic development of age-related neurodegenerative disorders. Oxidative stress occurs from an imbalance between reactive oxygen species (ROS) generation and antioxidant defense system. The oxidative stress theory of aging postulates that physical and functional losses in the aged are caused by ROS accumulation, their consequent reactivity and damage to cellular macromolecules [3]. Post-mortem brains of patients with neurodegenerative diseases have shown the presence of biomarkers of oxidative stress including protein carbonyl, *trans*-4-hydroxy-2-nonenal (4-HNE) and malondialdehyde (MDA) [4].

Moringa oleifera Lam. (Moringaceae family, commonly known as Horseradish tree) is a perennial herb tree that extensively grows in tropical and subtropical countries. *Moringa oleifera* is employed as vegetable, herbal tea and processed foods for its nutritional properties as a source of proteins and essential amino acids (i.e., cysteine, methionine, lysine and tryptophan) [5]. Moreover, the leaves of *Moringa oleifera* are rich in flavonoids, carotenoids and ascorbic acid [6]. Furthermore, this herbal product has demonstrated health benefits beyond its great nutritional value. Hence, in traditional medicine, ancient rules included the leaves of *Moringa oleifera* for its beneficial properties in mental health and smooth skin [7]. Moreover, *Moringa oleifera* leaves have been attributed numerous therapeutic applications in in-vitro and in-vivo studies such as antibacterial, antifungal, antiviral, cytotoxic, antihyperglycemic, antioxidant, anti-inflammatory, antiparasitic and cardioprotective activities [8]. In addition, there are several clinical studies on *Moringa oleifera* focused on its pharmacological role in metabolic syndrome, type 2 diabetes mellitus, osteoporosis, anemia and dyslipidemias [9]. However, despite its great nutritional and therapeutic value, *Moringa oleifera* leaves are not as popular as other leafy vegetables, and its potential pharmacological activities are still unexplored, particularly in terms of its role as neuroprotective agent.

Considering the growing consumption of *Moringa oleifera* in the world, the aim of this work was to investigate the *Moringa oleifera* ability to prevent and treat hydrogen peroxide-induced oxidative stress in neuroblastoma cells. The effect of methanol extract of moringa leaf powder on antioxidant/ROS imbalance and mitochondrial regulation was investigated in the human SH-SY5Y cell line.

2. Materials and Methods

2.1. Preparation of Moringa oleifera Extracts

Fresh leaves of *Moringa oleifera* were collected in Piribebuy, Paraguay between March 2016 and August 2016. After collection, the leaves were dried at room temperature and pulverized for further experimental analysis. Leaf powder of *Moringa oleifera* (over 50 mg) was macerated with methanol and acetone (2 mL) for 24 h at room temperature. The obtained extracts were then filtered through Whatman filter paper and evaporated until dry at room temperature. Extracts were kept in a freezer at $-20\ °C$ until use.

2.2. Nutritional Value

The nutritional value of *Moringa oleifera* was performed in triplicate to estimate fat, proteins, ash, carbohydrates, moisture, dietary fiber, energy, total carotenoids and vitamins B1 and C. The energy content in moringa was determined using Atwater factors. The protein content was determined based on the analysis of the total nitrogen content by the Kjeldahl method using a 6.25 correction factor [10]. Total available carbohydrates were analyzed based on an anthrone colorimetric technique; absorbance was measured at 630 nm [11]. Total dietary fiber content was quantified by the Association of Official Analytical Chemists (AOAC) enzymatic–non-gravimetric method (993.21) [10]. Moisture content was calculated by desiccation and ash content by combustion following the AOAC 984.25 method and 942.05 method, respectively [10]. Total fat was determined after petroleum ether extraction and consequent drying at 105 °C following the AOAC 983.23 procedure [10]. The total carotenoid content was determined by spectrophotometry (446 nm) according to the method described in AOAC [10]. The determination of vitamin B1 (thiamine), based on its oxidation to the fluorescent thiochrome with alkaline potassium hexacyanoferrate (III) (potassium ferricyanide), was performed following the AOAC 942.23 procedure [10]. Finally, vitamin C content was analyzed by high-performance liquid chromatography (HPLC) technique using Agilent 1260 equipment with a reversed-phase column and a diode array detector. The mobile phase was water acidified to pH 2.6 with sulfuric acid. The rate of flow was 0.9 mL/min. Detection wavelength for the UV-visible detector was set at 245 nm [12].

2.3. Total Phenolic Compounds

The Folin–Ciocalteu method was used to determine the total phenolic compounds presented in methanol and acetone extracts of moringa leaf powder. Extracts were incubated with Folin–Ciocalteu reagent (Sigma-Aldrich, St. Louis, MO, USA) for 5 min followed by 10% Na_2CO_3 incubation for 40 min. Absorbance was determined at 752 nm using a SPECTROstar BMG microplate reader (BMG Labtech Inc., Ortenberg, Germany) [13].

2.4. In-Vitro Antioxidant Assays

2.4.1. 1,1-Diphenyl-2-picrylhydrazyl (DPPH) Method

Extracts of moringa were incubated with 1,1-Diphenyl-2-picrylhydrazyl (DPPH) (50 µM) (Sigma-Aldrich) for 30 min. Absorbance was then measured at 517 nm using a SPECTROstar BMG microplate reader [14].

2.4.2. Oxygen Radical Absorbance Capacity (ORAC) Assay

Extracts of moringa were incubated with fluorescein (70 nm) for 10 min of darkness. Then, 2,2'-Azobis(2-amidinopropane) dihydrochloride (AAPH) solution (Sigma-Aldrich) was added to the 96-well plates. Fluorescence was recorded for 98 min at a 485 nm excitation wavelength and at a 520 nm emission wavelength in a FLUOstar OPTIMA fluorimeter (BMG Labtech, Ortenberg, Germany) [15].

2.4.3. Ferric Reducing Antioxidant Power (FRAP) Assay

Extracts of moringa were incubated with FRAP reagent for 30 min. Absorbance was measured at 595 nm using a SPECTROstar BMG microplate reader [16].

2.5. Cell Culture and Cell Treatments

The human neuroblastoma SH-SY5Y cell line was cultured in DMEM (Lonza, Walkersville, USA) supplemented with 10% heat-inactivated FBS and 1% penicillin-streptomycin solution in a humidified atmosphere with 5% CO_2 at 37 °C. The SH-SY5Y cells were pretreated with different concentrations of *Moringa oleifera* methanol extracts (5, 10 and 25 µg/mL) for 24 h before hydrogen peroxide exposure to induce oxidative stress (100 µM, 1 h).

2.6. Cell Viability

Cell viability was measured using the colorimetric MTT assay [17]. MTT solution (2 mg/mL) (Sigma-Aldrich) was added for 1 h and then formazan crystals were dissolved in DMSO. Absorbance was measured at 550 nm using a SPECTROstar BMG microplate reader. Cell viability was calculated as a percentage of no extract cells (100%).

2.7. Intracellular Reactive Oxygen Species (ROS)

Intracellular ROS production was measured by dichlorofluorescein assay [18]. After cell treatments, SH-SY5Y cells were incubated in the fluorogenic dye 2,7-di-chloro-dihydrofluorescein diacetate (DCFH-DA) (0.01 M) (Sigma-Aldrich) for 30 min at 37 °C. ROS convert DCFH-DA into 2'-7'dichlorofluorescein (DCF). The intensity of the fluorescent signal was measured in a microplate fluorescence reader (FL×800, Bio-TekInstrumentation) at a λ excitation of 480 nm and λ emission of 580.

2.8. Thiobarbituric Acid Reactive Species (TBARS)

Lipid peroxidation content was determined by TBARS assay [19]. Total extracts (50 µL) were mixture with TBA-TCA-HCl (100 µL) and then boiled at 100 °C for 10 min. Absorbance was read at 535 nm using a SPECTROstar Omega microplate reader.

2.9. Glutathione Assay

Total cell extracts were incubated with O-phthalaldehyde (OPT) (Sigma-Aldrich) and sodium phosphate buffer for 15 min. Fluorescence intensity was measured at an excitation wavelength of 528 nm and emission wavelength of 485 nm using a FLUOstar Omega microplate reader [20].

2.10. Antioxidant Enzymes Activity

For preparation of total cell extracts, pellets were resuspended in lysis buffer (TRIS 25 mM, NaCl 150 mM, EDTA 1 mM and Triton×100 (0.1%), pH 7.4) with antiproteases (phenylmethylsulfonyl fluoride, pepstatin and leupeptin).

2.10.1. Catalase Activity (CAT)

Total cell extracts were incubated with hydrogen peroxide (15 mM) and absorbance was measured at 240 nm for 1 min using a SPECTROstar Omega microplate reader [21].

2.10.2. Superoxide Dismutase Activity (SOD)

Total cell extracts were incubated with pyrogallol (0.15 mM) dissolved in HCl (10 mM) and Tris−DTPA (pH 8.2). Absorbance was measured at 420 nm for 1 min using a SPECTROstar Omega microplate reader [22].

2.10.3. Glutathione Peroxidase Activity (GPx)

Total cell extracts were incubated with EDTA, GSH, glutathione reductase, NADPH, sodium azide and phosphate buffer for 4 min. Then hydrogen peroxide was added and absorbance was measured at 340 nm for 3 min using a SPECTROstar Omega microplate reader [23].

2.11. Mitochondrial Membrane Potential

After treatments, cells were incubated with tetramethylrhodamine methyl ester (TMRM) (Gibco-Invitrogen, Grand Island, NY, USA) in Krebs medium and fluorescence was measured for 45 min at 37 °C with an emission wavelength and excitation wavelength of 549 nm and 573 nm, respectively, using a FLUOstar OPTIMA (BMG Labtech, Ortenberg, Germany) microplate reader. Then, oligomycin and trifluoromethoxy carbonylcyanide phenylhydrazone (FCCP) (Sigma-Aldrich) were added to induce mitochondrial depolarization. Fluorescence was measured for 15 min. The mitochondrial membrane potential value is the result of the difference between the maximum fluorescence and the baseline fluorescence [24].

2.12. Mitochondrial Calcium Levels

After treatments, cells were incubated with the cationic dye Rhod-2/AM (Gibco-Invitrogen) in Krebs normal calcium medium for 40 min. Then, cells were incubated in Krebs normal calcium medium for 30 min. Fluorescence was recorded for 4 min at 581 nm emission wavelength and 552 nm excitation wavelength using a FLUOstar OPTIMA (BMG Labtech, Ortenberg, Germany) microplate reader. Finally, the calcium ionophore A23187 (Sigma-Aldrich) was added, and fluorescence was measured for 15 min. Mitochondrial calcium levels were calculated as the ratio between the maximum fluorescence signal after the calcium ionophore A23187 addition and the basal fluorescence [25].

2.13. Cytosolic Calcium Levels

After treatments, cells were incubated with Indo-1/AM (Gibco-Invitrogen) in Krebs medium for 45 min at 37 °C. Then, cells were maintained in dye-free Krebs medium for 15 min at 37 °C. Fluorescence was measured for 4 min at 37 °C with an emission wavelength and excitation wavelength of 410 nm and 350 nm, respectively, using a FLUOstar OPTIMA microplate reader. Following this, ionomycin and $MnCl_2$ were added, and fluorescence was measured under identical conditions for 8 min and 4 min, respectively. Cytosolic calcium levels were measured using the following formula: $[Ca^{2+}]i = Kd \times [F - Fmin]/[Fmax - F]$, where Kd is the dissociation constant for Indo-1; F is the fluorescence signal for samples; Fmax is the maximum fluorescence signal after ionomycin addition and Fmin is calculated using this formula: Fmin = AF + 1/12 × (Fmax−AF), AF being the minimum fluorescence after adding MnCl$_2$ [26].

2.14. Statistical Analysis

Data are presented as mean ± standard deviation. Statistical analysis was performed by SigmaPlot version 11.0 (Systat Software Inc., San Jose, CA, USA). Data were analyzed by one-way analysis of variance (ANOVA) with Tukey's test. Statistical significance was set at $p < 0.05$.

3. Results and Discussion

Although *Moringa oleifera* has demonstrated numerous therapeutic activities, studies on its neuroprotective activity are still limited. The aim of the present work is to investigate the potential neuroprotective role of methanol extracts of *Moringa oleifera* leaf powder on antioxidant/ROS imbalance and mitochondrial regulation in a hydrogen peroxide-induced oxidative stress model in human neuroblastoma cells.

3.1. Nutritional Value

The nutritional value of the leaves of *Moringa oleifera* is shown in Table 1. The content of proteins is over 25%; this value is higher than that of other vegetables with high-protein content (potato, pumpkin) and is similar to other high-protein foods (i.e., milk, eggs and meat) [27]. Moreover, *Moringa oleifera* has a low–medium content in fat (over 10%) and carbohydrates (28.5%). Furthermore, moringa leaf powder has 12% of dietary fiber, 4% of ashes and 0.52% of moisture. Comparing the results of the nutritional composition of leaf powder of *Moringa oleifera* of our study with other previously published ones, there are certain differences in carbohydrates (25.5% versus 44.4%), fat (10% versus 7.1%) and ash content (4% *versus* 10.9%) [28]. It is especially worth highlighting the total carotenoid content (1.10 mg β-carotene), vitamin B1 (326 μg/100 g) and vitamin C (15.2 mg/100 g). Moringa leaves have more vitamin A than carrots and more vitamin C than oranges [29].

Table 1. Nutritional value of *Moringa oleifera* leaf powder.

	Moringa oleifera **Leaf Powder**
Ashes (%)	4.45 ± 0.33
Carbohydrates (%)	28.50 ± 0.45
Dietary fiber (%)	11.83 ± 1.19
Energy (kcal/100 g)	324.4 ± 2.89
Fat (%)	10.42 ± 0.63
Moisture (%)	0.52 ± 0.05
Proteins (%)	25.02 ± 0.37
Total carotenoids (mg β-carotene)	1.108 ± 0.12
Vitamin B1 (μg/100 g)	326.4 ± 1.28
Vitamin C (mg/100 g)	15.2 ± 0.78

Data are expressed as mean ± standard deviation (n = 3).

3.2. In-Vitro Antioxidant Assays

The results of the in-vitro antioxidants assays and phenolic content are shown in Table 2. The yield of moringa leaf powder was similar for both methanol extraction and acetone extraction (6.38% and 6.66%, respectively). The in-vitro antioxidant activity of methanol and acetone extracts was measured using DPPH assay, ORAC method and FRAP assay. These methods differ in the type of reaction: hydrogen atom transfer (HAT)-based assays and electron transfer (ET)-based assays. HAT assays measure the ability of antioxidants to scavenge free radicals by H-atom donation [i.e., ORAC assay]. ET assays measure the ability of antioxidants to reduce an oxidant, which changes color when reduced [i.e., FRAP and DPPH]. The results of the present work showed that methanol extract has significant antioxidant activity than acetone extract. Hence, DPPH values were 44.89 μg/mL and 305.44 μg/mL, ORAC value 8360 μmol TE/100 g sample and 866.1 μmol

TE/100 g sample and FRAP value 59.32 µmol Fe^{2+} eq/g sample and 27.91 µmol Fe^{2+} eq/g sample for methanol and acetone extracts, respectively.

Table 2. In-vitro assays for antioxidant activity evaluation and phenolic content of methanol and acetone extracts of *Moringa oleifera* leaf powder.

Extracts of *Moringa oleifera* Leaf Powder	Yield of Extract (% w/w)	DPPH EC$_{50}$ (µg/mL)	ORAC (µmol TE/100 g Sample)	FRAP (µmol Fe^{2+} eq/g Sample)	Total Phenol Content (mg gallic acid/g extract)
Methanol extract	6.38% ± 0.47	44.89 ± 1.01 *	8360 ± 0.05 *	59.32 ± 0.29 *	2.17 ± 0.03 *
Acetone extract	6.66% ± 0.09	305.44 ± 8.21	866.1 ± 0.01	27.91 ± 1.90	0.88 ± 0.005

Data are expressed as mean ± standard deviation (n = 3). * $p < 0.05$ versus acetone extract.

For the additional characterization of moringa extracts, total phenolic content was evaluated using Folin–Ciocalteu method. The amount of total phenolic content was high in methanol extract (2.17 mg gallic acid/g extract) than in acetone extract (0.88 mg gallic acid/g extract). The variations in the phenolic content are attributed to the time of harvesting of the leaves, the growing conditions, and the solvent of the extraction. Hence, the more mature the moringa leaves, the higher the phenolic content [30]. There are different phenolic compounds identified in *Moringa oleifera* leaves such as rutin, quercetin, isoquercetin, astragalin, kaempferol, apigenin, luteolin, genistein, myricetin, and vicenin-2, among others [8]. Epidemiological studies have shown a relationship between polyphenol-rich foods and a lower risk of suffering neurodegenerative diseases [31].

3.3. Effect on Cell Viability and Cell Morphology

Since the methanol extract of moringa leaf powder had greater antioxidant activity, we selected this extract to evaluate its potential neuroprotective activity in a cellular model of oxidative stress induced by hydrogen peroxide. Oxidative stress is one major pathway contributing to neurodegeneration. The brain has some characteristics that make it especially susceptible to oxidative stress, including high rate of oxygen consumption, low catalase content, neurotransmitters (dopamine) that can auto-oxidize and high content in redox active transition metals [32]. Medicinal plants with antioxidants properties can slow or stop the neurodegenerative processes through scavenging free radicals, metal chelation or upregulating endogenous antioxidant system. Polyphenolic compounds can pass across blood-brain barrier [33]. Earlier studies demonstrated that *Moringa oleifera* could have a neuroprotective effect against oxidative stress. Hence, the methanol leaf extract improved the homocysteine and AF64A induced oxidative stress, cognitive impairments and Aβ pathology in rats, being a promising candidate for Alzheimer's disease [34,35]. Moreover, the methanol extract of moringa leaves (250 mg/kg, 300 mg/kg) attenuated lead and aluminum-induced cerebral damage in rats by reducing oxidative stress, inflammation and apoptosis and by improving neurohistopathology [36,37]. Compounds identified as potential neuroprotective agents for moringa include isothiocyanate isolated from seeds [38].

In the current study, we initially investigated the effect of different concentration of *Moringa oleifera* methanol leaves extracts (from 5 to 500 µg/mL) on the human neuroblastoma SH-SY5Y cells. This cell line is widely used as a dopaminergic neuronal model for common neurodegenerative diseases such as Alzheimer's disease, Parkinson's disease, and Amyotrophic lateral sclerosis. SH-SY5Y cells express dopamine transporter and the enzymes tyrosine hydroxylase and dopamine-beta-hydroxylase [39]. As shown in Figure 1A, all assayed concentrations were non-toxic except for 250 and 500 µg/mL which significantly decreased cell viability. Next, an in-vitro oxidative stress model was established with hydrogen peroxide (100 µM, 1 h). Hydrogen peroxide passes across membranes using aquaporin-3 [40]. Hydrogen peroxide significantly reduced cell viability by around 32% compared to no extract cells. However, pretreatments with 5, 10 and 25 µg/mL significantly increased the viability of cells by over 25–30% compared to hydrogen peroxide-treated cells, as shown in Figure 1B. Moreover, hydrogen peroxide modified morphology towards round cells. *Moringa oleifera* extracts prevented these alterations in neuroblastoma cells morphology (Figure 1C). Previous studies demonstrated that the aqueous extract of moringa protected cell viability and ameliorated cytotoxicity against cadmium in colon and kidney cells [41].

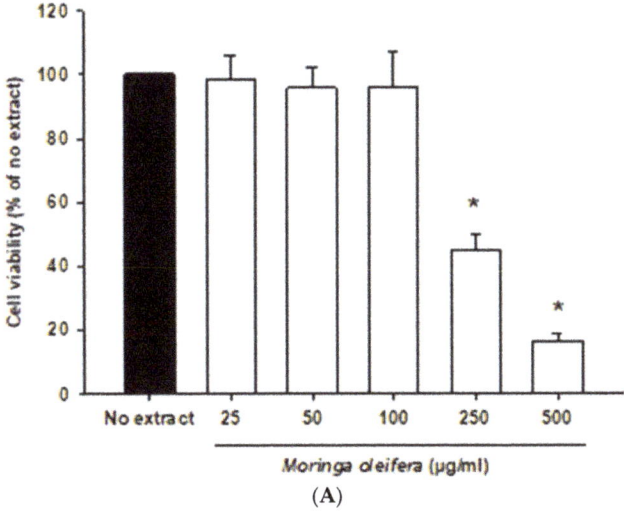

(A)

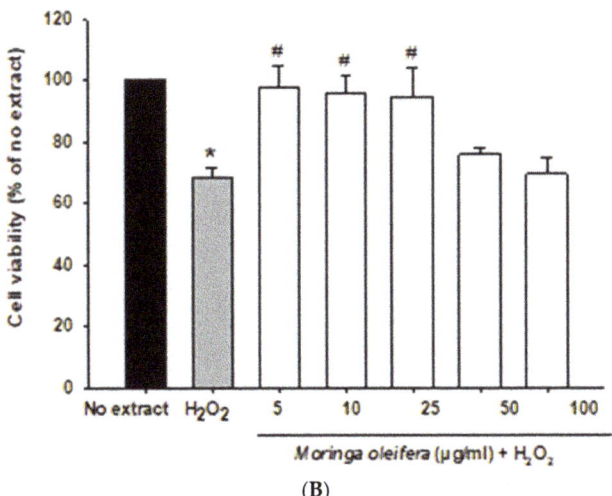

(B)

Figure 1. *Cont.*

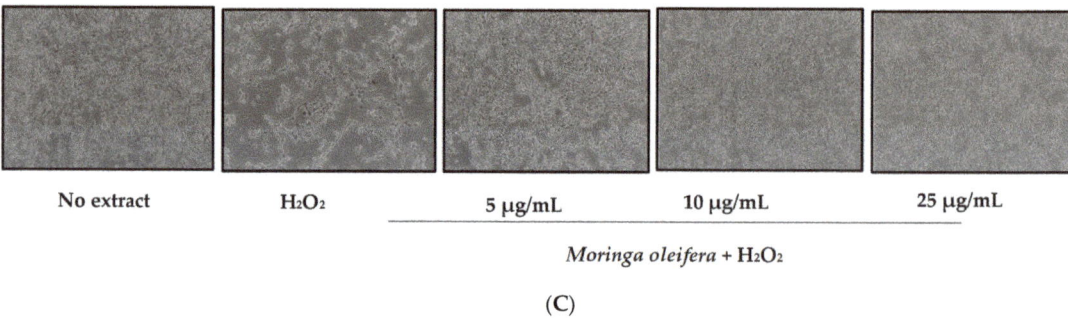

No extract | H₂O₂ | 5 µg/mL | 10 µg/mL | 25 µg/mL

Moringa oleifera + H₂O₂

(C)

Figure 1. Effect of methanol extracts of *Moringa oleifera* leaf powder on cell viability and cell morphology. (**A**) Effect of moringa on SH-SY5Y cell viability. Cells were treated with moringa from 5 to 500 µg/mL for 24 h. (**B**) Protective effect of moringa in a hydrogen peroxide-induced oxidative stress model. Cells were pretreated with moringa from 5 to 100 µg/mL for 24 h before 100 µM H$_2$O$_2$ for 1 h. (**C**) Effect of moringa on SH-SY5Y cell morphology. * $p < 0.05$ versus no extract, # $p < 0.05$ versus H$_2$O$_2$.

3.4. Effect on Intracellular ROS Production

The most cytoprotective and non-toxic concentrations (5, 10 and 25 µg/mL) of *Moringa oleifera* methanol extracts were selected for subsequent experiments. Hydrogen peroxide can be converted into hydroxyl radical (HO•) via Fenton reaction [42]. The intracellular production of ROS was measured using the DCFHA-DA assay. As shown in Figure 2, hydrogen peroxide significantly increased by 56% compared to no extract cells. However, pretreatments with the three assayed concentrations of *Moringa oleifera* significantly reduced hydrogen peroxide-induced ROS overproduction. Similar results were observed for moringa leaf flavonoids in bovine mammary epithelial cells against hydrogen peroxide and the compound 1-O-(4-hydroxymethylphenyl)-α-L-rhamnopyranoside from *Moringa oleifera* seeds against carbon against CCl$_4$ [43,44].

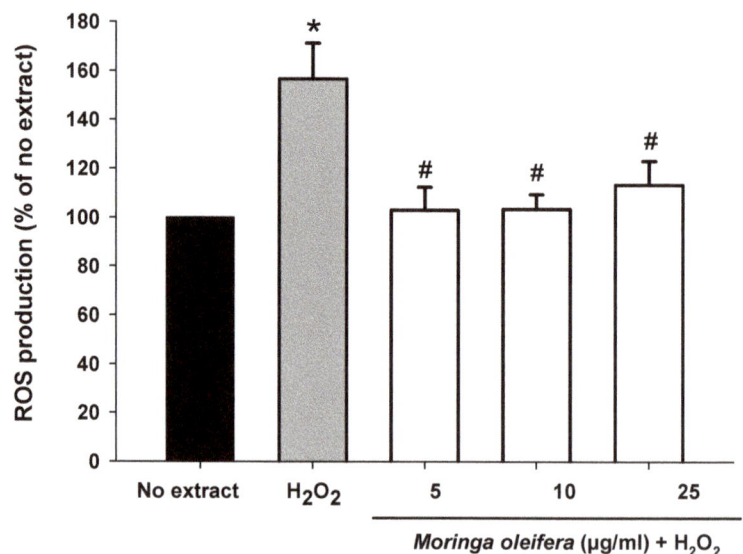

Figure 2. Effect of methanol extracts of *Moringa oleifera* leaf powder on intracellular ROS overproduction. Cells were pretreated with moringa (5, 10 and 25 µg/mL) for 24 h before 100 µM H$_2$O$_2$ for 1 h. * $p < 0.05$ versus no extract, # $p < 0.05$ versus H$_2$O$_2$.

3.5. Effect on Oxidative Stress Markers

An overproduction of ROS to the detriment of endogenous antioxidants leads to oxidative damage to biomolecules. Lipid peroxidation and GSH content are clinically significant biomarkers of oxidative stress in humans [45]. The double bonds of polyunsaturated fatty acids are highly vulnerable to ROS attack and consequently to lipid peroxidation. Malondialdehyde (MDA) is one the most investigated end product of lipid oxidation [42]. As shown in Figure 3A, hydrogen peroxide significantly increased the peroxidation of lipids by 229%. However, pretreatments with methanol extract of moringa leaf powder at 25 µg/mL significantly reduced TBARS levels (160% compared to 229% of hydrogen peroxide). Therefore, moringa leaf extract has a potent preventive effect against the peroxidation of lipids. As shown above, the methanol extract of moringa has scavenging capacity, so the effect on lipid peroxidation can be attributed to a direct action on free radicals process [33].

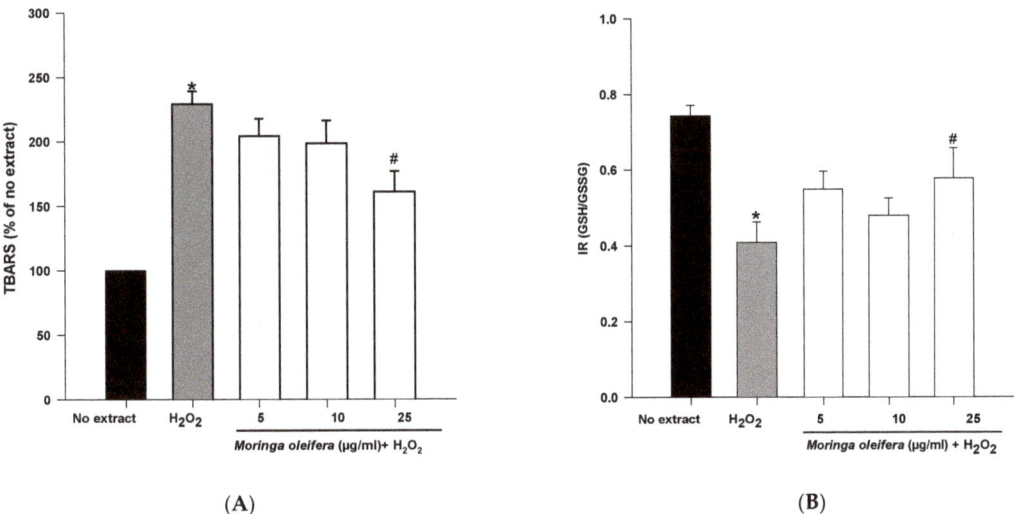

Figure 3. Effect of methanol extracts of *Moringa oleifera* leaf powder on (**A**) lipid peroxidation and (**B**) Index Redox (GSH/GSSG). Cells were pretreated with moringa (5, 10 and 25 µg/mL) for 24 h before 100 µM H_2O_2 for 1 h. * $p < 0.05$ versus no extract, # $p < 0.05$ versus H_2O_2.

Reduced glutathione is the major antioxidant compound in mammalian cells. The index redox (GSH/GSSG) was significantly decreased in hydrogen peroxide (IR = 0.41) compared to no extract cells (IR = 0.74). On the other hand, methanol extract of moringa at 25 µg/mL significantly increased IR to 0.578 compared to hydrogen peroxide-treated cells.

3.6. Effect on Antioxidant Enzymes Activities

The antioxidant enzymatic defense system plays a key role against free radicals. The enzymes catalase (CAT), superoxide dismutase (SOD) and glutathione peroxidase (GPx) constitute the first defense system against oxidative stress. Superoxide dismutase (SOD) converts the superoxide anion radical into hydrogen peroxide. Catalase (CAT) and glutathione peroxidase (GPx) catalyze the decomposition of hydrogen peroxide to water (GPx) and to water and oxygen (CAT) [46]. In Figure 4, our study demonstrated that there is a significant decrease in the activity of these antioxidant enzymes by 53% for CAT, 51% for SOD and 65% for GPx compared to no extract cells (100%). However, pretreatments with moringa extracts reversed this impairment in the defensive system. For catalase, there was a significant increase at 10 and 25 µg/mL (82.9% and 81.2%). For SOD and GPx, the three assayed concentrations markedly improved the activity of these enzymes. The ability of moringa to increase antioxidant enzymatic activity suggests that their polyphenols have a direct antioxidant effect [33].

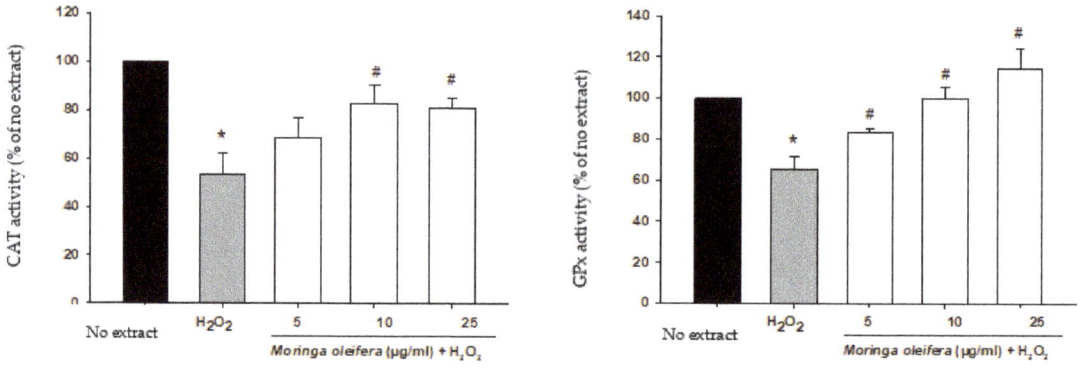

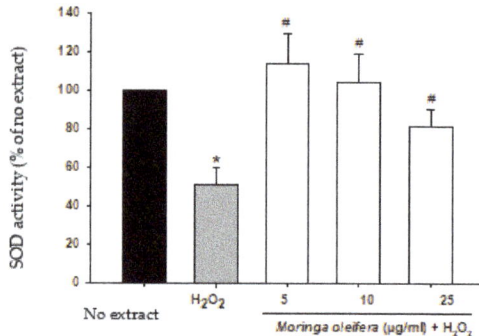

Figure 4. Effect of methanol extracts of *Moringa oleifera* leaf powder on antioxidant enzyme activity. Cells were pretreated with moringa (5, 10 and 25 µg/mL) for 24 h before 100 µM H_2O_2 for 1 h. * $p < 0.05$ versus extract, # $p < 0.05$ versus H_2O_2.

3.7. Effect on Mitochondrial Regulation

Mitochondria are double membrane-bound cell organelles presented in almost all cell eukaryotes. Mitochondria are involved in energy production [47]. The increased ROS generation can be associated with mitochondrial dysfunction. Mitochondria is a key target for the prevention and treatment of those oxidative stress-related neurodegenerative diseases [48]. As shown in Figure 5A, hydrogen peroxide reduced significantly mitochondrial membrane potential (MMP) by 55% compared to no extract cells (100%). However, pretreatments with 10 µg/mL and 25 µg/mL significantly increased MMP to 76% and 88%, respectively. Regarding calcium cytosolic, there was a significant increase (357 nM) after hydrogen peroxide-treated cells compared to no extract cells (88 nM). However, the pretreatment with 25 µg/mL almost reduced cytosolic calcium levels to no extract levels (95 nM) (Figure 5B). Furthermore, hydrogen peroxide significantly increased mitochondrial calcium level (1.18 relative to no extract). This increase in mitochondrial calcium level was markedly reduced after pretreatments with 10 µg/mL and 25 µg/mL of moringa extracts (1.01 and 1.03 relative to no extract, respectively) (Figure 5C). Hydrogen peroxide interacts with mitochondrial structure and function, leading to an impaired calcium level and a mitochondrial potential deficiency [49]. Altered calcium levels can affect mitochondrial function and integrity (i.e., depletion of mitochondrial DNA, release of cytochrome C, ultrastructural lesions, morphological changes) as well as to promote the production of more ROS (i.e., peroxidation of cardiolipin), contributing to the pathogenesis of many common neurodegenerative diseases [50]. The methanol extract of moringa leaves exerts a mitochondrial protective role in neurons, showing for the first time that the mitochondria is the target of action for this medicinal plant.

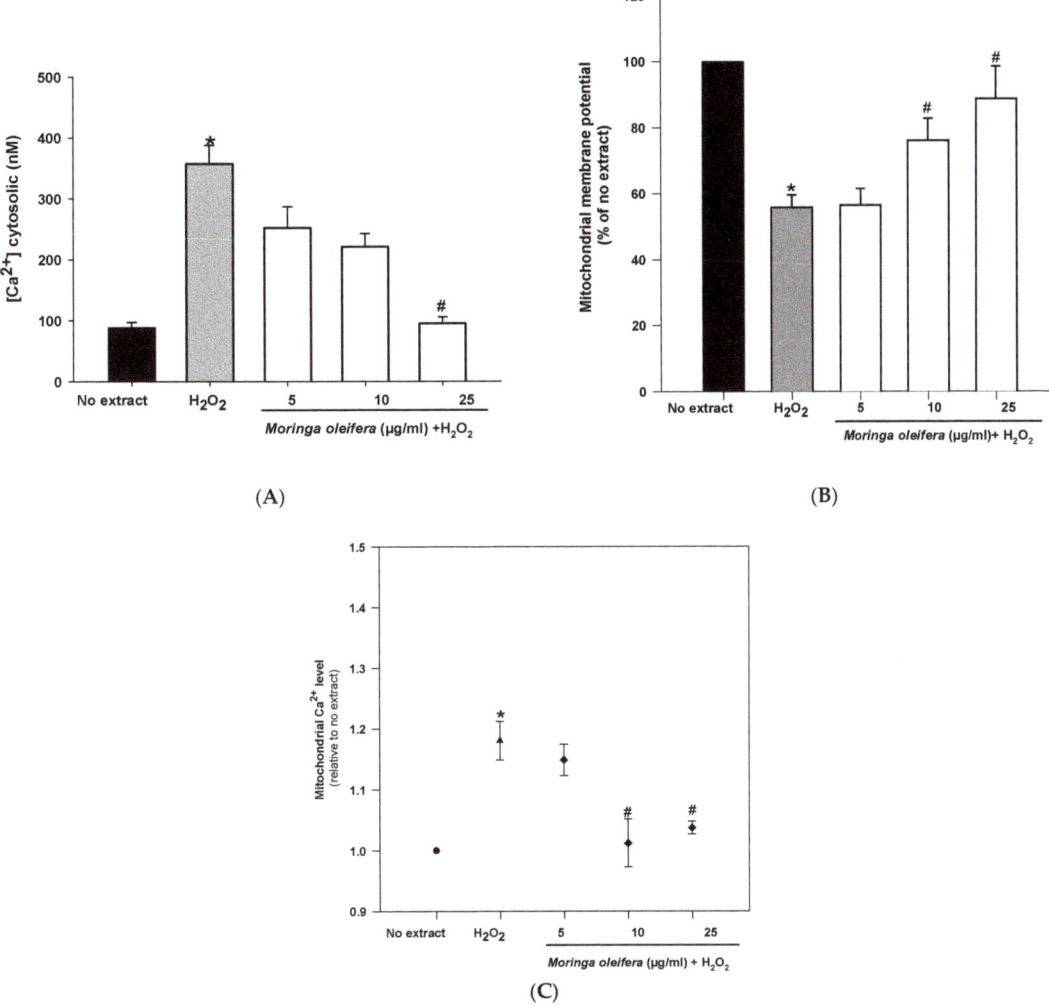

Figure 5. Effect of methanol extracts of *Moringa oleifera* leaf powder on (**A**) mitochondrial membrane potential (**B**) levels of cytosolic calcium and (**C**) levels of mitochondrial calcium. Cells were pretreated with moringa (5, 10 and 25 µg/mL) for 24 h before 100 µM H_2O_2 for 1 h. * $p < 0.05$ versus no extract, # $p < 0.05$ versus H_2O_2.

The major polyphenols identified in methanolic extract of leaves of *Moringa oleifera* include quercetin, kaempferol, apigenin and gallic acid [8]. Previous studies have demonstrated that, after intestinal absorption, polyphenols can reach bloodstream concentration to exert their action [51]. Particularly, these polyphenols presented in moringa have been detected and quantified in blood (quercetin at a concentration of 0.0723 ± 0.0810 µM; kaempferol at a concentration of 0.0579 ± 0.0609 µM; apigenin at a concentration of

0.0106 ± 0.0123 µM and gallic acid at a concentration of 0.007 ± 0.003 µM) [52–54]. Additionally, Nair et al. (2020) have recently demonstrated that compounds presented in moringa extracts are able to pass across Blood-brain-barrier (BBB) and to reach its pharmacological target [55]. Regarding the safe toxicological profile of moringa, doses of up to 2000 mg/kg of methanol and aqueous leaf extract were safe in animal studies [56,57].

Conversely, gallic acid is one of the most abundant phenolic compounds identified in the leaf extract [58]. Previous studies demonstrated that pretreatments with gallic acid protected SH-SY5Y cells against 6-Hydroxydopamine (6-OHDA) induced damage by attenuating mitochondrial dysfunction, reducing intracellular ROS level, and inhibiting apoptotic cell death [59]. Moreover, pretreatments with gallic acid also exerted a potent protection in a hydrogen peroxide-induced oxidative stress model in SH-SY5Y cells by decreasing intracellular ROS production, increasing REDOX activity, and inhibiting caspase-3 activation [60]. Apart from its neuroprotective effect in oxidative stress models in SH-SY5Y cells, gallic acid and its derivatives have shown to inhibit the aggregation of several amyloid proteins associated with the pathological process of many neurodegenerative diseases. Hence, the oral administration of gallic acid improved memory in an APP/PS1 transgenic mouse model by reducing Aβ1-42 aggregation [61]. Moreover, gallic acid also inhibited the insulin amyloid fibril formation in an in-vitro model [62]. Studies on the relationship between structure and inhibitors of amyloid formation have revealed that gallic acid owes its activity to both aromatic and hydroxyl groups and the presence of galloyl moiety [62,63]. In addition to gallic acid, epigallocatechin-3-gallate has shown to reduce Abeta generation in murine neuron-like cells (N2a) transfected with the human "Swedish" mutant amyloid precursor protein (APP) and in primary neurons derived from Swedish mutant APP-overexpressing mice (Tg APPsw line 2576) as well as to reduce the intensity of pancreatic amyloid fibrils in human islet amyloid polypeptide (hIAPP) in trasgenic mice [64,65]. Epigallocatechin-3-gallate exerts its action by binding transthyretin (TTR) and maintaining it in a non-aggregated soluble form [65–68]. Therefore, in our study, the neuroprotective effect of the methanol extract of moringa may be partly due to gallic acid and its derivatives.

4. Conclusions

In conclusion, the current work provides preliminary evidence of the antioxidant-mediated neuroprotective effects of the methanol extract of *Moringa oleifera* leaf powder. Moringa has shown to exert a protective effect against hydrogen peroxide in neuroblastoma cells by reducing ROS overproduction and lipid peroxidation levels, by increasing GSH content and antioxidant enzymes activity and by avoiding mitochondrial dysfunction. The most active concentration was 25 µg/mL. This work supports and deepens the therapeutic properties of a nutritionally rich plant. Particularly, this research delves into the molecular mechanisms by which *Moringa oleifera* methanol extract exerts its neuroprotective effect. These promising results create the need for in-vivo studies and even clinical trials to validate the physiological relevance of our in-vitro data.

Author Contributions: Conceptualization, E.G.-B. and M.P.G.-S.; methodology, E.G.-B., I.U.-V. and M.S.; formal analysis, E.G.-B., I.U.-V. and M.S.; investigation, E.G.-B., I.U.-V. and M.S.; writing—original draft preparation, E.G.-B.; writing—review and editing, E.G.-B., I.U.-V. and M.P.G.-S. All authors have read and agreed to the published version of the manuscript.

Funding: This research received no external funding.

Institutional Review Board Statement: Not applicable.

Informed Consent Statement: Not applicable.

Data Availability Statement: Not applicable.

Conflicts of Interest: The authors declare no conflict of interest.

References

1. World Health Organization. *WHO Monographs on Selected Medicinal Plants*; WHO Library: Geneva, Switzerland, 1999; Volume 1.
2. Committee on Herbal Medicinal Products. European Union Herbal Monograph on Ginkgobiloba L., Folium. EMA/HMPC/321097/2012. Available online: https://www.ema.europa.eu/en/documents/herbal-monograph/final-european-union-herbal-monograph-ginkgo-biloba-l-folium_en.pdf (accessed on 28 January 2015).
3. Liguori, I.; Russo, G.; Curcio, F.; Bulli, G.; Aran, L.; DELLA Morte, D.; Gargiulo, G.; Testa, G.; Cacciatore, F.; Bonaduce, D.; et al. Oxidative stress, aging, and diseases. *Clin. Interv. Aging* **2018**, *13*, 757–772. [CrossRef]
4. Jomova, K.; Vondrakova, D.; Lawson, M.; Valko, M. Metals, oxidative stress and neurodegenerative disorders. *Mol. Cell. Biochem.* **2010**, *345*, 91–104. [CrossRef]
5. Stadtlander, T.; Becker, K. Proximate Composition, Amino and Fatty Acid Profiles and Element Compositions of Four Different Moringa Species. *J. Agric. Sci.* **2017**, *9*, 46. [CrossRef]
6. Anwar, F.; Ashraf, M.; Bhanger, M.I. Interprovenance variation in the composition of *Moringa oleifera* oilseeds from Pakistan. *J. Am. Oil Chem. Soc.* **2005**, *82*, 45–51. [CrossRef]
7. Mahmood, K.T.; Mugal, T.; Haq, I.U. *Moringa oleifera*: A natural gift–A review. *J. Pharm. Sci. Res.* **2010**, *2*, 775–781.
8. Dhakad, A.K.; Ikram, M.; Sharma, S.; Khan, S.; Pandey, V.V.; Singh, A. Biological, nutritional, and therapeutic significance of *Moringa oleifera* Lam. *Phytotherapy Res.* **2019**, *33*, 2870–2903. [CrossRef]
9. ClinicalTrials.gov. Available online: http://clinicaltrials.gov/ (accessed on 12 May 2021).
10. Horwitz, W.; Latimer, G.W. Asociación de Químicos Analíticos Oficial Internacional AOAC. In *Official Methods of Analysis*, 18th ed.; AOAC International: Gaithersburg, MD, USA, 2006.
11. Osborne, D.R.; Voogt, P.; Barrado, A.M. *Análisis de Los Nutrientes de Los Alimentos*; Acribia: Zaragoza, Spain, 1986.
12. Sánchez-Mata, M.C.; Cámara-Hurtado, M.; Díez-Marqués, C.; Torija-Isasa, M.E. Comparison of high-performance liquid chromatography and spectrofluorimetry for vitamin C analysis of green beans (Phaseolus vulgaris L.). *Eur. Food Res. Technol.* **2000**, *210*, 220–225. [CrossRef]
13. Cásedas, G.; Les, F.; Gomez-Serranillos, M.P.; Smith, C.; López, V. Bioactive and functional properties of sour cherry juice (Prunus cerasus). *Food Funct.* **2016**, *7*, 4675–4682. [CrossRef]
14. Amarowicz, R.; Pegg, R.; Rahimi-Moghaddam, P.; Barl, B.; Weil, J. Free-radical scavenging capacity and antioxidant activity of selected plant species from the Canadian prairies. *Food Chem.* **2004**, *84*, 551–562. [CrossRef]
15. Dávalos, A.; Gómez-Cordovés, A.C.; Bartolomé, B. Extending Applicability of the Oxygen Radical Absorbance Capacity (ORAC–Fluorescein) Assay. *J. Agric. Food Chem.* **2004**, *52*, 48–54. [CrossRef]
16. Avan, A.N.; Çekiç, S.D.; Uzunboy, S.; Apak, R. Spectrophotometric Determination of Phenolic Antioxidants in the Presence of Thiols and Proteins. *Int. J. Mol. Sci.* **2016**, *17*, 1325. [CrossRef] [PubMed]
17. Mosmann, T. Rapid colorimetric assay for cellular growth and survival: Application to proliferation and cytotoxicity assays. *J. Immunol. Methods* **1983**, *65*, 55–63. [CrossRef]
18. LeBel, C.P.; Ischiropoulos, H.; Bondy, S.C. Evaluation of the probe 2′,7′-dichlorofluorescin as an indicator of reactive oxygen species formation and oxidative stress. *Chem. Res. Toxicol.* **1992**, *5*, 227–231. [CrossRef]
19. Mihara, M.; Uchiyama, M. Determination of malonaldehyde precursor in tissues by thiobarbituric acid test. *Anal. Biochem.* **1978**, *86*, 271–278. [CrossRef]
20. Hissin, P.J.; Hilf, R. A fluorometric method for determination of oxidized and reduced glutathione in tissues. *Anal. Biochem.* **1976**, *74*, 214–226. [CrossRef]
21. Aebi, H. Catalase in vitro. *Methods Enzymol.* **1984**, *105*, 121–126. [CrossRef]
22. Marklund, S.; Marklund, G. Involvement of the Superoxide Anion Radical in the Autoxidation of Pyrogallol and a Convenient Assay for Superoxide Dismutase. *Eur. J. Biochem.* **1974**, *47*, 469–474. [CrossRef]
23. Paglia, D.E.; Valentine, W.N. Studies on the quantitative and qualitative characterization of erythrocyte glutathione peroxidase. *J. Lab. Clin. Med.* **1967**, *70*, 158–169. [CrossRef]
24. Correia, S.C.; Santos, R.X.; Cardoso, S.M.; Santos, M.S.; Oliveira, C.R.; Moreira, P.I. Cyanide preconditioning protects brain endothelial and NT2 neuron-like cells against glucotoxicity: Role of mitochondrial reactive oxygen species and HIF-1α. *Neurobiol. Dis.* **2012**, *45*, 206–218. [CrossRef]
25. Arduíno, D.M.; Esteves, A.R.; Cardoso, S.M.; Oliveira, C. Endoplasmic reticulum and mitochondria interplay mediates apoptotic cell death: Relevance to Parkinson's disease. *Neurochem. Int.* **2009**, *55*, 341–348. [CrossRef] [PubMed]
26. Resende, R.; Ferreiro, E.; Pereira, C.M.F.; Oliveira, C. Neurotoxic effect of oligomeric and fibrillar species of amyloid-beta peptide 1-42: Involvement of endoplasmic reticulum calcium release in oligomer-induced cell death. *Neuroscience* **2008**, *155*, 725–737. [CrossRef]
27. Fuglie, L.J. *The Moringa Tree: A Local Solution to Malnutrition*; Church World Service: Dakar, Senegal, 2005.
28. Teixeira, E.M.B.; Carvalho, M.R.B.; Neves, V.A.; Silva, M.A.; Pereira, L. Chemical characteristics and fractionation of proteins from *Moringa oleifera* Lam. leaves. *Food Chem.* **2014**, *147*, 51–54. [CrossRef] [PubMed]
29. Ganatra, T.; Umang, J.; Payal, B.; Tusharbindu, D.; Tirgar, D.P. A Panoramic View on Pharmacognostic, Pharmacological, Nutritional, Therapeutic and Prophylactic Values of *Moringa Oleifera* Lam. *Int. Res. J. Pharm.* **2012**, *3*, 1–7.
30. Sreelatha, S.; Padma, P.R. Antioxidant Activity and Total Phenolic Content of *Moringa oleifera* Leaves in Two Stages of Maturity. *Plant Foods Hum. Nutr.* **2009**, *64*, 303–311. [CrossRef]

31. Alvariño, R.; Alonso, E.; Alfonso, A.; Botana, L.M. Neuroprotective Effects of Apple-Derived Drinks in a Mice Model of Inflammation. *Mol. Nutr. Food Res.* **2019**, *64*, 1901017. [CrossRef]
32. Cobley, J.N.; Fiorello, M.L.; Bailey, D.M. 13 reasons why the brain is susceptible to oxidative stress. *Redox Biol.* **2018**, *15*, 490–503. [CrossRef]
33. De Almeida, S.R.; Alves, M.G.; Sousa, M.; Oliveira, P.F.; Silva, B.M. Are Polyphenols Strong Dietary Agents Against Neurotoxicity and Neurodegeneration? *Neurotox. Res.* **2016**, *30*, 345–366. [CrossRef]
34. Sutalangka, C.; Wattanathorn, J.; Muchimapura, S.; Thukham-Mee, W. *Moringa oleifera* Mitigates Memory Impairment and Neurodegeneration in Animal Model of Age-Related Dementia. *Oxidative Med. Cell. Longev.* **2013**, *2013*, 1–9. [CrossRef] [PubMed]
35. Mahaman, Y.A.R.; Huang, F.; Wu, M.; Wang, Y.; Wei, Z.; Bao, J.; Salissou, M.T.M.; Ke, D.; Wang, Q.; Liu, R.; et al. Moringa Oleifera Alleviates Homocysteine-Induced Alzheimer's Disease-Like Pathology and Cognitive Impairments. *J. Alzheimer's Dis.* **2018**, *63*, 1141–1159. [CrossRef] [PubMed]
36. Ekong, M.B.; Ekpo, M.M.; Akpanyung, E.O.; Nwaokonko, D.U. Neuroprotective effect of *Moringa oleifera* leaf extract on aluminium-induced temporal cortical degeneration. *Metab. Brain Dis.* **2017**, *32*, 1437–1447. [CrossRef]
37. Alqahtani, W.S.; Albasher, G. *Moringa oleifera Lam.* extract rescues lead-induced oxidative stress, inflammation, and apoptosis in the rat cerebral cortex. *J. Food Biochem.* **2021**, *45*, e13579. [CrossRef] [PubMed]
38. Jaafaru, M.S.; Nordin, N.; Shaari, K.; Rosli, R.; Razis, A.F.A. Isothiocyanate from *Moringa oleifera* seeds mitigates hydrogen peroxide-induced cytotoxicity and preserved morphological features of human neuronal cells. *PLoS ONE* **2018**, *13*, e0196403. [CrossRef] [PubMed]
39. Xie, H.R.; Hu, L.S.; Li, G.Y. SH-SY5Y human neuroblastoma cell line: In vitro cell model of dopaminergic neurons in Parkinson's disease. *Chin. Med. J.* **2010**, *123*, 1086–1092. [CrossRef] [PubMed]
40. Miller, E.W.; Dickinson, B.C.; Chang, C.J. Aquaporin-3 mediates hydrogen peroxide uptake to regulate downstream intracellular signaling. *Proc. Natl. Acad. Sci. USA* **2010**, *107*, 15681–15686. [CrossRef]
41. Souid, G.; Sfar, M.; Timoumi, R.; Romdhane, M.H.; Essefi, S.A.; Majdoub, H. Protective effect assessment of *Moringa oleifera* against cadmium-induced toxicity in HCT116 and HEK293 cell lines. *Environ. Sci. Pollut. Res.* **2020**, *27*, 23783–23792. [CrossRef]
42. Marrocco, I.; Altieri, F.; Peluso, I. Measurement and Clinical Significance of Biomarkers of Oxidative Stress in Humans. *Oxidative Med. Cell. Longev.* **2017**, *2017*, 1–32. [CrossRef]
43. Sun, C.; Li, W.; Liu, Y.; Deng, W.; Adu-Frimpong, M.; Zhang, H.; Wang, Q.; Yu, J.; Xu, X. In vitro/in vivo hepatoprotective properties of 1-O-(4-hydroxymethylphenyl)-α-L-rhamnopyranoside from *Moringa oleifera* seeds against carbon tetrachloride-induced hepatic injury. *Food Chem. Toxicol.* **2019**, *131*, 110531. [CrossRef]
44. Liu, J.; Ma, G.; Wang, Y.; Zhang, Y. *Moringa oleifera* leaf flavonoids protect bovine mammary epithelial cells from hydrogen peroxide-induced oxidative stress in vitro. *Reprod. Domest. Anim.* **2020**, *55*, 711–719. [CrossRef]
45. Galasko, D.; Montine, T.J. Biomarkers of oxidative damage and inflammation in Alzheimer's disease. *Biomarkers Med.* **2010**, *4*, 27–36. [CrossRef]
46. Weydert, C.J.; Cullen, J.J. Measurement of superoxide dismutase, catalase and glutathione peroxidase in cultured cells and tissue. *Nat. Protoc.* **2009**, *5*, 51–66. [CrossRef]
47. Guo, R.; Gu, J.; Zong, S.; Wu, M.; Yang, M. Structure and mechanism of mitochondrial electron transport chain. *Biomed. J.* **2018**, *41*, 9–20. [CrossRef]
48. Filosto, M.; Scarpelli, M.; Cotelli, M.S.; Vielmi, V.; Todeschini, A.; Gregorelli, V.; Tonin, P.; Tomelleri, G.; Padovani, A. The role of mitochondria in neurodegenerative diseases. *J. Neurol.* **2011**, *258*, 1763–1774. [CrossRef] [PubMed]
49. Kirkinezos, I.G.; Moraes, C.T. Reactive oxygen species and mitochondrial diseases. *Semin. Cell Dev. Biol.* **2001**, *12*, 449–457. [CrossRef] [PubMed]
50. Duchen, M.R. Mitochondria, calcium-dependent neuronal death and neurodegenerative disease. *Pflügers Archiv Eur. J. Physiol.* **2012**, *464*, 111–121. [CrossRef] [PubMed]
51. Borges, G.; Lean, M.E.J.; Roberts, S.A.; Crozier, A. Bioavailability of dietary (poly)phenols: A study with ileostomists to discriminate between absorption in small and large intestine. *Food Funct.* **2013**, *4*, 754–762. [CrossRef]
52. Cao, J.; Zhang, Y.; Chen, W.; Zhao, X. The relationship between fasting plasma concentrations of selected flavonoids and their ordinary dietary intake. *Br. J. Nutr.* **2009**, *103*, 249–255. [CrossRef]
53. Loke, W.M.; Jenner, A.M.; Proudfoot, J.M.; McKinley, A.J.; Hodgson, J.M.; Halliwell, B.; Croft, K.D. A Metabolite Profiling Approach to Identify Biomarkers of Flavonoid Intake in Humans. *J. Nutr.* **2009**, *139*, 2309–2314. [CrossRef]
54. Zhang, Y.; Cao, J.; Chen, W.; Yang, J.; Hao, D.; Zhang, Y.; Chang, P.; Zhao, X. Reproducibility and relative validity of a food frequency questionnaire to assess intake of dietary flavonol and flavone in Chinese university campus population. *Nutr. Res.* **2010**, *30*, 520–526. [CrossRef]
55. Nair, D.A.; Joseph, J.; Sreelatha, S.; Kariyil, J.; Nair, S. *Moringa oleifera (Lam.)*: A natural remedy for ageing? *Nat. Prod. Res.* **2020**, *23*, 1–7. [CrossRef]
56. Adedapo, A.A.; Mogbojuri, O.M.; Emikpe, B.O. Safety evaluations of the aqueous extract of the leaves of *Moringa oleifera* in rats. *J. Med. Plant.* **2009**, *3*, 586–591.
57. Saleem, A.; Saleem, M.; Akhtar, M.F.; Baig, M.M.F.A.; Rasul, A. HPLC analysis, cytotoxicity, and safety study of *Moringa oleifera Lam.* (wild type) leaf extract. *J. Food Biochem.* **2020**, *44*, e13400. [CrossRef]

58. Oboh, G.; Ademiluyi, A.O.; Ademosun, A.O.; Olasehinde, T.A.; Oyeleye, S.I.; Boligon, A.A.; Athayde, M.L. Phenolic Extract from *Moringa oleifera* Leaves Inhibits Key Enzymes Linked to Erectile Dysfunction and Oxidative Stress in Rats' Penile Tissues. *Biochem. Res. Int.* **2015**, *2015*, 1–8. [CrossRef]
59. Chandrasekhar, Y.; Kumar, G.P.; Ramya, E.M.; Anilakumar, K.R. Gallic Acid Protects 6-OHDA Induced Neurotoxicity by Attenuating Oxidative Stress in Human Dopaminergic Cell Line. *Neurochem. Res.* **2018**, *43*, 1150–1160. [CrossRef]
60. González-Sarrías, A.; Núñez-Sánchez, M.Á.; Tomás-Barberán, F.A.; Espín, J.C. Neuroprotective Effects of Bioavailable Polyphenol-Derived Metabolites against Oxidative Stress-Induced Cytotoxicity in Human Neuroblastoma SH-SY5Y Cells. *J. Agric. Food Chem.* **2017**, *65*, 752–758. [CrossRef] [PubMed]
61. Yu, M.; Chen, X.; Liu, J.; Ma, Q.; Zhuo, Z.; Chen, H.; Zhou, L.; Yang, S.; Zheng, L.; Ning, C.; et al. Gallic acid disruption of $A\beta1$–42 aggregation rescues cognitive decline of APP/PS1 double transgenic mouse. *Neurobiol. Dis.* **2019**, *124*, 67–80. [CrossRef] [PubMed]
62. Jayamani, J.; Shanmugam, G. Gallic acid, one of the components in many plant tissues, is a potential inhibitor for insulin amyloid fibril formation. *Eur. J. Med. Chem.* **2014**, *85*, 352–358. [CrossRef] [PubMed]
63. Ferreira, N.; Pereira-Henriques, A.; Almeida, M.R. Transthyretin chemical chaperoning by flavonoids: Structure–activity insights towards the design of potent amyloidosis inhibitors. *Biochem. Biophys. Rep.* **2015**, *3*, 123–133. [CrossRef]
64. Rezai-Zadeh, K.; Shytle, D.; Sun, N.; Mori, T.; Hou, H.; Jeanniton, D.; Ehrhart, J.; Townsend, K.; Zeng, J.; Morgan, D.; et al. Green Tea Epigallocatechin-3-Gallate (EGCG) Modulates Amyloid Precursor Protein Cleavage and Reduces Cerebral Amyloidosis in Alzheimer Transgenic Mice. *J. Neurosci.* **2005**, *25*, 8807–8814. [CrossRef]
65. Franko, A.; Camargo, D.C.R.; Böddrich, A.; Garg, D.; Camargo, A.R.; Rathkolb, B.; Janik, D.; Aichler, M.; Feuchtinger, A.; Neff, F.; et al. Epigallocatechin gallate (EGCG) reduces the intensity of pancreatic amyloid fibrils in human islet amyloid polypeptide (hIAPP) transgenic mice. *Sci. Rep.* **2018**, *8*, 1116. [CrossRef] [PubMed]
66. Ferreira, N.; Cardoso, I.; Domingues, M.R.; Vitorino, R.; Bastos, M.; Bai, G.; Saraiva, M.J.; Almeida, M.R. Binding of epigallocatechin-3-gallate to transthyretin modulates its amyloidogenicity. *FEBS Lett.* **2009**, *583*, 3569–3576. [CrossRef]
67. Ferreira, N.; Saraiva, M.J.; Almeida, M.R. Epigallocatechin-3-Gallate as a Potential Therapeutic Drug for TTR-Related Amyloidosis: "In Vivo" Evidence from FAP Mice Models. *PLoS ONE* **2012**, *7*, e29933. [CrossRef] [PubMed]
68. Ferreira, N.; Saraiva, M.J.; Almeida, M.R. Natural polyphenols inhibit different steps of the process of transthyretin (TTR) amyloid fibril formation. *FEBS Lett.* **2011**, *585*, 2424–2430. [CrossRef] [PubMed]

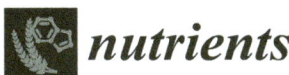

Article

Reversal of Insulin Resistance in Overweight and Obese Subjects by *trans*-Resveratrol and Hesperetin Combination—Link to Dysglycemia, Blood Pressure, Dyslipidemia, and Low-Grade Inflammation

Naila Rabbani [1], Mingzhan Xue [2], Martin O. Weickert [3] and Paul J. Thornalley [2,*]

1. Department of Basic Medical Science, College of Medicine, QU Health, Qatar University, Doha P.O. Box 2713, Qatar; n.rabbani@qu.edu.qa
2. Diabetes Research Center, Qatar Biomedical Research Institute, Hamad Bin Khalifa University, Qatar Foundation, Doha P.O. Box 34110, Qatar; mxue@hbku.edu.qa
3. Endocrinology & Metabolism, Warwickshire Institute for the Study of Diabetes, University Hospitals of Coventry & Warwickshire NHS Trust, Coventry CV2 2DX, UK; Martin.Weickert@uhcw.nhs.uk
* Correspondence: pthornalley@hbku.edu.qa; Tel.: +974-7090-1635

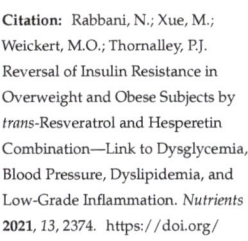

Citation: Rabbani, N.; Xue, M.; Weickert, M.O.; Thornalley, P.J. Reversal of Insulin Resistance in Overweight and Obese Subjects by *trans*-Resveratrol and Hesperetin Combination—Link to Dysglycemia, Blood Pressure, Dyslipidemia, and Low-Grade Inflammation. *Nutrients* 2021, 13, 2374. https://doi.org/10.3390/nu13072374

Academic Editors: Elena González-Burgos and M. Pilar Gómez-Serranillos Cuadrado

Received: 30 May 2021
Accepted: 7 July 2021
Published: 11 July 2021

Publisher's Note: MDPI stays neutral with regard to jurisdictional claims in published maps and institutional affiliations.

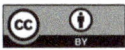

Copyright: © 2021 by the authors. Licensee MDPI, Basel, Switzerland. This article is an open access article distributed under the terms and conditions of the Creative Commons Attribution (CC BY) license (https://creativecommons.org/licenses/by/4.0/).

Abstract: The dietary supplement, *trans*-resveratrol and hesperetin combination (tRES-HESP), induces expression of glyoxalase 1, countering the accumulation of reactive dicarbonyl glycating agent, methylglyoxal (MG), in overweight and obese subjects. tRES-HESP produced reversal of insulin resistance, improving dysglycemia and low-grade inflammation in a randomized, double-blind, placebo-controlled crossover study. Herein, we report further analysis of study variables. MG metabolism-related variables correlated with BMI, dysglycemia, vascular inflammation, blood pressure, and dyslipidemia. With tRES-HESP treatment, plasma MG correlated negatively with endothelial independent arterial dilatation ($r = -0.48$, $p < 0.05$) and negatively with peripheral blood mononuclear cell (PBMC) quinone reductase activity ($r = -0.68$, $p < 0.05$)—a marker of the activation status of transcription factor Nrf2. For change from baseline of PBMC gene expression with tRES-HESP treatment, Glo1 expression correlated negatively with change in the oral glucose tolerance test area-under-the-curve plasma glucose (ΔAUCg) ($r = -0.56$, $p < 0.05$) and thioredoxin interacting protein (TXNIP) correlated positively with ΔAUCg ($r = 0.59$, $p < 0.05$). Tumor necrosis factor-α (TNFα) correlated positively with change in fasting plasma glucose ($r = 0.70$, $p < 0.001$) and negatively with change in insulin sensitivity ($r = -0.68$, $p < 0.01$). These correlations were not present with placebo. tRES-HESP decreased low-grade inflammation, characterized by decreased expression of CCL2, COX-2, IL-8, and RAGE. Changes in CCL2, IL-8, and RAGE were intercorrelated and all correlated positively with changes in MLXIP, MAFF, MAFG, NCF1, and FTH1, and negatively with changes in HMOX1 and TKT; changes in IL-8 also correlated positively with change in COX-2. Total urinary excretion of tRES and HESP metabolites were strongly correlated. These findings suggest tRES-HESP counters MG accumulation and protein glycation, decreasing activation of the unfolded protein response and expression of TXNIP and TNFα, producing reversal of insulin resistance. tRES-HESP is suitable for further evaluation for treatment of insulin resistance and related disorders.

Keywords: polyphenol; insulin resistance; methylglyoxal; obesity; glyoxalase; low-grade inflammation

1. Introduction

Epidemiological studies suggest a diet rich in polyphenols decreases the risk of developing type 2 diabetes mellitus (T2DM) [1]. This has led to the evaluation of polyphenol dietary supplements for improvement of metabolic health and improved prevention of T2DM. *trans*-Resveratrol (tRES), a polyphenolic stilbenoid, improved metabolic health and survival of mice on a high-calorie diet [2]. Similar effects have been difficult to translate clinically with meta-analysis of intervention studies concluding that tRES does not affect glycemic status in overweight and obese human subjects [3]. A barrier to effective clinical translation of expected health benefits of polyphenols is limited clinical potency when given individually [4]. We therefore explored synergistic combination of tRES with other polyphenols and targeted insulin resistance for treatment—the driver of development of T2DM [5].

Preclinical and clinical studies suggest a role of increased protein glycation by the endogenous reactive dicarbonyl metabolite, methylglyoxal (MG), in the development of insulin resistance and T2DM [6]. MG modifies proteins to form the major advanced glycation endproduct (AGE), arginine-derived hydroimidazolone, MG-H1 [7,8]. MG-modified proteins are misfolded and activate the unfolded protein response (UPR) and downstream inflammatory signaling [9,10]. MG is metabolized by glyoxalase 1 (Glo1), the first enzyme of the glyoxalase pathway which metabolizes MG, to D-lactate [11] (Figure 1). Plasma D-lactate concentration is a surrogate indicator of flux of formation of MG [6,9,12]. Decrease of MG concentration, related protein glycation and alleviation of the UPR-linked inflammation may offer a route to novel insulin sensitizing agents [13]. Inducers of expression of Glo1, Glo1 inducers, may support this by suppressing MG concentration [6]. We developed a pharmacological strategy to induce Glo1 expression, through activation of transcriptional factor Nrf2 and its binding of a functional antioxidant response element (ARE) in the GLO1 gene [14]. In a screen of dietary bioactive compounds that activate Nrf2, we found the synergistic combination of tRES and hesperetin (HESP), tRES-HESP, was the most effective Glo1 inducer [15]. In a randomized, placebo-controlled crossover study in overweight and obese subjects—the Healthy Aging Through Functional Food (HATFF) study—treatment with tRES-HESP reversed insulin resistance, with an improvement of insulin sensitivity in obese subjects comparable to outcomes of metabolic surgery. The placebo had no effect. There were also improvements in dysglycemia and low-grade inflammation [15]. The aim of this study was to explore evidence for association of target pharmacology of Glo1 inducer, tRES-HESP, to clinical variables of insulin resistance, dysglycemia, blood pressure, dyslipidemia, and low-grade inflammation assessed in the HATFF study—including established mediators of insulin resistance, thioredoxin interacting protein (TXNIP), and tumor necrosis factor-α.

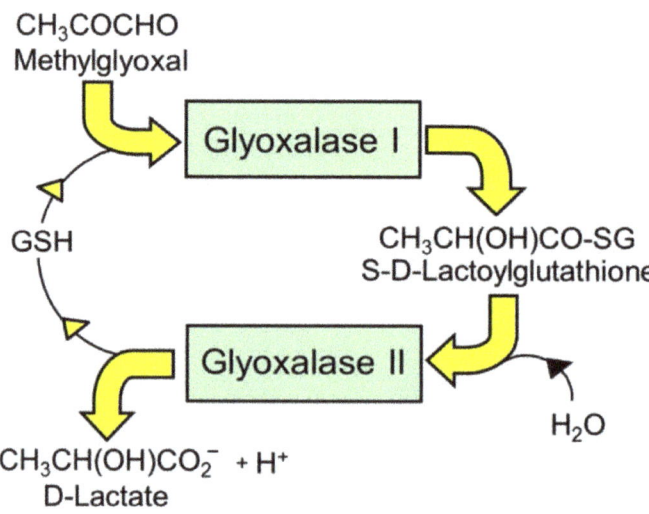

Figure 1. Metabolism of methylglyoxal by the glyoxalase pathway.

Herein, we present further analysis of clinical and biochemical variables of the HATFF study, particularly correlation analysis of glyoxalase pathway, clinical variables and peripheral blood mononuclear cell (PBMC) gene expression. The outcome reveals, for the first time, a link of target pharmacology to insulin resistance, dysglycemia, blood pressure, dyslipidemia, and low-grade inflammation—including key mediators of insulin resistance, TXNIP, and TNFα.

2. Materials and Methods

2.1. HATFF Study Design and Methods

HATFF is a randomized, double-blind, placebo-controlled crossover study evaluating treatment with tRES-HESP against insulin resistance in healthy overweight and obese subjects. Subject recruitment, including inclusion and exclusion criteria, power analysis, and pharmacological target validation (increase of Glo1 activity and decrease of plasma MG and MG-mediated protein glycation) have been described previously [15]. tRES-HESP was evaluated in 29 subjects with impaired metabolic health; 9 subjects meeting criteria of prediabetes. Twenty participants were highly overweight and obese (BMI $\geq$ 27.5 kg/m^2) and 11 were obese (BMI $\geq$ 30 kg/m^2). Subjects made 4 study visits for clinical assessments; one visit at the start and end of each treatment period. Treatment was by daily oral capsule before breakfast, containing with tRES-HESP (90 mg tRES, 120 mg HESP) or placebo, for 8 weeks, with 6 weeks washout between crossover treatment periods [15]. The study was approved by the National Research Ethics Service Committee West Midlands—Coventry & Warwickshire, U.K. (project number 13/WM/0368) and registered on the Clinicaltrials.gov (identifier: NCT02095873). The procedures followed were in accordance with institutional guidelines and the Declaration of Helsinki.

The primary endpoint was insulin sensitivity measured by oral glucose insulin sensitivity (OGIS) index in oral glucose tolerance tests (OGTTs) at the start and end of each treatment period. The OGIS index correlates very strongly with reference method assessment of insulin resistance by the hyperinsulinemic glucose clamp method [16]. Secondary endpoints were brachial artery flow-mediated dilatation response, also including brachial artery dilatation response to a sub-therapeutic dose of glyceryl trinitrate (FMD-GTN). Variables characterizing clinical status, glyoxalase pathway-linked metabolism, dysglycemia—including fasting plasma glucose (FPG), area-under-the-curve of the OGTT (AUCg), fasting insulin, and 90 min OGTT plasma insulin (plasma insulin OGTT)—vascular inflammation, blood pressure, and dyslipidemia were recorded and determined, as described [15]. Gene expression in PBMCs was assessed in a custom focussed 50-gene array, including 47 response and 3 reference genes, by the Nanostring method assessing relative mRNA copy number; RNA was extracted and quantified in-house with sample analysis out-sourced to the Nanostring Facility Service, University College, London, UK [15]. All sample analysis was performed with the investigator blinded to the subject and study group origin.

2.2. Target Pharmacology of Glyoxalase 1 Inducer

Glo1 activity and mRNA of PBMCs were assayed by spectrophotometric and Nanostring methods, respectively [17,18]. The plasma concentration of MG and plasma protein and urine content of MG-derived AGE, MG-H1, were measured by stable isotopic dilution analysis liquid chromatography-tandem mass spectrometry [19,20]. Plasma D-lactate was assayed by endpoint enzymatic assay by microplate fluorimetry [21]. Total tRES and HESP urinary metabolites were determined by stable isotopic LC-MS/MS after deconjugation of glucuronides and sulfates, as described [15].

2.3. Correlation Analysis

For glyoxalase pathway and clinical variables, we assessed the correlation between variables: (i) throughout the study, combining data from all time points and different treatments; and (ii) within treatment periods, tRES-HESP and placebo—exploring correlations of the established hypothesis linking MG metabolism to BMI, dysglycemia, insulin resistance, vascular inflammation, blood pressure, and dyslipidemia. We also assessed correlations of gene expression in PBMCs in treatment periods wherein we explored correlations with statistically significant major changes of gene expression in the tRES-HESP treatment:

namely, for monocyte chemoattractant protein-1 (MCP-1, gene CCL2), interleukin-8 (IL-8), cyclo-oxygenase-2—also known as prostaglandin synthase-2 (COX-2, gene PTGS2), and the receptor for advanced glycation endproducts (RAGE, gene AGER). Analysis was made for two study groups: all subjects, and highly overweight and obese subject groups—as previously described [15].

2.4. Statistical Analysis

Correlation analysis was by the non-parametric Spearman method. For correlations of gene expression in PBMCs in treatment periods without prior established hypothesis, a Bonferroni correction of 47 was applied. Where change in variable was analyzed, this referred to change from the start to the end of the 8-week treatment period. Statistical analysis was performed using IBM SPSS Statistics for Windows, version 24 (IBM Corp., Armonk, NY, USA).

3. Results

3.1. Correlation Analysis of Glyoxalase Pathway and Clinical Variables throughout the Study

The outcomes of the HATFF study were found in highly overweight and obese subjects where the following changes were recorded in the tRES-HESP treatment period: target pharmacology—increased in PBMC activity of Glo1 (+27%, $p < 0.05$) and decreased plasma MG concentration (-37%, $p < 0.05$); clinical endpoint-related variables—decreased FPG (-5%, $p < 0.010$), decreased AUCg (-8%, $p < 0.05$) and increased OGIS (+54 mlmin^{-1}m^{-2}, $p < 0.05$); and other—decreased expression of MCP-1, IL-8, COX-2, and RAGE in PBMCs. The placebo had no effect [15]. tRES-HESP treatment increased urinary excretion of tRES and HESP metabolites by > 2000- and > 100-fold, respectively, compared to the placebo.

Induction of expression and activity of Glo1 with related change in target pharmacology provided the opportunity to explore the association by correlation analysis of glyoxalase system-linked variables with clinical characteristics of dysglycemia and insulin resistance, vascular inflammation, blood pressure, and dyslipidemia. Statistics were maximized by assessing correlation analysis throughout the intervention study, including data from the 4 study visits for clinical assessment. For all subjects throughout the study, there were negative correlations of PBMC Glo1 activity with plasma protein MG-H1 and plasma D-lactate, suggesting that the increase of Glo1 may suppress both protein glycation by MG and, after improvement in metabolic health, flux of formation of MG as well. For clinical variables, BMI and AUCg correlated positively with plasma D-lactate, and the OGIS index correlated negatively with plasma D-lactate. This suggests that flux of MG is positively associated with dysglycemia, insulin resistance, and BMI.

For vascular inflammation markers, plasma MCP-1, sVCAM1, and sICAM1 correlated negatively with PBMC Glo1 activity and plasma soluble E-selectin (sE-selectin) correlated positively with plasma D-lactate. For blood pressure, systolic and diastolic blood pressure correlated positively with plasma MG concentration. Diastolic blood pressure and plasma endothelin-1 (ET-1) correlated negatively to PBMC Glo1 activity and positively with plasma D-lactate. For variables of clinical dyslipidemia, HDL correlated negatively and LDL-VLDL and TG positively with urinary MG-H1—a measure of total body MG glycation [15]; and plasma D-lactate correlated positively with TC, LDL-VLDL, and TG and negatively with HDL. This suggests increasing Glo1 expression may have health benefits through decreasing vascular inflammation and improving hemodynamics and dyslipidemia (Table 1). There was also a strong positive correlation of total urinary metabolites of tRES and total urinary metabolites of HESP (r = 0.84, p = 2 × 10^{-7}).

3.2. Correlation Analysis of Changes from Baseline of Glyoxalase Pathway and Clinical Variables in tRES-HESP and Placebo Treatment Periods

To assess clinical variables linked to pharmacological responses of tRES-HESP, we performed correlation analysis of glyoxalase pathway and clinical variables significantly changed from baseline in tRES-HESP treatment period, comparing these changes with placebo. In the tRES-HESP treatment period only, change in plasma MG correlated negatively with change in FMD-GTN and change in PBMC quinone reductase (NQO1) activity in highly overweight and obese subjects. This suggests decrease of plasma MG is associated with improved arterial dilatation response and increased NQO1 activity—a marker of Nrf2 activation [22]. For dysglycemia/insulin resistance linked variables, there were negative correlations of OGIS index with FPG, AUCg, and plasma insulin OGTT in all and the highly overweight and obese subject group. For change in AUCg, there was a positive correlation with change in sE-selectin in all subjects. In highly overweight and obese subjects, there was also a positive correlation of OGIS with urinary pentosidine. There was also a negative correlation of change in FPG with change in PBMC NQO1 in all subjects; and in highly overweight and obese subjects, there was a negative correlation of change in FPG with change in urinary pentosidine.

Several correlations between OGIS index, AUCg, and plasma insulin OGTT were found in both tRES-HESP treatment and placebo periods, as expected for the inverse relationship of insulin sensitivity to dysglycemia and hyperinsulinemia in subjects independent of treatment (Table 2).

Table 1. Correlation of variables throughout the HATFF study in all subjects.

Variable Class	Correlate	PBMC Glo1	MG$_{Plasma}$	MG-H1$_{urine}$	D-Lactate$_{Plasma}$
Glyoxalase pathway	Plasma protein MG-H1	−0.21 *			
	Plasma D-lactate	−0.34 ***			
Anthropometric	BMI				0.38 ***
Dysglycemia/	AUCg				0.25 **
insulin resistance	OGIS				−0.23 *
Vascular inflammation	Plasma MCP-1	−0.28 **			
	Plasma sVCAM1	−0.18 *			
	Plasma sICAM1	−0.22 *			
	Plasma sE-selectin				0.24 **
Blood pressure	Systolic BP		0.26 **		
	Diastolic BP		0.23 *		0.23 *
	Plasma ET-1	−0.24 **			0.25 **
Dyslipidemia	TC				0.19 *
	HDL			−0.20 *	−0.19 *
	LDL-VLDL			0.39 ***	0.26 **
	TG			0.28*	0.20 *

Spearman correlation coefficients; $n = 116$. Significance: *, $p < 0.05$; **, $p < 0.01$, and ***, $p < 0.001$. Estimates of variables at all four study visits and both tRES-HESP and placebo treatments were included in the analysis.

3.3. Correlation Analysis of PBMC Gene Expression Changed in tRES-HESP and Placebo Treatment Periods

To assess PBMC gene expression changes linked to pharmacological responses of tRES-HESP, we performed correlation analysis of genes with expression changed from baseline in tRES-HESP treatment period with other gene expression assessed in the Nanostring expression array, comparing these to the placebo. In the tRES-HESP treatment period, most significant changes in PBMC gene expression were found in the highly overweight and obese subjects. Exploring the correlation of change in PBMC gene expression with clinical and metabolic variables, we found change in Glo1 expression correlated negatively with change in AUGg (r = −0.56, $p < 0.05$) and change in thioredoxin interacting protein (TXNIP) correlated positively with change in AUGg (r = 0.59, $p < 0.05$); and change in expression of tumor necrosis factor-α (TNFα) correlated positively with change in FPG (r = 0.70, $p < 0.001$) and negatively with change in OGIS (r = −0.68, $p < 0.01$). These correlations were not present with the placebo (Figure 2).

Table 2. Correlation of changes of glyoxalase and dysglycemia/insulin resistance-related variables in the tRES-HESP and placebo treatment periods of the HATFF study.

Variable Class	Variable	Study Group	Correlate
Glyoxalase pathway	Plasma MG	Highly overweight and obese	FMD-GTN (−0.48 *), PBMC NQO1 (−0.68 **)
Dysglycemia/insulin resistance	OGIS index	All	<u>FPG</u> (−0.79 ***), <u>AUCg</u> (−0.50 **), <u>plasma insulin OGTT</u> (−0.63 ***)
		Highly overweight and obese	<u>FPG</u> (−0.80 ***), <u>AUCg</u> (−0.57 **), <u>plasma insulin OGTT</u> (−0.57 **), urinary pentosidine (0.54 *)
	FPG	All	<u>OGIS index</u> (−0.79 ***), PBMC NQO1 (−0.50 *)
		Highly overweight and obese	<u>OGIS index</u> (−0.80 ***), urinary pentosidine (−0.56 *)
	AUCg	All	<u>OGIS</u> (−0.46 **), sE-selectin (0.47 *)
		Highly overweight and obese	<u>OGIS</u> (−0.57 **)

Spearman correlation coefficients; $n = 20$ (highly overweight and obese) and $n = 29$ (all). Significance: *, $p < 0.05$; **, $p < 0.01$ and ***, $p < 0.001$. Underlined correlates indicate correlation is also found in both tRES-HESP and placebo treatment periods of the HATFF study.

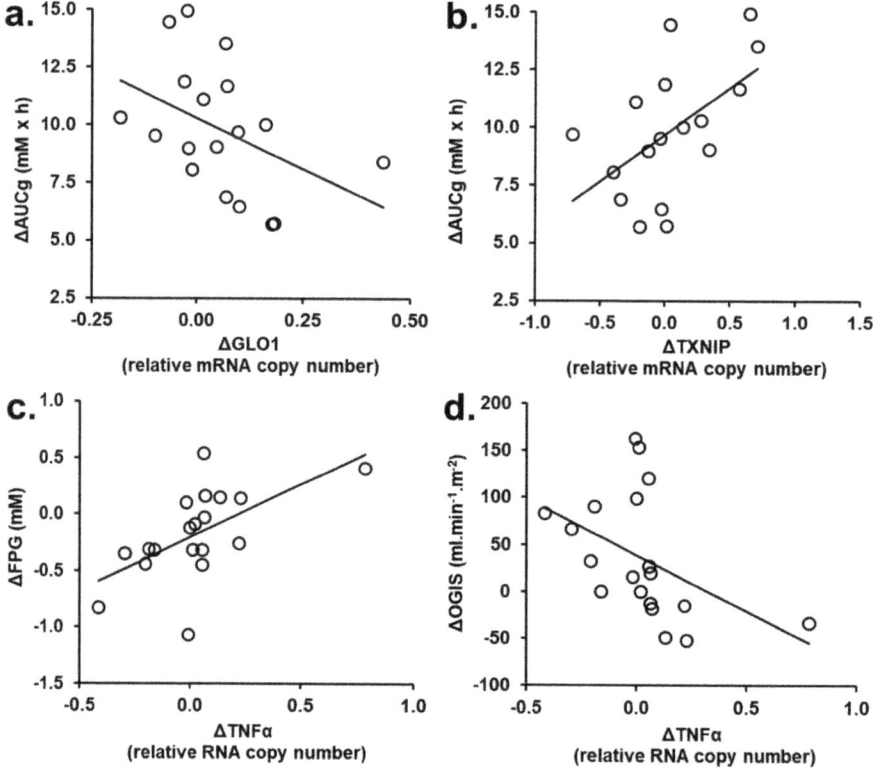

Figure 2. Correlation of variables of metabolic health with change in PBMC gene expression in highly overweight and obese subjects of the HATFF study during treatment with tRES-HESP. (**a**) Change of AUCg (ΔAUCg) on change expression of Glo1 (ΔGLO1); $r = -0.56$, $p < 0.05$. Regression equation: ΔAUCg = $(-8.8 \times$ ΔGLO1$) + 10.3$. (**b**) Change of AUCg (ΔAUCg) on change in expression of TXNIP (ΔTXNIP); $r = 0.59$, $p < 0.05$. Regression equation: ΔAUCg = $(4.1 \times$ ΔTXNIP$) + 9.7$. (**c**) Change in FPG (ΔFPG) on change in expression of TNFα (ΔTNFα); $r = 0.70$, $p < 0.001$. Regression equation: ΔFPG = $(0.94 \times$ ΔTNFα$) - 0.20$. (**d**) Change in OGIS (ΔOGIS) on ΔTNFα; $r = -0.68$, $p < 0.01$. Regression equation: ΔOGIS = $(-119 \times$ ΔTNFα$) + 39$. $n = 20$.

Major changes in gene expression in the tRES-HESP treatment period were: CCL2, −49%; IL-8, −39%; COX-2, −31%; and RAGE, −37%—as reported previously [15]. Change in expression of COX-2 correlated positively with change in expression of IL-8. Change in expression of CCL2, IL-8, and RAGE were intercorrelated and also all correlated with change in expression of the following genes: positive correlation—Mondo A (MLXIP), small maf protein, isoforms F and G (MAFF and MAFG), neutrophil cytosol factor-1 (NCF1, p47phox), and ferritin (FTH1); and negative correlation—heme oxygenase-1 (HMOX1) and transketolase (TKT). Change in expression of CCL2 correlated positively with change in expression of a further 11 genes: aldoketo reductase 1C1 (AKR1C1), glucose-6-phosphate dehydrogenase (G6PD), γ-glutamylcysteine ligase-modulatory subunit (GCLM), glutathione peroxidases, isoforms 1 and 4 (GPX1 and GPX4), glutathione reductase (GSR), interleukin-6 (IL-6), transcription factor Nrf2 (NFE2L2), NF-κB inhibitor-alpha (NFKBIA), NQO1 and superoxide dismutase-1 (SOD1); and correlated negatively with glutathione S-transferase P1 (GSTP1). Change in expression of IL-8 correlated positively with change in expression of a further 3 genes: AKR1C1, NQO1, and SOD1. Change in expression of RAGE correlated positively with change in expression of a further 7 genes: catalase (CAT), G6PD, GCLM, GPX4, Kelch-like ECH-associated protein 1 (KEAP1), NFKBIA, and SOD1; and correlated negatively with change in expression of CCL2 receptor (CCR2). Several of these correlations were found in the placebo arm of the study (Table 3).

Table 3. Correlation of changes of peripheral blood mononuclear gene expression in highly overweight and obese subjects in the tRES-HESP and placebo treatment periods of the HATFF study.

Gene	Gene Correlate (Correlation Coefficient)
COX-2	IL-8 (0.74 *)
CCL2	AKR1C1 (0.80 **), CCR2 (−0.83***), FTH1 (0.89 ***), G6PD (0.77 **), GCLM (0.93 ***), GPX1 (0.77 **), GPX4 (0.85 ***), GSR (0.70 *), GSTP1 (−0.69 *), HMOX1 (−0.88 ***), IL-6 (0.79 **), IL-8 (0.74 *), MAFF (0.76 **), MAFG (0.81 **), MLXIP (0.92 ***), NCF1 (0.74 *), NFE2L2 (0.75 *), NFKBIA (0.70 *), NQO1 (0.79 **), RAGE (0.87 ***), SOD1 (0.86 ***), TKT (−0.88 **).
IL-8	AKR1C1 (0.73 *), CCL2 (0.74 *), COX-2 (0.74 *), FTH1 (0.88 ***), MAFG (0.71 *), MLXIP (0.69 *), NCF1 (0.72 *), NQO1 (0.76 **), RAGE (0.70 *), SOD1 (0.73 *).
RAGE	CAT (−0.71 *), CCL2 (0.87 **), CCR2 (−0.74 *), FTH1 (0.84 ***), G6PD (0.86 ***), GCLM (0.76 **), GPX4 (0.71*), HMOX1 (−0.80 **), IL-8 (0.70 *), KEAP1 (0.69 *), MAFF (0.83 ***), MAFG (0.91 ***), NFKBIA (0.75 **), MLXIP (0.92 ***), NCF1 (0.88 ***), SOD1 (0.86 ***), TKT (−0.81 **).

Spearman correlation coefficients; $n = 20$. Significance: * $p < 0.05$; ** $p < 0.01$; and *** $p < 0.001$ (Bonferroni correction of 47 applied). Gene name correlates underlined had changes correlated similarly in the placebo arm. Gene expression assessed was: AGER, AKR1B1, AKR1C1, AKR1C3, CAT, CBR1, CCL2, CCR2, CD36, FTH1, G6PD, GCLC, GCLM, GPX1, GPX4, GSR, GSTA4, GSTP1, HIF1A, HMOX1, IL-6, IL-8, KEAP1, MAFF, MAFG, MAFK, MIF, MLX, MLXIP, NCF1, NFE2L2, NFKB1, NFKBIA, NQO1, PRDX1, PSMA1, PSMB5, PTGS2, SOD1, SQSTM1, SREBF1, TALDO1, TKT, TNFA, TXN, TXNIP, TXNRD1. Housekeeping reference genes: ACTB, CLTC, and GUSB.

4. Discussions

Reversal of insulin resistance in overweight and obese subjects with tRES-HESP treatment in the HATFF study was associated with decreased dysglycemia, blood pressure, vascular inflammation, and dyslipidemia—a remarkable multiplicity of pathogenic processes. Moreover, health improvement was linked to two established mediators of insulin resistance: TXNIP and TNFα. TXNIP is a mediator of insulin resistance in liver, skeletal muscle and adipose tissue, and impaired pancreatic beta-cell insulin secretion [23–25] and TNFα decreases insulin receptor signaling in adipose tissue and skeletal muscle, particularly prior to development of T2DM [26–28]. tRES-HESP treatment produced a decrease of PBMC TNFα expression in the obese subject subgroup of the HATFF study [15]. Reversal of insulin resistance by tRES-HESP was not achieved by tRES and HESP individually in clinical evaluation [3,29], suggesting pharmacological synergism of tRES-HESP. The dose of HESP given was likely sufficient to inhibit intestinal glucuronosyl transferase and facilitate uptake of unconjugated tRES and HESP [6]. The outcomes of the HATFF study may provide a pointer to effective synergistic combinations of dietary polyphenols to counter insulin resistance.

In consideration of the correlation analysis of glyoxalase pathway and clinical variables throughout the HATFF study, increased Glo1 activity decreases the cellular and extracellular concentration of MG in *in vitro* studies [9,14]. Hence, increased Glo1 expression in PBMCs and other cells in response to tRES-HESP treatment *in vivo* is expected to decrease plasma MG and plasma protein glycation by MG. Consistent with this, we found a negative correlation of PBMC Glo1 activity to plasma protein MG-H1. PBMC Glo1 activity also correlated negatively with markers of vascular inflammation and blood pressure. A hypertensive effect of increased MG glycation may be mediated through activation of the UPR by MG-modified proteins and associated inflammatory signaling through the heat shock factor-1 and NF-κB pathways, with increased expression and secretion of ET-1 [9,30]. Hypertension in obesity was linked to enhanced vascular activity of endogenous ET-1 [31]. tRES decreased ET-1 expression in endothelial cells *in vitro* [32]. Increased peripheral resistance to blood flow may also contribute to a hypertensive response. The negative correlation of change in plasma MG with FMD-GTN, an indicator of nitric oxide-independent arterial dilatation, suggests increased MG may support this. Indeed, plasma MG was an independent risk factor of increased arterial intimal-medial thickness, pulse-wave velocity and systolic blood pressure in patients with T2DM [33]. Urinary excretion of MG-H1 correlated positively with LDL-VLDL and TG and negatively with HDL. Urinary flux of MG-H1 reflects total body flux of protein glycation by MG, with a contribution from MG-H1 free adduct absorbed from digested glycated proteins in food [15,34]. These associations are consistent with formation of pro-atherogenic small, dense TG-rich LDL by MG modification of LDL, and decreased stability and half-life of HDL when modified by MG [35,36].

For changes from the baseline of clinical variables in the tRES-HESP treatment period, the positive correlation of change in the OGIS index with change in urinary pentosidine may reflect formation of pentosidine as a marker of pentosephosphate pathway metabolism [37]. Induction of the ARE-linked gene, G6PD, by tRES-HESP increases the flux through the pentosephosphate pathway and may thereby increase formation of pentose precursors of pentosidine; this also decreases glucose-6-phosphate-dependent carbohydrate response element/Mondo A (MLXIP) transcriptional response [9], which may contribute to reversal of insulin resistance [38].

For changes in gene expression of PBMCs, there was a strong anti-inflammatory response induced by tRES-HESP—characterized by decreased expression of COX-2, MCP-1, IL-8, and RAGE [15]. This anti-inflammatory effect has not been achieved in clinical studies with tRES alone: for example, 150 mg tRES daily for 4 weeks in obese men had no effect on IL-8 [39] and 500 mg tRES daily for 4 weeks in obese men had no effect on MCP-1 [40]. Change in expression of MCP-1, IL-8 and RAGE correlated strongly with change in expression of Mondo A. Increased expression of Mondo A in skeletal muscle is linked to lipid accumulation and insulin resistance [38]. A similar positive correlation with FTH1 and a negative correlation with HMOX1 suggested there may be decreased availability of iron and increased metabolism of heme iron during treatment with tRES-HESP. Iron metabolism has an important role in immunity [41], increasing inflammatory activity of macrophages and correlating with BMI increase in the healthy population [42]. The positive correlation with expression of NCF-1 of the NADPH oxidase system may relate to its regulation by MCP-1 and priming of NADPH oxidase by IL-8 [43], contributing to systemic oxidative stress in clinical obesity [44]. Several genes with positive correlations to MCP-1, IL-8, and RAGE—AKR1C1, G6PD, GCLM, GPX1, GPX4, GSR, MAFFF, MAFG, NFE2L2, and NQO1 are cytoprotective genes regulated by Nrf2—including autoregulation of Nrf2 itself [45]. This may reflect a host counter-response to low-grade inflammation sustained by these inflammatory mediators.

Decrease of MCP-1 and IL-8 by tRES-HESP may be a downstream effect of improved insulin sensitivity rather than an upstream mediator of it. Plasma MCP-1 concentration was not associated with insulin resistance clinically and overexpression of MCP-1 in mice induced inflammation without insulin resistance or dysglycemia [46,47]. However, adipose tissue levels of MCP-1 and IL-8 were increased by hyperinsulinemic clamp [48]. If the anti-inflammatory effects of tRES-HESP on gene expression in PBMCs translate to tissues, there may be additional health benefits through a decrease of insulin resistance-associated low-grade inflammation in development of non-alcoholic fatty liver disease [49–51], chronic kidney disease [52,53], decline of respiratory function [54–56], cardiovascular disease, and aging [57–59]. COX-2 may be decreased through its regulation by MCP-1 [60]; and decreased expression and *in situ* activity of RAGE through decrease of MG-H1 which is a ligand for RAGE [61].

Upstream signaling of MCP-1, IL-8, RAGE, and COX-2 may be linked to activation of the UPR by increased MG-modified misfolded proteins [9,10] (Figure 3). In UPR activation, IRE1α stabilizes TXNIP mRNA to increase its expression and activity [62]. TXNIP decreases glucose uptake by skeletal muscle and pancreatic beta-cell mass and insulin secretion and increases hepatic gluconeogenesis [23,63,64]. Inflammatory signaling may be mediated through X box-binding protein 1 (XBP1), increasing histone H3 lysine 4 methyltransferase, SET7/9, increasing expression of p65 of the NF-κB system and inflammatory mediators [65,66], including TNFα as key contributor to insulin resistance in skeletal muscle [13,67]. Treatment with tRES-HESP alleviates these UPR-mediated responses [9,10]; tRES-HESP may also decrease expression of TXNIP directly via Nrf2 and ARE-linked suppression [68]. tRES-HESP may thereby be a potent inducer of reversal of insulin resistance with applications for both prevention and treatment of T2DM.

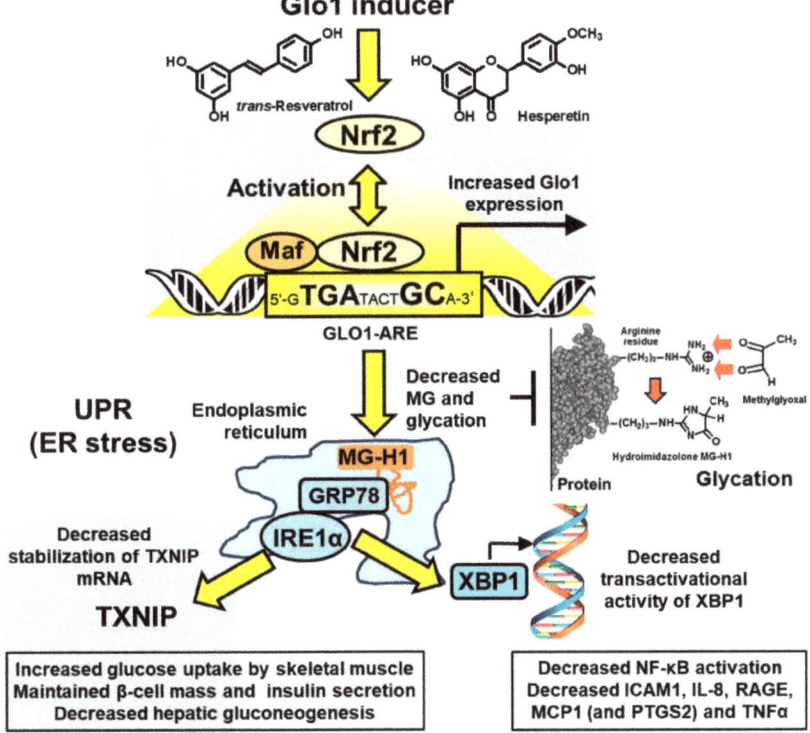

Figure 3. Proposed mechanism of action of Glo1 inducer, tRES-HESP, through suppression of the unfolded protein response. Key: yellow filled arrows—mechanism of health improvement; red filled arrows—damaging processes suppressed. See text for details.

Interestingly, since conducting the HATFF study, studies with human aortal endothelial cells and periodontal ligand fibroblasts in primary culture and model hyperglycemia have indicated that tRES-HESP may correct endothelial dysfunction and periodontal ligament dysfunction associated with hyperglycemia in prediabetes and diabetes [9,10]. tRES-HESP also corrected dysfunction of bone marrow progenitor cell in experimental diabetes, improving wound closure and angiogenesis in diabetic mice [69]. Suppression of activation of the UPR was implicated in these responses.

In conclusion, correlation analysis of data from the HATFF study indicates that the responses of optimised Glo1 inducer, tRES-HESP, are linked to improvements in dysglycemia, blood pressure, dyslipidemia, and low-grade inflammation. The reversal of insulin resistance induced by tRES-HESP was related inversely to expression of TNFα and TXNIP and may reflect countering of MG accumulation and protein glycation, with consequent decreased activation of the UPR [70].

Author Contributions: Conceptualization, P.J.T.; methodology, M.X., M.O.W., N.R., and P.J.T.; investigation, M.X., M.O.W., N.R., and P.J.T.; writing—original draft preparation, P.J.T.: writing—review and editing, M.X., M.O.W., and N.R. All authors have read and agreed to the published version of the manuscript.

Funding: The HATFF study was mainly funded by Unilever and Innovate UK (Project no 101129). N.R. and P.J.T. thank Qatar University and Qatar Foundation for funding for their glycation research.

Institutional Review Board Statement: The HATFF study was conducted in accordance with the guidelines of the Declaration of Helsinki, and approved by National Research Ethics Service Committee West Midlands—Coventry & Warwickshire (project number 13/WM/0368) and registered on the Clinicaltrials.gov (identifier: NCT02095873).

Informed Consent Statement: Informed consent was obtained from all subjects involved in the study.

Data Availability Statement: The data presented in this study are available on request from the corresponding author.

Conflicts of Interest: M.X., N.R., and P.J.T. are inventors/owners of a composition patent of tRES-HESP dietary supplement.

References

1. Williamson, G. The role of polyphenols in modern nutrition. *Nutr. Bull.* **2017**, *42*, 226–235. [CrossRef]
2. Baur, J.A.; Pearson, K.J.; Price, N.L.; Jamieson, H.A.; Lerin, C.; Kalra, A.; Prabhu, V.V.; Allard, J.S.; Lopez-Lluch, G.; Lewis, K.; et al. Resveratrol improves health and survival of mice on a high-calorie diet. *Nature* **2006**, *444*, 337–342. [CrossRef] [PubMed]
3. Liu, K.; Zhou, R.; Wang, B.; Mi, M.-T. Effect of resveratrol on glucose control and insulin sensitivity: A meta-analysis of 11 randomized controlled trials. *Am. J. Clin. Nutr.* **2014**, *99*, 1510–1519. [CrossRef] [PubMed]
4. Chimento, A.; De Amicis, F.; Sirianni, R.; Sinicropi, M.S.; Puoci, F.; Casaburi, I.; Saturnino, C.; Pezzi, V. Progress to Improve Oral Bioavailability and Beneficial Effects of Resveratrol. *Int. J. Mol. Sci.* **2019**, *20*, 1381. [CrossRef] [PubMed]
5. DeFronzo, R.A.; Eldor, R.; Abdul-Ghani, M. Pathophysiologic approach to therapy in patients with newly diagnosed type 2 diabetes. *Diabetes Care* **2013**, *36* (Suppl. 2), S127–S138. [CrossRef] [PubMed]
6. Rabbani, N.; Thornalley, P.J. Glyoxalase 1 modulation in obesity and diabetes. *Antioxid. Redox Signal.* **2018**, *30*, 354–374. [CrossRef]
7. Ahmed, N.; Dobler, D.; Dean, M.; Thornalley, P.J. Peptide mapping identifies hotspot site of modification in human serum albumin by methylglyoxal involved in ligand binding and esterase activity. *J. Biol. Chem.* **2005**, *280*, 5724–5732. [CrossRef]
8. Ahmed, N.; Babaei-Jadidi, R.; Howell, S.K.; Beisswenger, P.J.; Thornalley, P.J. Degradation products of proteins damaged by glycation, oxidation and nitration in clinical type 1 diabetes. *Diabetologia* **2005**, *48*, 1590–1603. [CrossRef]
9. Irshad, Z.; Xue, M.; Ashour, A.; Larkin, J.R.; Thornalley, P.J.; Rabbani, N. Activation of the unfolded protein response in high glucose treated endothelial cells is mediated by methylglyoxal. *Sci Rep.* **2019**, *9*, 7889. [CrossRef]
10. Ashour, A.; Xue, M.; Al-Motawa, M.; Thornalley, P.J.; Rabbani, N. Glycolytic overload-driven dysfunction of periodontal ligament fibroblasts in high glucose concentration, corrected by glyoxalase 1 inducer. *BMJ Open Diabetes Res. Care* **2020**, *8*, e001458. [CrossRef]
11. Rabbani, N.; Xue, M.; Thornalley, P.J. Methylglyoxal-induced dicarbonyl stress in aging and disease: First steps towards glyoxalase 1-based treatments. *Clin. Sci.* **2016**, *130*, 1677–1696. [CrossRef] [PubMed]
12. McLellan, A.C.; Thornalley, P.J.; Benn, J.; Sonksen, P.H. The glyoxalase system in clinical diabetes mellitus and correlation with diabetic complications. *Clin. Sci.* **1994**, *87*, 21–29. [CrossRef] [PubMed]

13. Hotamisligil, G.S. Endoplasmic reticulum stress and the inflammatory basis of metabolic disease. *Cell* **2010**, *140*, 900–917. [CrossRef]
14. Xue, M.; Rabbani, N.; Momiji, H.; Imbasi, P.; Anwar, M.M.; Kitteringham, N.R.; Park, B.K.; Souma, T.; Moriguchi, T.; Yamamoto, M.; et al. Transcriptional control of glyoxalase 1 by Nrf2 provides a stress responsive defence against dicarbonyl glycation. *Biochem. J.* **2012**, *443*, 213–222. [CrossRef] [PubMed]
15. Xue, M.; Weickert, M.O.; Qureshi, S.; Ngianga-Bakwin, K.; Anwar, A.; Waldron, M.; Shafie, A.; Messenger, D.; Fowler, M.; Jenkins, G.; et al. Improved glycemic control and vascular function in overweight and obese subjects by glyoxalase 1 inducer formulation. *Diabetes* **2016**, *65*, 2282–2294. [CrossRef]
16. Mari, A.; Pacini, G.; Brazzale, A.R.; Ahrén, B. Comparative evaluation of simple insulin sensitivity methods based on the oral glucose tolerance test. *Diabetologia* **2005**, *48*, 748–751. [CrossRef]
17. Arai, M.; Nihonmatsu-Kikuchi, N.; Itokawa, M.; Rabbani, N.; Thornalley, P.J. Measurement of glyoxalase activities. *Biochem. Soc. Trans.* **2014**, *42*, 491–494. [CrossRef]
18. Fortina, P.; Surrey, S. Digital mRNA profiling. *Nat. Biotechnol.* **2008**, *26*, 293–294. [CrossRef]
19. Rabbani, N.; Thornalley, P.J. Measurement of methylglyoxal by stable isotopic dilution analysis LC-MS/MS with corroborative prediction in physiological samples. *Nat. Protoc.* **2014**, *9*, 1969–1979. [CrossRef] [PubMed]
20. Rabbani, N.; Shaheen, F.; Anwar, A.; Masania, J.; Thornalley, P.J. Assay of methylglyoxal-derived protein and nucleotide AGEs. *Biochem. Soc. Trans.* **2014**, *42*, 511–517. [CrossRef] [PubMed]
21. McLellan, A.C.; Phillips, S.A.; Thornalley, P.J. Fluorimetric assay of D-lactate. *Anal. Biochem.* **1992**, *206*, 12–16. [CrossRef]
22. Xue, M.; Momiji, H.; Rabbani, N.; Barker, G.; Bretschneider, T.; Shmygol, A.; Rand, D.A.; Thornalley, P.J. Frequency modulated translocational oscillations of Nrf2 mediate the ARE cytoprotective transcriptional response *Antioxid. Redox Signal.* **2015**, *23*, 613–629. [CrossRef]
23. Jo, S.H.; Kim, M.Y.; Park, J.M.; Kim, T.H.; Ahn, Y.H. Txnip contributes to impaired glucose tolerance by upregulating the expression of genes involved in hepatic gluconeogenesis in mice. *Diabetologia* **2013**, *56*, 2723–2732. [CrossRef]
24. Xu, G.; Chen, J.; Jing, G.; Shalev, A. Thioredoxin-interacting protein regulates insulin transcription through microRNA-204. *Nat. Med.* **2013**, *19*, 1141–1146. [CrossRef]
25. Parikh, H.; Carlsson, E.; Chutkow, W.A.; Johansson, L.E.; Storgaard, H.; Poulsen, P.; Saxena, R.; Ladd, C.; Schulze, P.C.; Mazzini, M.J.; et al. TXNIP Regulates Peripheral Glucose Metabolism in Humans. *PLoS Med.* **2007**, *4*, e158. [CrossRef] [PubMed]
26. Hotamisligil, G.S.; Murray, D.L.; Choy, L.N.; Spiegelman, B.M. Tumor necrosis factor alpha inhibits signaling from the insulin receptor. *Proc. Natl. Acad. Sci. USA* **1994**, *91*, 4854–4858. [CrossRef] [PubMed]
27. Miyazaki, Y.; Pipek, R.; Mandarino, L.J.; DeFronzo, R.A. Tumor necrosis factor-alpha and insulin resistance in obese type 2 diabetic patients. *Int. J. Obes. Relat. Metab. Disord.* **2003**, *27*, 88–94. [CrossRef] [PubMed]
28. Plomgaard, P.; Bouzakri, K.; Krogh-Madsen, R.; Mittendorfer, B.; Zierath, J.R.; Pedersen, B.K. Tumor Necrosis Factor-α Induces Skeletal Muscle Insulin Resistance in Healthy Human Subjects via Inhibition of Akt Substrate 160 Phosphorylation. *Diabetes* **2005**, *54*, 2939–2945. [CrossRef]
29. Rizza, S.; Muniyappa, R.; Iantorno, M.; Kim, J.-a.; Chen, H.; Pullikotil, P.; Senese, N.; Tesauro, M.; Lauro, D.; Cardillo, C.; et al. Citrus Polyphenol Hesperidin Stimulates Production of Nitric Oxide in Endothelial Cells while Improving Endothelial Function and Reducing Inflammatory Markers in Patients with Metabolic Syndrome. *J. Clin. Endocrinol. Metab.* **2011**, *96*, E782–E792. [CrossRef]
30. Padilla, J.; Jenkins, N.T. Induction of endoplasmic reticulum stress impairs insulin-stimulated vasomotor relaxation in rat aortic rings: Role of endothelin-1. *J. Physiol. Pharmacol. Off. J. Pol. Physiol. Soc.* **2013**, *64*, 557–564.
31. Cardillo, C.; Campia, U.; Iantorno, M.; Panza Julio, A. Enhanced Vascular Activity of Endogenous Endothelin-1 in Obese Hypertensive Patients. *Hypertension* **2004**, *43*, 36–40. [CrossRef] [PubMed]
32. Liu, J.-C.; Chen, J.-J.; Chan, P.; Cheng, C.-F.; Cheng, T.-H. Inhibition of Cyclic Strain-Induced Endothelin-1 Gene Expression by Resveratrol. *Hypertension* **2003**, *42*, 1198–1205. [CrossRef] [PubMed]
33. Ogawa, S.; Nakayama, K.; Nakayama, M.; Mori, T.; Matsushima, M.; Okamura, M.; Senda, M.; Nako, K.; Miyata, T.; Ito, S. Methylglyoxal Is a Predictor in Type 2 Diabetic Patients of Intima-Media Thickening and Elevation of Blood Pressure. *Hypertension* **2010**, *56*, 471–476. [CrossRef] [PubMed]
34. Masania, J.; Faustmann, G.; Anwar, A.; Hafner-Giessauf, H.; Rajpoot, R.; Grabher, J.; Rajpoot, K.; Tiran, B.; Obermayer-Pietsch, B.; Winklhofer-Roob, B.M.; et al. Urinary metabolomic markers of protein glycation, oxidation and nitration in early-stage decline in metabolic, vascular and renal health. *Oxid. Med. Cell. Longev.* **2019**, *2019*, 4851323. [CrossRef]
35. Rabbani, N.; Godfrey, L.; Xue, M.; Shaheen, F.; Geoffrion, M.; Milne, R.; Thornalley, P.J. Conversion of low density lipoprotein to the pro-atherogenic form by methylglyoxal with increased arterial proteoglycan binding and aortic retention. *Diabetes* **2011**, *60*, 1973–1980. [CrossRef] [PubMed]
36. Godfrey, L.; Yamada-Fowler, N.; Smith, J.A.; Thornalley, P.J.; Rabbani, N. Arginine-directed glycation and decreased HDL plasma concentration and functionality. *Nutr. Diabetes* **2014**, *4*, e134. [CrossRef] [PubMed]
37. Wang, F.; Zhao, Y.; Niu, Y.; Wang, C.; Wang, M.; Li, Y.; Sun, C. Activated glucose-6-phosphate dehydrogenase is associated with insulin resistance by upregulating pentose and pentosidine in diet-induced obesity of rats. *Horm. Metab. Res.* **2012**, *44*, 938–942. [CrossRef]

38. Ahn, B.; Wan, S.; Jaiswal, N.; Vega, R.B.; Ayer, D.E.; Titchenell, P.M.; Han, X.; Won, K.J.; Kelly, D.P. MondoA drives muscle lipid accumulation and insulin resistance. *JCI Insight* **2019**, *5*, e129119. [CrossRef]
39. Timmers, S.; Konings, E.; Bilet, L.; Houtkooper, R.H.; van de Weijer, T.; Goossens, G.H.; Hoeks, J.; van der Krieken, S.; Ryu, D.; Kersten, S.; et al. Calorie Restriction-like Effects of 30 Days of Resveratrol Supplementation on Energy Metabolism and Metabolic Profile in Obese Humans. *Cell Metab.* **2011**, *14*, 612–622. [CrossRef]
40. Poulsen, M.M.; Vestergaard, P.F.; Clasen, B.F.; Radko, Y.; Christensen, L.P.; Stødkilde-Jørgensen, H.; Møller, N.; Jessen, N.; Pedersen, S.B.; Jørgensen, J.O.L. High-dose resveratrol supplementation in obese men: An investigator-initiated, randomized, placebo-controlled clinical trial of substrate metabolism, insulin sensitivity, and body composition. *Diabetes* **2013**, *62*, 1186–1195. [CrossRef]
41. Soares, M.P.; Hamza, I. Macrophages and Iron Metabolism. *Immunity* **2016**, *44*, 492–504. [CrossRef] [PubMed]
42. Abraham, N.G.; Junge, J.M.; Drummond, G.S. Translational Significance of Heme Oxygenase in Obesity and Metabolic Syndrome. *Trends Pharmacol. Sci.* **2016**, *37*, 17–36. [CrossRef]
43. Tan, J.H.; Ludeman, J.P.; Wedderburn, J.; Canals, M.; Hall, P.; Butler, S.J.; Taleski, D.; Christopoulos, A.; Hickey, M.J.; Payne, R.J.; et al. Tyrosine sulfation of chemokine receptor CCR2 enhances interactions with both monomeric and dimeric forms of the chemokine monocyte chemoattractant protein-1 (MCP-1). *J. Biol. Chem.* **2013**, *288*, 10024–10034. [CrossRef] [PubMed]
44. Keaney, J.F., Jr.; Larson, M.G.; Vasan, R.S.; Wilson, P.W.; Lipinska, I.; Corey, D.; Massaro, J.M.; Sutherland, P.; Vita, J.A.; Benjamin, E.J. Obesity and systemic oxidative stress: Clinical correlates of oxidative stress in the Framingham Study. *Arterioscler. Thromb. Vasc. Biol.* **2003**, *23*, 434–439. [CrossRef]
45. Malhotra, D.; Portales-Casamar, E.; Singh, A.; Srivastava, S.; Arenillas, D.; Happel, C.; Shyr, C.; Wakabayashi, N.; Kensler, T.W.; Wasserman, W.W.; et al. Global mapping of binding sites for Nrf2 identifies novel targets in cell survival response through ChIP-Seq profiling and network analysis. *Nucleic Acids Res.* **2010**, *38*, 5718–5734. [CrossRef]
46. Chacón, M.R.; Fernández-Real, J.M.; Richart, C.; Megía, A.; Gómez, J.M.; Miranda, M.; Caubet, E.; Pastor, R.; Masdevall, C.; Vilarrasa, N.; et al. Monocyte Chemoattractant Protein-1 in Obesity and Type 2 Diabetes. Insulin Sensitivity Study. *Obesity* **2007**, *15*, 664–672. [CrossRef]
47. Evers-van Gogh, I.J.A.; Oteng, A.-B.; Alex, S.; Hamers, N.; Catoire, M.; Stienstra, R.; Kalkhoven, E.; Kersten, S. Muscle-specific inflammation induced by MCP-1 overexpression does not affect whole-body insulin sensitivity in mice. *Diabetologia* **2016**, *59*, 624–633. [CrossRef]
48. Bruun, J.M.; Verdich, C.; Toubro, S.; Astrup, A.; Richelsen, B. Association between measures of insulin sensitivity and circulating levels of interleukin-8, interleukin-6 and tumor necrosis factor-alpha. Effect of weight loss in obese men. *Eur. J. Endocrinol.* **2003**, *148*, 535–542. [CrossRef] [PubMed]
49. Glass, O.; Henao, R.; Patel, K.; Guy, C.D.; Gruss, H.J.; Syn, W.-K.; Moylan, C.A.; Streilein, R.; Hall, R.; Mae Diehl, A.; et al. Serum Interleukin-8, Osteopontin, and Monocyte Chemoattractant Protein 1 Are Associated With Hepatic Fibrosis in Patients With Nonalcoholic Fatty Liver Disease. *Hepatol. Commun.* **2018**, *2*, 1344–1355. [CrossRef]
50. Haukeland, J.W.; Damås, J.K.; Konopski, Z.; Løberg, E.M.; Haaland, T.; Goverud, I.; Torjesen, P.A.; Birkeland, K.; Bjøro, K.; Aukrust, P. Systemic inflammation in nonalcoholic fatty liver disease is characterized by elevated levels of CCL2. *J. Hepatol.* **2006**, *44*, 1167–1174. [CrossRef]
51. Ajmera, V.; Perito, E.R.; Bass, N.M.; Terrault, N.A.; Yates, K.P.; Gill, R.; Loomba, R.; Diehl, A.M.; Aouizerat, B.E. Novel plasma biomarkers associated with liver disease severity in adults with nonalcoholic fatty liver disease. *Hepatology* **2017**, *65*, 65–77. [CrossRef]
52. Spoto, B.; Pisano, A.; Zoccali, C. Insulin resistance in chronic kidney disease: A systematic review. *Am. J. Physiol. Ren. Physiol.* **2016**, *311*, F1087–F1108. [CrossRef]
53. Haller, H.; Bertram, A.; Nadrowitz, F.; Menne, J. Monocyte chemoattractant protein-1 and the kidney. *Curr. Opin. Nephrol. Hypertens.* **2016**, *25*, 42–49. [CrossRef]
54. Reynolds, C.J.; Quigley, K.; Cheng, X.; Suresh, A.; Tahir, S.; Ahmed-Jushuf, F.; Nawab, K.; Choy, K.; Walker, S.A.; Mathie, S.A.; et al. Lung Defense through IL-8 Carries a Cost of Chronic Lung Remodeling and Impaired Function. *Am. J. Respir. Cell Mol. Biol.* **2018**, *59*, 557–571. [CrossRef]
55. Valentine, M.S.; Link, P.A.; Herbert, J.A.; Kamga Gninzeko, F.J.; Schneck, M.B.; Shankar, K.; Nkwocha, J.; Reynolds, A.M.; Heise, R.L. Inflammation and Monocyte Recruitment Due to Aging and Mechanical Stretch in Alveolar Epithelium are Inhibited by the Molecular Chaperone 4-Phenylbutyrate. *Cell. Mol. Bioeng.* **2018**, *11*, 495–508. [CrossRef]
56. Lee, Y.B.; Kim, Y.S.; Lee, D.-H.; Kim, H.Y.; Lee, J.-I.; Ahn, H.-S.; Sohn, T.S.; Lee, T.-K.; Song, J.Y.; Yeo, C.D.; et al. Association between HOMA-IR and Lung Function in Korean Young Adults based on the Korea National Health and Nutrition Examination Survey. *Sci. Rep.* **2017**, *7*, 11726. [CrossRef] [PubMed]
57. Moreno Velásquez, I.; Gajulapuri, A.; Leander, K.; Berglund, A.; de Faire, U.; Gigante, B. Serum IL8 is not associated with cardiovascular events but with all-cause mortality. *BMC Cardiovasc. Disord.* **2019**, *19*, 34. [CrossRef] [PubMed]
58. Piemonti, L.; Calori, G.; Lattuada, G.; Mercalli, A.; Ragogna, F.; Garancini, M.P.; Ruotolo, G.; Luzi, L.; Perseghin, G. Association Between Plasma Monocyte Chemoattractant Protein-1 Concentration and Cardiovascular Disease Mortality in Middle-Aged Diabetic and Nondiabetic Individuals. *Diabetes Care* **2009**, *32*, 2105–2110. [CrossRef] [PubMed]
59. Ausk, K.J.; Boyko, E.J.; Ioannou, G.N. Insulin resistance predicts mortality in nondiabetic individuals in the U.S. *Diabetes Care* **2010**, *33*, 1179–1185. [CrossRef]

60. Futagami, S.; Hiratsuka, T.; Shindo, T.; Hamamoto, T.; Tatsuguchi, A.; Nobue, U.; Shinji, Y.; Suzuki, K.; Kusunoki, M.; Tanaka, S.; et al. COX-2 and CCR2 induced by CD40 ligand and MCP-1 are linked to VEGF production in endothelial cells. *Prostaglandins Leukot. Essent. Fat. Acids* **2008**, *78*, 137–146. [CrossRef]
61. Xue, J.; Ray, R.; Singer, D.; Böhme, D.; Burz, D.S.; Rai, V.; Hoffmann, R.; Shekhtman, A. The Receptor for Advanced Glycation End Products (RAGE) Specifically Recognizes Methylglyoxal-Derived AGEs. *Biochemistry* **2014**, *53*, 3327–3335. [CrossRef]
62. Lerner, A.G.; Upton, J.-P.; Praveen, P.V.K.; Ghosh, R.; Nakagawa, Y.; Igbaria, A.; Shen, S.; Nguyen, V.; Backes, B.J.; Heiman, M.; et al. IRE1α induces thioredoxin-interacting protein to activate the NLRP3 inflammasome and promote programmed cell death under irremediable ER stress. *Cell Metab.* **2012**, *16*, 250–264. [CrossRef]
63. Waldhart, A.N.; Dykstra, H.; Peck, A.S.; Boguslawski, E.A.; Madaj, Z.B.; Wen, J.; Veldkamp, K.; Hollowell, M.; Zheng, B.; Cantley, L.C.; et al. Phosphorylation of TXNIP by AKT Mediates Acute Influx of Glucose in Response to Insulin. *Cell Rep.* **2017**, *19*, 2005–2013. [CrossRef]
64. Oslowski, C.M.; Hara, T.; O'Sullivan-Murphy, B.; Kanekura, K.; Lu, S.; Hara, M.; Ishigaki, S.; Zhu, L.J.; Hayashi, E.; Hui, S.T.; et al. Thioredoxin-interacting protein mediates ER stress-induced β cell death through initiation of the inflammasome. *Cell Metab.* **2012**, *16*, 265–273. [CrossRef]
65. Li, Y.; Reddy, M.A.; Miao, F.; Shanmugam, N.; Yee, J.-K.; Hawkins, D.; Ren, B.; Natarajan, R. Role of the Histone H3 Lysine 4 Methyltransferase, SET7/9, in the Regulation of NF-κB-dependent Inflammatory Genes: Relevance to diabetes and inflammation. *J. Biol. Chem.* **2008**, *283*, 26771–26781. [CrossRef]
66. Chen, J.; Guo, Y.; Zeng, W.; Huang, L.; Pang, Q.; Nie, L.; Mu, J.; Yuan, F.; Feng, B. ER stress triggers MCP-1 expression through SET7/9-induced histone methylation in the kidneys of db/db mice. *Am. J. Physiol. Ren. Physiol.* **2014**, *306*, F916–F925. [CrossRef] [PubMed]
67. Hotamisligil, G.S. Mechanisms of TNF-alpha-induced insulin resistance. *Exp. Clin. Endocrinol. Diabetes* **1999**, *107*, 119–125. [CrossRef] [PubMed]
68. He, X.; Ma, Q. Redox Regulation by Nuclear Factor Erythroid 2-Related Factor 2: Gatekeeping for the Basal and Diabetes-Induced Expression of Thioredoxin-Interacting Protein. *Mol. Pharmacol.* **2012**, *82*, 887–897. [CrossRef] [PubMed]
69. Li, H.; O'Meara, M.; Zhang, X.; Zhang, K.; Seyoum, B.; Yi, Z.; Kaufman, R.J.; Monks, T.J.; Wang, J.-M. Ameliorating Methylglyoxal-Induced Progenitor Cell Dysfunction for Tissue Repair in Diabetes. *Diabetes* **2019**, *68*, 1287–1302. [CrossRef]
70. Rabbani, N.; Xue, M.; Thornalley, P.J. Dicarbonyl stress, protein glycation and the unfolded protein response. *Glycoconj. J.* **2021**, *38*, 331–334. [CrossRef]

MDPI
St. Alban-Anlage 66
4052 Basel
Switzerland
Tel. +41 61 683 77 34
Fax +41 61 302 89 18
www.mdpi.com

Nutrients Editorial Office
E-mail: nutrients@mdpi.com
www.mdpi.com/journal/nutrients

www.ingramcontent.com/pod-product-compliance
Lightning Source LLC
LaVergne TN
LVHW070417100526
838202LV00014B/1478